RENEWING THE STUFF OF LIFE

Renewing the Stuff of Life

Stem Cells, Ethics, and Public Policy

CYNTHIA B. COHEN

OXFORD
UNIVERSITY PRESS
2007

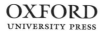

OXFORD
UNIVERSITY PRESS

Oxford University Press, Inc., publishes works that further
Oxford University's objective of excellence
in research, scholarship, and education.

Oxford New York
Auckland   Cape Town   Dar es Salaam   Hong Kong   Karachi
Kuala Lumpur   Madrid   Melbourne   Mexico City   Nairobi
New Delhi   Shanghai   Taipei   Toronto

With offices in
Argentina   Austria   Brazil   Chile   Czech Republic   France   Greece
Guatemala   Hungary   Italy   Japan   Poland   Portugal   Singapore
South Korea   Switzerland   Thailand   Turkey   Ukraine   Vietnam

Copyright © 2007 by Oxford University Press, Inc.

Published by Oxford University Press, Inc.
198 Madison Avenue, New York, New York 10016

www.oup.com

Oxford is a registered trademark of Oxford University Press

Library of Congress Cataloging-in-Publication Data
Cohen, Cynthia B.
Renewing the stuff of life : stem cells, ethics, and public policy /
Cynthia B. Cohen.
    p. cm.
ISBN 978-0-19-530524-1 ✓
1. Stem cells—Moral and ethical aspects.
2. Stem cells—Government policy—
United States. I. Title.

QH588.S83C46 2007
174.2'8—dc22   2006047800

9 8 7 6 5 4 3 2 1

Printed in the United States of America
on acid-free paper

For Pete,
Love never fails . . .

Acknowledgments

I owe thanks to several colleagues and friends for reading one or more draft chapters of this book and providing me with extremely valuable insights and comments about them. Of course, they are not responsible for the final versions of the chapters that they read and, indeed, may disagree with them.

They are:

Bruce P. Brandhorst, R. Alta Charo, Peter J. Cohen, Holly C. Cooper, George Q. Daley, Q. Todd Dickinson, Donald Evans, Jan C. Heller, Rosario M. Isasi, Rudolf Jaenisch, Albert R. Jonsen, Phillip Karpowicz, Bartha M. Knoppers, Arthur Leader, Margaret O. Little, Bernard Lo, Ruth Macklin, Mary Anderlik Majumder, Margaret E. Mohrmann, Madison Powers, Melinda A. Roberts, Hans-Martin Sass, David A. Scott, Timothy F. Sedgwick, David H. Smith, Davor Solter, Clive Svendson, Carol A. Tauer, Derek van der Kooy, and LeRoy Walters.

I also thank the staff of the National Reference Center for Bioethics Literature at the Kennedy Institute of Ethics at Georgetown University for their unfailing and invaluable assistance with many of the thorny research questions that arose as I was writing this book.

I am grateful to Roberta A. Heisterkamp of Denver, Colorado, whose artistic talents have added a special note of beauty and interest to this book.

Finally, I owe my greatest debt of gratitude to my husband, Peter J. Cohen, without whose moral support this book would never have been written.

Contents

RENEWING THE STUFF OF LIFE

Introduction

Human embryonic stem cells burst from the obscurity of the research lab into public view almost a decade ago. We had known for some before then that these cells exist and that they are extremely versatile, for they can be converted into almost any type of cell found in the human body—heart, liver, blood, pancreas, and muscle among them. These stem cells can also reproduce themselves, sustaining the organs and tissues of the human body throughout an individual's lifetime. We were also familiar with adult stem cells that are found in various parts of the human body, including bone marrow, blood, and body fat cells. Although we had started down the path of developing adult stem cells, we had not been able to culture and grow human embryonic stem cells, even though the lure of these sorts of stem cells, in particular, was immense.

That changed in 1998, when stem cell investigators successfully developed human embryonic stem cells in vitro (in a laboratory dish). In doing so, they initiated a new era of what is called "regenerative medicine" in which we hope to learn how and why stem cells of both major types grow and proliferate throughout the human body and, on the basis of the knowledge that we obtain, develop ways in which to use stem cells to replace diseased and injured cells hidden away in the bodies of those with serious illnesses. Stem cell investigators, patients afflicted with debilitating diseases, families who assist them, and many others look for the day when a host of diseases and injuries will be treated more readily and permanently through research that promises to renew the very stuff of life.

Yet as stem cell research has proceeded, it has raised compelling ethical issues. Its offer to restore parts of the human body that have gone awry has come up against serious moral and religious questions related to the use of human embryos. This is because applying human embryonic stem cell transplants in attempts to develop treatments for those with certain diseases involves destroying human embryos, and this is deeply offensive to some. Others, however, do not share their moral reservations about this research use of human embryos and believe, to the contrary, that it is morally wrong not to proceed with stem cell research in attempts to treat the millions of human beings with debilitating diseases.

This disagreement about the moral significance of early human embryos as the very source of the stuff of life has been the focus of ethical and policy discussions of stem cell research ever since these cells first emerged in the laboratory. The question has captured the attention of the presidents of the United States, members of Congress, state legislators, patient interest groups, religious bodies, major universities, private biotech companies, and "ordinary" citizens in the street. What we owe to early human embryos in the way of support and protection is an extremely important question that calls for further inquiry. We urgently need to work toward an answer to the question of whether human embryos are of such immense moral significance that we should never destroy them, even in research that might treat and perhaps save the lives of human beings.

However, in all the furor about whether we should engage in embryonic stem cell research, especially whether we should do so with federal funds, we have tended to overlook other important ethical and public policy questions raised by stem cell research, such as the following: Should we use dead embryos to treat living persons and, if so, how could we tell whether they were dead? Should we create human-nonhuman chimeras in order to test how both human adult and embryonic stem cells spread throughout the bodies of living organisms? Might the introduction of research cloning tempt some maverick scientists to steal cloned embryos and use them to create babies by means of reproductive cloning? Would it be wrong to alter human neural stem cells genetically in order to use them as vehicles for treating or even enhancing the human brain? Will those who are economically well-off be the sole beneficiaries of stem cell research? Indeed, what, if any, are the limits of our search to renew the very stuff of life? Who should decide this and how stringent should the guidelines be that we impose on the conduct of stem cell research?

The central thesis of this book is that we need to expand and transform the debate about stem cell research to address a much wider range of ethical and policy issues than are currently being taken into account. We have been so intent on taking the initial steps necessary to get stem cell research off the ground in ways that are ethically sound that we have not looked further downstream. As a result, we have not considered in much depth a host of ethical and policy questions that we will face in the future if and when stem cell research begins to realize its scientific and therapeutic promise. Many of these questions are new, and we have no ready answers to them at hand. To begin to remedy this situation, this book explores a range of scientific, ethical, religious, policy, and regulatory issues raised by stem cell research and offers responses to them that are in keeping with our shared values and are supported by what I believe are reasoned arguments.

We need to begin by developing an understanding of just what stem cells are, how they function within the bodies of human beings, and how we might apply them to treat those with damaged or diseased cells. In chapter 1 of this book, I delve into these questions, exploring them in terms that are accessible to nonscientists. I offer explanations of how adult stem cells develop and how they are distinguished from embryonic stem cells in their makeup and functions. The thrust of the discussion is on what sorts of research might be undertaken with adult stem cells and what the ultimate purpose of such research might be. I go on to explore the world of human embryonic stem cell research, detailing how these cells were discovered and grown in culture and the ways in which they are being developed in the laboratory and studied in living organisms today. In particular, I consider the scientific and medical issues raised by the possibility of transplanting these cells to patients in attempts to restore them to a baseline of good health. I conclude this chapter with a comparison of the advantages and disadvantages of using human adult stem cells and human embryonic stem cells in research and possible future therapies.

Scientists and policy makers have been trying to ferret out new ways to develop human pluripotent cells (cells that can specialize and become almost any cell of the human body) with the same characteristics as human embryonic stem cells for two main reasons. Either (1) they find the number of human embryonic stem cell lines that are currently available insufficient for research purposes or (2) they hope to avoid any methods of developing these cells that involve the destruction of human embryos; both reasons can also motivate their efforts. In chapter 2, I consider the various methods that have been proposed for developing sources for human pluripotent stem cells in addition to those involving the use of human embryos that remain at in vitro fertilization (IVF) clinics. These include such measures as cloning, parthenogenesis, recovering stem cells from dead embryos, "altered nuclear transfer," and dedifferentiating specialized cells back to a pluripotent state. I assess these proposed new sources of pluripotent cells in terms of their scientific promise and ethical soundness and conclude that only some of them pass muster on both counts.

Both secular and religious thinkers have grappled with the question that has stirred the most intense public debate to date—the moral significance of early human embryos—in varying ways. In chapter 3, I consider this question from the perspective of those who have developed arguments about the question within secular contexts in our society. I explain the view underlying current federal policy—that these embryos are full-fledged living human beings and consequently are owed all the protections offered to already born human beings. I go on to set out the positions of those who do not see these embryos at five or six days after fertilization as the moral equivalent of you or me. This leads us to explore the strengths and weaknesses of five major arguments that have provided the basis for several different views of the moral significance of human embryos. The position that emerges as the most reasonable and best supported in terms of the most recent science, in my view, is that the human embryo at fourteen days after fertilization (or some would maintain even later) starts on its journey toward developing into an individual human being and, because of this, has certain moral significance starting at that time. I then turn to the vexed question of whether we ought to create human embryos for use in stem cell research that might lead to treatments for those who are seriously ill, finding that the restorative and preservative value of human embryos renders it appropriate to create them for research in certain clearly defined contexts.

In a pluralistic society such as ours, with citizens of many different religious persuasions, it can be difficult to reach agreement about a contentious issue such as what we owe morally to early human embryos. Yet a democratic republic cannot and should not ignore the religious voices of its citizens or hear only the voices of those within one tradition at the expense of others. In a liberal (in the broad sense) democracy such as ours, it is morally important to gain various religious insights into issues of public concern as we strive to reach common ground in addressing them. Consequently, in chapter 4, I review the beliefs of several different religious traditions concerning the moral significance of early human embryos. These include the Christian, Jewish, Islamic, Buddhist, and Hindu traditions—with apologies to those traditions omitted. No attempt is made in this chapter to reconcile these varied religious beliefs into one grand, but vacuous, religious view. Instead, I seek to understand their similarities and their differences and to capture beliefs and values they share that are relevant to making decisions about proceeding with stem cell research.

Stem cell research has brought to the fore yet another novel ethical issue with which scientists, ethicists, and members of the public have been grappling: Should we develop human-nonhuman chimeras—animals into whose innermost depths researchers have inserted human stem cells? Scientists are exploring the ways in which human stem cells, both specialized and unspecialized, behave once they are transferred into living organic systems. The problem is that they cannot test this in human beings, for the risks of transferring human stem cells or their progeny to humans are unknown. The solution to which several stem cell investigators have turned is to insert these human stem cells into animals at various points in their development and then trace the travels of these cells through their bodies. How human might these chimeric animals become if they were to carry human embryonic stem cells, which can be transformed into almost any cell of the body— including brain and germ (reproductive) cells? Might such experiments result in the creation of animals with human minds trapped inside them or animals that gave birth to humans?

In chapter 5, I address such troubling ethical issues, which rival the question of the moral significance of early human embryos in their depth and intensity. I consider the main ethical arguments that have been raised against such chimeric research and adopt one in particular, the human dignity argument, questioning how far we should go in transferring human neural stem cells and human embryonic stem cells into nonhumans. In the conclusion to this chapter, I propose ethical guidelines for the transfer of differentiated neural stem cells and human embryonic stem cells into nonhuman hosts that place certain limits on such transfers.

International measures that have been adopted to regulate stem cell research provide the underlying focus of chapter 6. After a brief survey of international stem cell research policies, I consider the development of stem cell research legislation and policy in three countries: the United Kingdom, Germany, and Japan. I explore how the views of the moral significance of early human embryos held by various religious, feminist, ecological, and other groups within each of these countries have influenced their laws and policies regarding stem cells. With this discussion, it becomes clear that it is not only the moral significance of early human embryos that has been at stake in debates about stem cell research policy in these countries but also a set of cultural, religious, ecological, economic, and scientific concerns that carry different weight in each of them. These concerns include those revolving around the potential for eugenic misuse that powerful new biotechnologies such as stem cell research represent, the role that this research might have in retaining each country's economic and scientific competitiveness vis-à-vis the rest of the world, and the desire to uphold traditional values in addition to those connected to the moral significance of human embryos that seem threatened by novel research areas such as stem cell research. In the conclusion of this chapter, I consider whether it is realistic to expect to develop one common international policy regarding this research in view of such national differences.

In chapter 7, I bring the varied insights that have been derived from examining the policies of these other countries to a review of the development of stem cell research policy in the United States. This country as of this writing finds itself in an odd position with regard to stem cell research. It strictly limits the pursuit of federally funded human embryonic stem cell research but allows this research to proceed virtually unimpeded in the states and in the private sector. As a result, we face a patchwork of varied and sometimes conflicting guidelines for stem cell research across the country. How did this situation develop? What were the theological and political considerations that led to this current pastiche of guidelines?

I give special attention in this chapter to the ethical and political reasoning used by the Clinton and Bush administrations to reach decisions about whether to provide federal support for human embryonic stem cell research. The interpretation given to the theory of complicity by the Bush administration comes in for special review, as it provides the basis for the human embryonic stem cell research policy that has been in place on the federal level since August 2001. I then go on to trace how stem cell research policies have lurched into place in some states. This leads to an exploration of the mixed response of the business community to the possibility of carrying out this research in the private sector, along with the way in which patent policies regarding stem cell research are evolving in this country. I conclude by emphasizing that current stem cell research policy across the country is fundamentally incoherent, despite the best efforts of certain professional groups to establish voluntary guidelines for those carrying out this research.

In chapter 8, I consider how to remedy this conflicted situation. As of this writing, it seems possible that federal legislation might be passed that would expand the scope of federally funded human embryonic stem cell research in this country. If this legislation were to survive, that would heighten the force of a question originally raised by the National Bioethics Advisory Commission in 1999: Do we need a national stem cell review and oversight panel to provide guidelines that embody a coherent national policy for stem cell research?

I argue in this chapter that we need a coherent national response—not only to the spate of ethical questions that are currently arising about stem cell research but also to certain novel ethical questions and justice issues that are bound to arise in the future as this research moves ahead to improve and enhance human bodies. The current forms of federal regulation of stem cell research are limited in several significant ways, I point out, that preclude them from providing the broad sort of ethical overview and review of this research that is needed on the national level. New guidelines set out by the National Academies, which attempt to move into this public policy gap, conflict in certain respects with the guidelines followed by those in reproductive medicine, leaving stem cell investigators and their colleagues who treat infertility and who provide embryos and gametes for the pursuit of embryonic stem cell research and therapy in a state of uncertainty about how to proceed.

This confusion provides the impetus for exploring in this chapter five different models for a stem cell research review and oversight panel that have been either proposed or developed by various groups. Drawing on their proposals, I provide a distinctive model for a federally sponsored national stem cell review and oversight panel that would develop guidelines for stem cell research and offer a coherent national policy regarding this research. I recommend functions and membership for such a panel and emphasize the importance of a method of democratic deliberation and public consultation for its work. There is an ever more pressing need to establish such a national stem cell research panel to set out clear, carefully developed, and ethically sound stem cell research guidelines and national policy in view of the move that is currently emerging across the country and in the halls of Congress to expand the scope of stem cell research in the United States.

This book is intended to go beyond sound bites to provide readers with a sense of the broad scope and complexity of the ethical and policy issues raised by stem cell research—and to offer ways of resolving these issues that do not soft-pedal significant ethical differences among us. In it, I develop an approach to these issues that is not radically new, but, to the contrary, is embedded in our ordinary ways of moral reasoning, as well as shared values at the foundation of our constitutional democracy. I believe that it is time to draw back from the bitter infighting and name-calling that have characterized public debate about the development of stem cell research policy in recent years to attend more carefully to these ways of reasoning and these shared values in order to develop an approach to this research that is both ethically responsible and supported by reason and reflection. We need to devote more time to thinking coolly about the difficult ethical and policy issues that stem cell research raises if we are to grasp the points of view of others and find ways to resolve our differences without hatred or strife. I hope that this book makes some contribution to mutual understanding and even to mutual agreement about the difficult and sometimes tragic issues raised by stem cell research.

1

What Are Stem Cells? How Do They Function? What Might They Do?

The prospect of human stem cell research has emerged as a frontier scientific and bioethical issue. Ever since investigators reported that they had succeeded in isolating and culturing human embryonic stem cells in 1998,[1] research into these cells has attracted immense scientific and public interest. This newfound ability to grow human stem cells has opened the door to the generation of brand new cells and tissues that might be used to treat those with such serious diseases as Parkinson's, heart disease, and diabetes. Moreover, it has improved our prospects for understanding the processes of early human development and offers a novel way of testing drugs for their safety and effectiveness without involving human subjects. Given the immense promise of stem cell research, it is important to understand just what stem cells are, where they come from, and what they might do before we go on to explore several major ethical and public policy issues that their application to human beings raises.

Stem cells exhibit two characteristics found in no other cells of the human body: they can renew themselves by cell division and, although they are unspecialized, can differentiate into various cell types, such as those of bone, muscle, and blood.[2] These cells are central to human development and health for two main reasons: they have a role in the formation and maintenance of our bodily organs and they travel to diseased or injured tissue sites to inject a stream of new cells to replace those that have gone awry.[3] Stem cells have been discovered in human adults and infants, as well as in human embryos, fetuses, placentas, and umbilical cord blood. They are also found in a wide variety of animals, including mice, rabbits, monkeys, and fruit flies.

Scientific investigators are growing human stem cells in cultures in the laboratory with several different goals in mind. Their first aim is to use stem cells as the basis of new therapies for those with serious diseases. Medical researchers hope to learn how to guide the differentiation of stem cells into specific types of cells and then transfer these stem cell offshoots to patients to provide lifelong treatments for such conditions as diabetes, spinal cord injury, and heart failure.[4] Researchers are also exploring the use of stem cells for the treatment of degenerative diseases associated with aging, such as Alzheimer's disease and Parkinson's disease. The transferred cells would not just stop the progression of disease, as do current methods of medical treatment, but would also restore lost cellular, tissue, and organ functions. Such cell-based therapy is therefore often referred to as "regenerative medicine."[5]

In their efforts to develop stem cell–based therapies, some scientists are attempting to pair stem cell research with research into human genes. This involves taking stem cells from patients, modifying them genetically to correct genes associated with inherited disorders, and then reintroducing them into these patients. Inserting modified genes into stem cells would provide a more precise way to repair tissue in patients than current methods of direct gene transfer by means of viral vectors or other means.[6] Medical researchers could, for instance, insert a normal copy of a gene into differentiating stem cells that are missing that gene or in which that gene is malfunctioning in the laboratory and, when satisfied that the genetically modified cells meet appropriate tests for safety and efficacy, could then transfer them to the bodies of patients with such conditions as hemophilia and muscular dystrophy.[7] Indeed, some predict that, in the future, it will be possible through the combined use of stem cells, gene transfer, and tissue engineering not only to provide patients with treatments that will last a lifetime but also to create whole organs to replace those that fail.[8]

A second major aim of stem cell researchers is to gain increased understanding of the processes of human development. They hope to learn how a single cell, the early embryo, divides, grows, and gives rise to the trillions of cells and hundreds of tissues that make up the human body. Gaining a more complete grasp of how the human organism develops could open the door to understanding how healthy cells replace damaged cells and how cellular proliferation is regulated in space and time. Since many cancers arise from disturbances of normal developmental processes, the study of human stem cells is already informing cancer research. Further, studies of how abnormal cell divisions that may occur during the first few days of embryonic growth lead to chromosomal and developmental disorders in newborn children could lead medical researchers to develop treatments for such birth anomalies.[9] Stem cell research could also advance knowledge about the causes of infertility and help diminish premature pregnancy loss.

A third goal of stem cell research, scientists point out, is to provide new ways to test drugs for efficacy, toxicity, and safety. Investigators currently assess new pharmaceuticals in animals before they begin trials of these drugs in human beings. Yet there are significant differences between animal and human physiology. Consequently, animal studies do not necessarily reveal how these new drugs will affect humans. Indeed, some assays performed on animals may overstate the toxicity of drugs.[10] For such reasons, it has been proposed that human stem cells could be used for drug screening and testing. Drugs would be applied to specialized cells derived from human stem cells, such as those of the heart and liver, and these cells would then be evaluated for evidence of drug efficacy and toxicity. This would help weed out dangerous compounds before they were used in clinical testing in humans. If results indicated that further testing was warranted, human trials of such drugs could be initiated.[11]

A word of caution is in order. The field of stem cell research is fraught with challenges. There are many issues related to the derivation, expansion, manipulation, characterization, and testing of stem cells for efficacy, toxicity, disposition to tumor and cancer formation, and immune responses that must be resolved before these cells or cells derived from them can be used to treat patients.[12] It is important to realize that, as things stand as of this writing, few stem cells progeny are ready for safe and ethical use in treating human beings. Some believe that in another five years, clinical researchers will be ready to transplant specialized stem cells or their offshoots into patients to replace cells that are diseased or carry deleterious mutations. Others argue that it will take much longer to achieve these goals, since considerably more information about the basic biology of human stem cells needs to be developed before they can be used more broadly to treat human beings safely.[13]

Brief History of the Discovery and Derivation of Stem Cells

The groundwork for the 1998 development of the first embryonic stem cell lines was provided in the early 1960s when James Till and Ernest McCulloch and their colleagues at the University of Toronto came across reservoirs of cells in mice with the properties of stem cells: the abilities to self-renew and to differentiate into specialized cells.[14] They found that these stem cells, which they had discovered in the bone marrow of mice, had the remarkable capacity to make all the cell types found in blood.

Researchers applied these findings to humans and in the late 1960s began to infuse hematopoietic stem cells from human adult bone marrow into patients to treat such blood diseases as leukemia and sickle cell anemia. They also developed more advanced techniques of harvesting hematopoietic stem cells to counteract non-Hodgkin's lymphoma and other inherited blood disorders. In 1988, investigators introduced umbilical cord blood transplants into clinical practice; these also involved the infusion of hematopoietic stem cells into patients with diseases related to the blood. More recently, they have discovered additional stem cells that reside in such diverse tissues of the human body as brain, muscle, and skin.[15] These sorts of stem cells have been dubbed "adult" stem cells, because they are found in human adults (this is a misnomer, because these cells are also found in infants, fetuses, placentas, and umbilical cord blood).

Meanwhile, work continued in mice, and in 1981 scientists isolated embryonic stem cells from the inner cell mass of mouse embryos.[16] They discovered that these cells could give rise to all the tissues that eventually make up a normal mouse, such as blood, brain, liver, kidney, and bone. In the mid-1990s, scientists went on to derive embryonic stem cells from monkeys and found that stem cells from these primates had similar properties.[17] The first documentation of the isolation of embryonic stem cells from human embryos, although not their culture, was by Ariff Bongso and colleagues in 1994.[18] These findings, taken together, suggested that embryonic stem cells could be used to develop new ways to repair or regenerate a wide variety of damaged cells and tissues in seriously ill patients and paved the way for the derivation and culture of human embryonic stem cells.

In 1998, James Thomson and colleagues at the University of Wisconsin announced that they had completed the first successful isolation and culture of human embryonic stem cells from five-day-old embryos. These embryos had been donated by couples who had embryos remaining after they had completed in vitro fertilization (IVF) procedures.[19] (See chapter 2.) In that same year, a group directed by John Gearhart of Johns Hopkins University isolated and cultured human embryonic germ cells (cells that can grow into sperm and eggs) from cadaveric fetuses five to nine weeks old. These fetuses had been donated for research after elective abortions.[20] Embryonic germ cells, they found, have properties similar to those of embryonic stem cells. These studies were of tremendous scientific interest, for such stem cells are pluripotent, meaning that they can develop into almost all of the more than 200 different known cell types of the body. Their isolation meant that scientists could study them in detail to learn how they differentiate into specific types of cells. However, embryonic germ cells have not proven as useful in research as embryonic stem cells, since they do not tend to proliferate in the same large numbers as embryonic stem cells. Therefore, when "embryonic stem cells" are mentioned, this is usually taken to refer to the sort of stem cells developed by Thomson rather than to human embryonic germ cells.

Stem cell investigators today face the critical question of whether one of the two major sorts of human stem cells, adult or embryonic, might prove more effective in developing therapies for those with serious conditions or whether research on both should be pursued. Before we consider this question, however, it is important to gain a better understanding of how each sort of stem cell functions and what prospects each offers for opening fruitful lines of research and therapy.

Kinds of Stem Cells

The two major kinds of stem cells that are of interest to stem cell researchers are adult stem cells and embryonic stem cells. Although they exhibit the same defining properties, the two types differ in their ability to renew themselves and to produce a wide range of specialized cells. A third category of stem cells, fetal stem cells has also been sorted out by some investigators; although they can be expanded in greater numbers than adult stem cells can, this occurs only within a limited range of more specialized cells since their lineage is restricted to the region from which they are taken.[21] For the sake of simplicity, I focus here on the first two kinds of stem cell.

Human Adult Stem Cells

Most of the cells of the human body are terminally differentiated. That is, the cells of our organs, such as those of the lung, liver, kidney, and brain, have reached their final specialized state. However, there are some cells that hold back and remain stem cells; they continue to deliver new specialized cells to the bodies of humans that they need to continue living. These cells share the two main characteristics of stem cells: they can renew themselves, and they can give rise to new specialized cells. They are known as "adult" stem cells because, as noted, they are found in the bodies of adults—although they also can be found in infants, fetuses, placentas, and umbilical cord blood.[22] The primary role of these cells is to replace cells in the body that deteriorate because of injury or disease.

Although adult stem cells are rare, they have been found in bone marrow, blood vessels, peripheral blood, cornea, retina, brain, spinal cord, skeletal muscle, dental pulp, liver, skin, gastrointestinal tract, and pancreas.[23] Scientists are attempting to grow these cells in culture and direct them to generate specific cell types that can be used to treat disease and injury in humans. For example, they hope to develop insulin-producing cells from adult stem cells found in the pancreas to treat those with type I diabetes and to produce cardiac muscle cells from adult stem cells dwelling in the heart to repair heart muscles that have been damaged by heart attacks. Because adult stem cells tend to lose their ability for self-renewal as the body ages, some investigators have used adult stem cells derived from the donated tissue of miscarried and aborted fetuses in studies. For instance, researchers at the University of California have transplanted human neural fetal stem cells into mice with spinal cord injuries, producing some improvements.[24] Such investigations may pave the way for future testing in humans.[25]

Debate about Adult Stem Cell Versatility ("Plasticity")

It had long been thought that adult stem cells are prone to become only a few of the specialized cell types of the body. Each type of adult stem cell, it was maintained, could only generate cell types derived from the layer of the developing embryo in which it originates. It was believed that the middle layer of the embryo, for instance, could only generate blood, muscle, cartilage, endothelial cells, and cardiac cells. Moreover, it was thought that a cell fated to make blood cells could not make pancreatic or liver cells, and a cell fated to make neurons could not make blood or muscle cells.

Some investigators have recently challenged this view. In the last decade, a number of published studies have suggested that adult stem cells from one tissue are capable of developing into cell types characteristic of other tissues.[26] Scientists have reported finding that

Neural stem cells became blood cells[27] and muscle cells;[28]
Bone marrow stem cells generated cells akin to neurons[29] and heart tissue;[30]
Bone marrow and hematopoietic stem cells gave rise to muscle cells.[31]

Indeed, investigators in one study found that a single cell from the bone marrow of an adult mouse had contributed not only to the bone and blood but also to the lung tissue, liver, intestine, and skin of experimental mice.[32] Such studies supported the newly emerging view that a stem cell from one adult tissue can generate the differentiated cell types of certain other tissues when given the opportunity through experimental interventions. This phenomenon has been termed stem cell "plasticity."[33]

The concept of the plasticity of human adult stem cells came to greater public attention in 2002 when Catherine Verfaillie of the University of Minnesota and her colleagues reported finding that rare adult bone marrow progenitor stem cells of mice could differentiate into a wider variety of specialized cells than had been previously been found, although not all of the specialized cells of the human body.[34] When these adult bone marrow stem cells were transplanted into host animals, they entered into many different tissue types, including liver, lung, and intestine, where they differentiated into cell types appropriate to that tissue or organ. This report and others seemed to signify that adult stem cells are pluripotent and can produce almost any cell of the body. In short, this work suggested that an adult stem cell may be able to become any other cell, given certain permissive or instructive conditions.

The new thesis of the plasticity of adult stem cells was startling, for it went against some thirty-five years of previous research and thought. Not surprisingly, it was greeted with both excitement and skepticism. The versatility of certain adult stem cells that this new research displayed made them attractive as therapeutic agents. Taking stem cells from healthy tissue in one part of an individual's body to repair and regenerate diseased tissue in another part, it was speculated, would avoid the immunological rejection problem that can arise when transplanting cells, tissue, and organs from one individual to another.

Other studies questioned these novel claims about the plasticity of adult stem cells, however. Some investigators could not reproduce the results of certain studies that had been said to demonstrate such plasticity in adult stem cells. For instance, Derek van der Kooy and colleagues reported that they were unable to reproduce studies exhibiting a contribution of adult neural stem cells to blood cells.[35] Several other investigators who found that earlier reports of adult stem cell plasticity could not be repeated called into question their experimental design.[36] These findings, although not without critics of their own,[37] put into question several previous studies that had been heralded as exhibiting the plasticity of adult stem cells.

Some investigators who questioned the plasticity of adult stem cells explained this phenomenon in terms of cell fusion, hypothesizing that the inserted adult stem cells had simply merged with already existing differentiated cells in the recipients.[38] Thus, these investigators proposed that fusion, rather than differentiation across cell types, explained the seeming plasticity of adult stem cells. They concluded that the potential of adult stem cells to generate cells of other types is limited.

The debate about the plasticity of adult stem cells has not yet been resolved. The question of whether adult stem cells can differentiate into cell types outside their own lineage is one of the most important issues that stem cell scientists face today.[39] Just what occurs when adult stem cells transform into other sorts of cells, how efficient this process is, whether it is rare or common, and whether it has a role in the repair of tissue are still open questions. Many of the studies cited were carried out in mouse cells, which exhibit considerable plasticity. However, there are fewer cases in which human adult stem cells have exhibited such plasticity and have transdifferentiated into cells outside their lineage.

Current Therapeutic Uses of Adult Stem Cells

Although some adult stem cell applications have led to documented therapeutic results, the vast majority of possible uses of many different kinds of adult stem cells to treat patients is largely untested or is in the early stages.[40] The adult stem cell therapies developed thus far have primarily used hematopoietic stem cells. These kinds of cells, which are derived from bone marrow, have been employed for decades to treat patients with leukemia and other blood disorders.[41] Umbilical cord hematopoietic stem cells have been used for therapeutic purposes, primarily in children.[42] Transplants of stem cells derived from bone marrow are currently being carried out to treat certain forms of cancer, diseases that involve bone failure (such as aplastic anemia), and autoimmune diseases.[43] Although recent research has raised the possibility that adult stem cells derived from bone marrow could be used to treat a wider range of diseases, progress thus far has been slow and spotty.

The case of attempted cardiac repair using several different sorts of adult stem cells found in bone marrow is instructive. Attempts to use such stem cells in patients with heart disease, although initially hailed as life-saving, have produced ambiguous findings.[44] Some researchers, prompted by findings that stem cells derived from bone marrow had apparently changed into heart cells in mice with heart injuries,[45] used human stem cells derived from bone marrow to study heart repair in patients.[46] In some of these studies, patients showed modest improvement in heart function and provided some evidence that their heart tissue had been restored.[47] However, in other studies, cardiac patients who received such bone marrow-derived stem cells showed no significant long-term improvement or no improvement at all.[48] It is unclear whether the cells inserted into patients actually transformed into cardiac cells, or instead stimulated a repair mechanism within the patients themselves. The consensus at this time appears to be that such studies do not offer convincing evidence to support claims of cardiac muscle regeneration through the use of bone-marrow derived stem cell transplants.

Some scientists maintain that before proceeding further with clinical trials of adult stem cells, it is necessary to gain a greater understanding of the processes of adult stem repair.[49] Researchers need to comprehend how stem cells multiply, which renewal factors are at work, and which pathways these cells take in living systems. Some add that research with human embryonic stem cells will enable researchers to isolate authentic progenitors of different types of cells and to define the specific factors that drive their renewal.[50] Further down the road, stem cell investigators will need to develop ways of maximizing grafts in human subjects and identifying potential adverse effects that such subjects might experience. Many additional attempts will need to be made in animals and in humans (in double-blinded, placebo-controlled studies) if research using adult stem cells is to fulfill its promise for patients with chronic degenerative diseases.

Advantages and Limitations of Using Human Adult Stem Cells

Although stem cells in adult tissues in general may not be pluripotent, there is some evidence, as noted, that some of these cells can change course and differentiate into tissue of another type from that in which they originate. These findings suggest that adult stem cells may have therapeutic potential beyond their original lineage. This would be a significant advantage offered by the use of these types of stem cells.

However, research into adult stem cells faces several stumbling blocks. It is difficult to identify adult stem cells and separate them from other cells, since their presence in a tissue or mixture of cells currently must be inferred from experimental observations, rather than indicated by specific biochemical markers. Furthermore, when adult stem cells have been identified, it has been difficult to grow them in an unspecialized state and to direct them to become specialized, functionally useful cells in tissue culture.[51] Research is needed to show, for example, that adult neural stem cells injected into the brain will make brain cells and not bone or muscle cells, that they will produce sufficient numbers of neural cells to be effective, and that these brain cells will function properly. It is generally believed that stem cells used for therapies should be at least partially differentiated to reduce the possibility that they will proliferate uncontrollably to form a tumor. Adult stem cells generally do not proliferate well in culture, restricting the numbers available to use in therapies.

A major factor restricting attempts to use adult stem cells to replace damaged cells in the body is that the human body contains only minute quantities of adult stem cells to transplant into patients. Further, there is a dearth of reports indicating that adult stem cells can be purified to a point where no other cell types are present. It may be that some adult stem cells retain many of their characteristics as a result of the presence of signals from the cells surrounding them and that this explains why it is difficult to maintain them in culture apart from a living organism.

Scientists will not only have to overcome such basic experimental issues, but also to address certain safety issues that arise related to the therapeutic use of adult stem cells in humans. These cells may exhibit DNA abnormalities caused by sunlight and toxins, as well as by errors in DNA copies found within the bodies of humans in which they reside.[52] Moreover, some adult stem cells may become malignant if they are allowed to multiply for long periods of time, especially outside the body. For instance, one form of leukemia has been shown to be associated with adult bone marrow stem cells that have malfunctioned.[53] In culture, rapidly proliferating adult stem cells may be transformed into cancerous cells. Scientists are hoping to learn how to inactivate the proliferation of these aberrant adult stem cells before they cause damage.

More broadly, there is uncertainty about just what the scientific and therapeutic potential of adult stem cells might be. There are huge gaps between growing a set of adult stem cells in culture, controlling their differentiation into specific cell types (such as heart or nerve cells), injecting such cells into patients in order to treat disease, and ensuring that uncontrolled development of cancerous tumors does not occur. If such stem cells are to be of therapeutic use, it will be necessary to learn how to isolate them, grow them in culture, and differentiate them into normal new cell types.[54]

Human Embryonic Stem Cells

Human embryonic stem cells exhibit the two major characteristics of stem cells: they can renew themselves and can also give rise to specialized cells of the body.[55] What is distinctive about these sorts of stem cells is that they can develop into almost all of the cell types of the body. They have been shown to transform in culture into blood,[56] skin,[57] heart,[58] neural progenitor,[59] skeletal muscle,[60] and insulin-producing cells.[61] In addition, they multiply rapidly and can be grown in great abundance in culture.[62] Thus, they provide a large-scale source of stem cells, which makes them of tremendous interest to those seeking treatments for a wide variety of diseases.

Human embryonic stem cells are derived from the early embryo, generally at or before four to six days after sperm and egg merge. (See figure 1.1.) At this stage, the embryo is a microscopic ball composed of approximately 200–250 cells and is smaller than a pinpoint. Within it is an inner cell mass of some 30–40 cells that is surrounded by an outer ring. The primitive undifferentiated cells of this inner cell mass can be cultured into human embryonic stem cells. In the course of the delicate process of removing the cells of the inner cell mass to derive stem cells from them, the embryo is destroyed.

In 1998, Thomson and his team cultured embryonic stem cells by transferring them to laboratory dishes that held nutrients and growth factors.[63] There the cells divided and spread over the surface of the dishes. After several days, when the multiplying stem cells began to crowd the culture dishes, the scientists removed them and placed them in fresh dishes, a process that they repeated many times. Gradually, they were able to expand these cells into stem cell lines, which are colonies of millions of stem cells that continue to multiply but retain

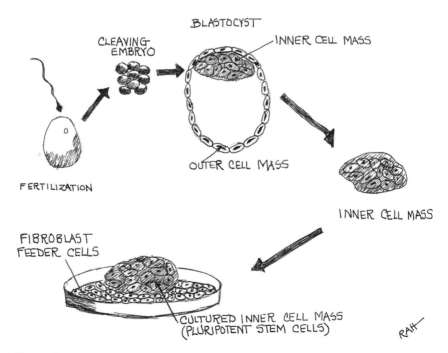

Figure 1.1. Derivation of human embryonic stem cells. Stem cells are removed from the inner cell mass of a blastocyst (early embryo) and placed in a culture of feeder cells to grow and divide.

their original undifferentiated state. Once these cell lines were established, batches of them were frozen; most of them recovered after thawing. This method has been used with some modifications in subsequent studies in which human embryonic stem cells have been cultured.[64] This work has been extremely fruitful. By mid-2005 there were approximately 150 embryonic stem cell lines worldwide.[65]

Human embryonic germ cells, which were also isolated in 1998, are derived from cells in the gonadal ridge of the embryo or fetus; this is the area from which eggs and sperm develop. These cells have some of the same characteristics as human embryonic stem cells. Both are capable of long-term self-renewal.[66] However, as noted, embryonic stem cells have a greater capacity than embryonic germ cells for proliferation in culture. Human embryonic stem cells can proliferate for two years through 300 population doublings,[67] whereas those grown from human germ cells can increase their numbers for around twenty-one days at most, with only 40–80 population doublings.[68] This capacity for proliferation is one of the features of human embryonic stem cells that makes them of greater interest to investigators. Another factor leading researchers to focus on human embryonic stem cells, rather than germ cells, is that attempts to derive specialized cells from embryonic germ cells in mice have led to abnormalities in the resulting cells.[69]

Human embryonic stem cells not only offer great potential for therapeutic advances but also can be used to increase knowledge about very early human development. The study of such stem cells could lead researchers to identify the genetic, molecular, and cellular events that are responsible for congenital birth anomalies and placental abnormalities. From there, clinical investigators could go on to develop methods for preventing such conditions and treating those that they cannot avert. Research on embryonic stem cells should lead to better understanding of the basis for their greater pluripotency and proliferative capacity in comparison with adult stem cells. It might then be possible to engineer those crucial capacities into adult stem cells derived from patients for subsequent therapeutic uses.

Several reports have documented that genes can be introduced into human embryonic stem cells[70] and even targeted to specific sites. This provides scientists with a way to analyze gene function and regulation in human embryonic stem cells as they differentiate, as well as the opportunity to study cells with genetic abnormalities in those instances in which the gene associated with a specific disease is known. It lays the groundwork for future efforts to genetically alter such cells for therapeutic purposes based on the information gained in such studies.[71] That is, targeted gene replacement provides an opportunity to replace a defective mutant gene with a functional gene, a first step in genetic therapy.

However, researchers using embryonic stem cells face a significant challenge, for they must come to understand the mechanisms by which these cells differentiate into specific cell types. (See figure 1.2.) Multiple signaling networks orchestrate the development and differentiation of these stem cells, and scientists must separate these networks from one another and come to understand the functions of each.[72] They know that some signals for cell differentiation come from chemicals secreted by other cells, physical contact with neighboring cells, and molecules in their immediate environment[73] and therefore hypothesize that these cells are probably responding to complex mixtures of signaling molecules. Stem cell investigators are attempting to identify such signals more specifically in order to develop methods for controlling embryonic stem cell differentiation in the laboratory and then in living systems. They must complete this effort before they can attempt to insert embryonic stem cells or their progeny into humans in order to overcome diseases and debilitating conditions.[74]

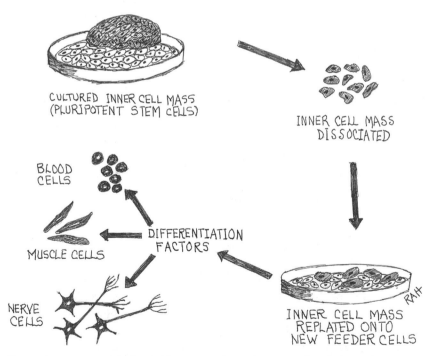

Figure 1.2. Differentiation of human embryonic stem cells. Embryonic stem cells are removed from culture and directed to develop into specialized cells, such as blood, muscle, and nerve cells. These specialized stem cell offshoots might be used for transplantation into a patient's body for therapy or for research.

Therapeutic Uses of Human Embryonic Stem Cells

Human embryonic stem cells and their derivatives have many of the same potential therapeutic uses as adult stem cells. They could be used to replace or restore tissue damaged by disease or injury. However, at this point in time, human therapies based on the application of embryonic stem cells are still experimental. Those working in the field generally maintain that research on these sorts of stem cells has not reached the stage at which it can be attempted in humans. Even so, many current embryonic stem cell investigations are geared toward exploring possible future cures for certain diseases. For instance, some researchers are attempting to produce neurons from human embryonic stem cells in order to treat persons with Parkinson's disease and to elicit pancreatic cells producing insulin to transplant into those with diabetes.[75] However, many scientists agree that clinical trials of human embryonic stem cells for these conditions and others, such as amyotrophic lateral sclerosis and multiple sclerosis, are not likely to take place for at least five or—more likely—ten years.[76]

Other scientists argue that animal studies indicate that certain human embryonic stem cell treatments might be effective for repairing damaged cells in patients sooner than that. Geron Corporation in Menlo Park, California, plans to begin treatment of those with spinal cord injuries by means of human embryonic stem cells sometime in 2007.[77] This work, based on research by Hans Keirstead of the University of California at Irvine and his colleagues,[78] is designed to ameliorate but not cure such injuries. One of its purposes is to display the safety of using human embryonic stem cell therapies in humans. However, as was the case with adult stem cell research, here, too, researchers disagree about whether sufficient work has been done in animals to justify moving this research to clinical efforts with human beings.

Advantages and Limitations of Using Human Embryonic Stem Cells

A significant advantage that human embryonic stem cells offer is that they can be multiplied over long periods of time in the laboratory—in principle, indefinitely. One group of embryonic stem cells, after proliferating in the laboratory for several months, can provide millions of cells. Moreover, embryonic stem cells can differentiate into a wide range of cell types and can regenerate all normal cell types found in the body. Their extreme flexibility and capacity for growth appear to make them ideal for producing large quantities of cells to treat many diseases and injuries.

Yet research on human embryonic stem cells is at a relatively early stage, and there are still numerous barriers that stem cell investigators must overcome before the promise of this research might be realized. It is difficult to derive and maintain embryonic stem cells. The molecular mechanisms that underlie their self-renewal are unknown. They can be hard to study in a living system;[79] when tested in animals, these cells have at times differentiated into the wrong cells or migrated away from the insertion site.[80] Perhaps the most serious problem associated with the therapeutic use of embryonic stem cells in humans is that, if they are transferred to patients, these cells might grow into unwanted tissue or cancerous tumors.[81] Studies indicate that if embryonic stem cells that have not begun to differentiate are injected into mice with compromised immune systems, a benign tumor known as a teratoma with rapidly growing cells of several differentiated cell types can develop.[82] This would clearly be undesirable if such stem cells were transplanted into patients. Since it is undifferentiated embryonic stem cells (but not the specialized cells that are developed from them) that have been shown to induce teratomas, it has been hypothesized that such tumor formation might be avoided by removing any undifferentiated embryonic cells from the groups of such cells that are to be inserted into patients. Only the more specialized cells into which embryonic stem cell differentiate, such as skin and pancreas cells, stem cell scientists currently think, should be considered for therapy in humans. This would reduce the risk that tumors might develop in patients.

Another significant problem that those attempting to use embryonic stem cells for therapeutic purposes have to confront is that of immune rejection. Because embryonic stem cells will not ordinarily have been derived from the specific patient to be treated, there is a risk that they will be rejected by that patient's immune system. Scientists have proposed several different ways of avoiding this difficulty. These include using research cloning (somatic cell nuclear transfer) procedures to generate human embryonic stem cells that are genetically identical to those of the person receiving the transplant, genetically engineering the embryonic stem cells to express certain antigens of the recipient that would counter any possible immune reaction, or developing "universal" donor stem cell lines that could be used in many different patients.[83] However, each of these methods has its drawbacks. (See chapter 2.)

Many of the embryonic stem cell lines currently available for research, including all of those approved for use in federally funded research under the Bush policy as of this writing, were cultured on mouse feeder cells layers that promote proliferation.[84] However, there is significant evidence that these lines are contaminated with sialic acid from mice, which produces an immune reaction,[85] and with mouse viruses. These factors could make them unsafe to use in clinical applications in human beings.[86] In 2005, scientists tested five human embryonic stem cell lines that had been nurtured on mouse feeder cells, along with several cultures of mouse feeder cells for signs of mouse retroviruses and found no evidence of such viruses.[87] Although their study suggests that stem cell lines established on mouse feeder layers might be free from viruses, it does not overcome the problem of the contamination of human embryonic stem cell lines cultured on mouse feeders with sialic acid. Therefore, it is preferable to use feeder cells that do not contain animal products to avoid this difficulty.[88]

Scientists have attempted to overcome the contamination problem by developing new methods of culturing human embryonic stem cells that do not require mouse feeder cells.[89] Some have developed human components for this purpose,[90] while others have employed cells derived from differentiated human embryonic stem cells.[91] Still others have used mouse extracellular matrix components, rather than whole mouse cells, to culture human embryonic stem cells.[92] Such measures have allowed them to develop some human embryonic stem cell lines that are free of animal contamination.[93]

Comparing Human Embryonic Stem Cells with Human Adult Stem Cells

There are significant biological differences between human embryonic and adult stem cells. Embryonic stem cells can be isolated from embryos with relative ease and have an unlimited ability to self-renew and proliferate in culture in huge numbers for many generations. Further, they are the only stem cell lines known to be undifferentiated and pluripotent that are available for study. This means that they are more likely to generate a wider range of cell types. Such characteristics, in combination, give embryonic stem cells a remarkably broad therapeutic potential. Yet the availability of human embryos for the production of stem cells is limited and subject to considerable ethical controversy and legal restrictions. Many of the existing stem cell lines are incompletely characterized and may not be robust or stable in their properties.

Adult stem cells, in contrast, are found in low numbers in the human body, can be difficult to obtain, do not expand readily in culture, and may be capable of differentiation into only a limited number of cell types. It seems likely that a few known adult stem cells exhibit stem cell plasticity and can differentiate into cell types outside their usual path. Such adult stem cells would need somehow to be isolated, expanded, and then efficiently reprogrammed onto a new pathway of differentiation if they were to be used to treat patients. This extra reprogramming step makes the development of specialized cells from adult stem cells more complicated than from embryonic stem cells. All of these factors seem to give embryonic stem cells an edge over adult stem cells for research and therapy, based on the current state of scientific knowledge.

Consequently, some stem cell scientists and research experts consider human embryonic stem cell research more promising than adult stem cell research and, ultimately, more promising for patient treatment. Yet most in the field appear to see both kinds of stem cells as providing complementary avenues for research and therapy.[94] The National Research Council of the National Academies maintains that the "best available scientific and medical evidence indicates that research on both embryonic and adult human stem cells will be needed."[95] The National Institutes of Health has come to a similar conclusion.[96]

The extent to which these two different stem cell types will be useful in generating replacement cells and tissues in patients with disease and injury is unknown at this point in time.[97] Substantially more research on both sorts of stem cells is needed before it can be definitively determined whether one provides a better route to therapies than the other. There are multiple technical hurdles that must first be overcome. Over the next several years, it will be important to continue to compare these two sorts of stem cells in terms of their ability to proliferate, differentiate, survive and function after transplant, and avoid immune rejection.[98] If stem cell therapies of either kind are to be of clinical benefit and of demonstrated safety, a much clearer understanding of the processes of differentiation and dedifferentiation will be needed. It will also be important to develop clear and rigorous standards for evaluating embryonic and adult stem cells so that their potential uses can be accurately compared. There is increasing evidence that stem cells, like other cells, accumulate mutations as they are maintained in culture and may become transformed into cancerous cells. Sensitive methods for testing cells used for therapies must be developed. Since few animal studies have looked at results much longer than a year after transplantation, the long-term consequences of both of these sorts of stem cell therapies need to be studied. In short, continued intensive research on both sorts of stem cells is needed before one kind can be said to be overwhelmingly superior to the other for research and therapy.

Future Outlook for Stem Cell Research in the United States

Additional research on human embryonic stem cells in the United States and abroad will undoubtedly require the development and characterization of new lines of these cells. The existing lines that have been approved for public funding in the United States, stem cell scientists and others maintain, are insufficient in number and genetic variety for the research that many federally funded stem cell investigators maintain it is necessary and important to pursue.[99] Moreover, state and private funding of this research are proceeding slowly. (See chapter 6.) A 2006 survey of publication rates of U.S. and non-U.S. stem cell research groups indicates that "the United States is falling behind in the international race to make fundamental discoveries in hES cell-related fields."[100] This has been and still is a source of consternation for scientists, patients, and others concerned about the treatment of those with serious disease and those who recognize the need to develop a more fulsome basic understanding of the processes of human development.[101] Significant questions are being raised about whether the United States, if the current federal stem cell research policy continues in force, will continue to play a role as a scientific powerhouse at the forefront of cutting-edge scientific research, such as that involving human stem cells, or will have to cede that role to scientists working abroad. These are important and troubling questions to which we will return in several subsequent chapters.

2

The Search for New Sources
of Pluripotent Stem Cells

The number of human embryonic stem cell lines currently available for research in the United States, some scientists, legislators, and commentators maintain, is insufficient for research and therapeutic efforts.[1] They find that the policy of President George W. Bush of providing federal funding only for research on twenty-two embryonic stem cell lines derived before August 2001 has left researchers with too small a number of stem cell lines with which to go forward at a rapid pace. Furthermore, cells that are maintained in culture for a significant length of time tend to deteriorate, including those listed on the National Institutes of Health (NIH) registry. Many of these stem cell lines, although some say not all,[2] have been cultured with nonhuman cells or serum that would pose health risks to patients who received differentiated offshoots from them in research or therapy.[3] For such reasons, stem cell investigators are attempting to develop a larger pool of human pluripotent stem cells—cells that can transform into almost any cell of the body except placental tissue—by expanding the use of certain currently available sources of these cells and developing new sources.

Meanwhile, other scientists, legislators, and commentators—many of whom are convinced of the therapeutic promise of embryonic stem cell research but object to the destruction of human embryos that it currently entails—are looking for new sources of pluripotent stem cells that are free of what they view as the ethical taint of embryo destruction.[4] Finding additional sources of these stem cells, they believe, would lift the major ethical barrier to the successful pursuit of such research and encourage greater federal and private support for this field.

For such reasons, a search for additional sources of embryonic stem cells is under way in the United States. Although those pursuing it are motivated by different concerns, they are not entirely at odds. They agree that certain proposed additional sources might prove fruitful and might also avoid raising ethical concerns for those who object to the destruction of human embryos in stem cell research. However, they disagree about whether it is scientifically feasible to develop certain of these sources of pluripotent stem cells and whether it is ethically necessary and defensible to do so.

In this chapter, I launch the exploration of the search for new techniques for developing pluripotent stem cells by first examining the current situation, which primarily involves the use of spare embryos remaining after in vitro fertilization (IVF) treatment for research and the creation of embryos for research by means of IVF. I consider several significant scientific, practical, and ethical issues that each of these sources of embryonic stem cells raises and then turn to certain new strategies that have been proposed for obtaining pluripotent stem cells, examining the major scientific, practical, and ethical questions evoked by each of these. Additional sources of pluripotent stem cells are being proposed at a rapid pace, and it is probable that even more than those discussed here—those that are incipient in the minds of inventive scientists and commentators—will see the light of day in the coming years.

Using Spare Embryos Remaining after In Vitro Fertilization for Research and Therapy

Many embryonic stem cells currently available for research and eventual therapy have been derived from spare embryos remaining at IVF centers. These embryos exist because IVF treatment can result in the development of more of them than are ultimately needed by those attempting to have children. This means that some embryos remain at infertility treatment centers that will never be used for the reproductive purposes of those who had them developed. To understand how and why this occurs, it is important to grasp how the IVF process works. (See chapter 8 for further discussion.)

IVF involves joining a human egg and sperm in a laboratory dish where they can fuse to form an embryo. The eggs that figure in this process come from women who have undergone ovarian stimulation and egg extraction.[5] Since women ordinarily develop only one or two mature eggs a month, they are usually advised to improve their chances of pregnancy by increasing the number of eggs they produce. They can do so by injecting themselves with ovulation-stimulating drugs for eight to twelve days.[6] The use of such drugs poses certain health risks to those receiving them. The multiple eggs produced are then removed from the bodies of these women in a procedure known as ultrasound transvaginal egg retrieval, which also carries certain physical risks for women.[7] (See chapter 8 for further discussion.)

Many embryos that are not used for the first IVF round are frozen. Should the initial IVF attempt prove unsuccessful or should patients succeed in a first try and want to have additional children in the future, these frozen embryos would be available to them. The main advantage of such freezing is that there would be no need for women to undergo the risks of egg retrieval again in future IVF attempts. As a result of this practice, it was estimated that in 2002 there were nearly 400,000 frozen embryos stored in the United States.[8]

Those with frozen embryos remaining after IVF treatment may decide that they no longer need them for procreation for a variety of reasons, such as that they now have sufficient children, they no longer have the heart to undergo additional IVF treatments, or they are not able to develop viable embryos. They face a choice of discarding them, donating them to another couple for procreative attempts, donating them for research, or keeping them frozen indefinitely. Some among them choose to donate these spare embryos for research.[9] Others have fresh embryos remaining that they do not plan to use for reproductive purposes in the future and that they do not wish to cryopreserve. They choose not to freeze them for varying reasons, such as that they do not want to use embryos that might be damaged by freezing or that their religious tradition proscribes embryo freezing.[10] Those who choose against cryopreserving spare embryos may also decide to donate them for research.

Some spare embryos remaining at IVF clinics are not considered viable and could not be used in reproductive efforts.[11] Bernard Lo and colleagues point out that "embryos may be of poor quality or otherwise fail to develop sufficiently for implantation or freezing. In these situations, the...embryos cannot be used in ART [assisted reproductive technology]."[12] Some couples decide that instead of discarding such embryos they would rather donate them for research that might aid those who are seriously ill. Three of the seventeen new human embryonic stem cell lines derived in 2004 by Douglas Melton and his team at Harvard University were derived from IVF embryos with poor morphological characteristics; these embryos would otherwise have been discarded. Four of them were of "intermediate" quality and would also probably not have been used in attempts at IVF.[13]

Thus there are many reasons why embryos remain at IVF clinics in both frozen and fresh states that will not be used in attempts to have a child. Some who object to the destruction of these embryos in stem cell research maintain that they should be donated to others in order to initiate pregnancies. Yet some couples and individuals do not wish to have such embryos used to create children who would be biologically theirs but who would exist somewhere else in the world, children who would be raised by people about whom they know nothing. For this reason, many among them choose not to donate their spare embryos to others for procreative purposes. Rather than discard these embryos, they decide to donate them for research that might help others overcome serious diseases.

Whether It Is Wrong to Use Spare Embryos for Research and Therapy

Since these spare embryos will no longer be used for a procreative end, some commentators maintain, it is ethically sound to use them for research that has a therapeutic end.[14] They argue that the ultimate goal of such research, to treat those who are sick and suffering, is as worthy as the goal of reproduction and justifies using, rather than discarding, these remaining embryos. (See chapter 3 for further discussion.) Early human embryos do not have the same moral significance as individual living human beings, they maintain, and are not owed protection from destruction in such research. Consequently, it is ethically acceptable, in their view, to use these spare embryos in stem cell research.

Others believe that human embryos are individual living human beings and that it is wrong to create embryos and then destroy them in research, no matter how beneficial that research might be. For instance, Robert George, of the President's Council on Bioethics, and Patrick Lee declare:

> No one would object to the use of embryonic stem cells in biomedical research or therapy if they could be harvested without killing or harming the embryos from whom they were obtained. . . . The point of the controversy is the ethics of deliberately destroying human embryos for the purpose of harvesting their stem cells. The threshold question is whether it is unjust to kill members of a certain class of human beings—those in the embryonic stage of development—to benefit others.[15]

They argue that the lives of some human beings should not be sacrificed in order to develop cures for others. Every spare embryo should be used for a procreative end, in their view. They do not address what should be done with those embryos developed by means of IVF that are not viable and therefore are not suitable for procreative purposes.

The key issue here is how we should view the moral significance of early human embryos. If all early embryos were individual human beings, that would close this discussion. However, there are serious reasons to question whether this is the case and to argue that both procreation and regeneration are ethically sound ends to which to direct the use of early human embryos. (See chapter 3 for further discussion.)

Possibility of Deliberately Overproducing Spare Embryos

An ethical and policy concern that has been raised about the use of spare human embryos in stem cell research is that some infertility specialists might deliberately develop more embryos than it is reasonable to produce in IVF treatment without the knowledge of their patients.[16] They might do so, on this hypothesis, in order to provide these embryos to colleagues who are stem cell investigators for research. Although infertility specialists indicate that such overproduction does not occur, there is currently no way to verify that this is the case in the United States. Professional guidelines promulgated by the American Society for Reproductive Medicine (ASRM) recognize this possibility in passing but offer no proposal to address it.[17]

This issue surfaces because little is known in a systematic way about what goes on as a matter of practice during the course of IVF treatments.[18] Few methods have been developed in common by assisted reproduction clinics across the country to cope with the wide range of informed consent and other patient care issues that arise in IVF. This is the situation despite persistent calls for better ways of ensuring that patients are appropriately informed about what IVF and egg retrieval involve and for improved methods of discouraging infertility specialists from overproducing embryos in attempts to increase the pregnancy rates at their clinics and thereby attract greater numbers of prospective patients.[19] (See chapter 8 for further discussion.)

Developing Embryos through In Vitro Fertilization for Research and Therapy

Embryos have been developed specifically for stem cell research by means of IVF.[20] In such instances, the IVF procedure described above is carried out with eggs and sperm that are donated for research. The resulting embryos are grown in culture, and at about five or six days after fertilization, when they have reached the blastocyst stage, stem cells are removed from their inner cell mass. Researchers then use these stem cells in various forms of stem cell research.

Whether It Is Wrong to Create Embryos through IVF for Research and Eventual Therapy

Once again, this time in the context of the creation of embryos for research, the question of the moral significance of early human embryos comes to the fore. It is especially heated in this context just because procreation, the most familiar end for which embryos have been created historically, is not at issue here. Some view it as ethically sound to develop human embryos for research because this might lead to the development of treatments for those with serious diseases.[21] Here too, as when procreation is the end sought, they contend, early human embryos do not have the same moral significance as individual living human beings. Others maintain that human embryos are individual living human beings and should not be used for any purpose other than procreation. It is especially egregious ethically, in their view, to develop human embryos specifically for research and therapy, knowing that they will be destroyed. (See chapter 3 for further discussion.)

Altruism and the Risks of Gamete Retrieval to Donors

The health risks that women who go through egg retrieval procedures face, briefly described above in the context of creating embryos through IVF, are more difficult to justify, some maintain, when women undertake them solely to aid unknown others in the future.[22] Although women who provide eggs for research receive the altruistic satisfaction of knowing that they might assist others to overcome serious disease, they gain such satisfaction only at some risk to themselves. Consequently, some critics of the creation of embryos for research have raised a basic ethical question about gamete donation: Is it ethically acceptable to ask women to put themselves in some degree of danger by donating eggs for research when there is no individual or group of individuals who would be the direct beneficiaries of their donation?

Male gametes are also needed to create embryos for research. The procedure of sperm donation is not as onerous and risky for men as egg donation is for women. However, the same question arises with regard to sperm donors: Is it ethically acceptable to ask them to donate gametes for research that will benefit no specific persons?

We have as a society answered this question in the affirmative in contexts in which individuals volunteer to participate as research subjects. That is, we allow individuals to contribute to the development of generalizable knowledge at some risk to themselves—within reasonable limits—if they are fully informed about what the proposed research in which they might participate involves and make a voluntary choice to go forward with their role in that research . It is difficult to defend the view that women and men who are well informed about the risks of gamete donation and who understand the nature of the research project in which their gametes would be used should not be allowed to do the same. Altruism, even when directed toward those who might not yet experience serious disease, balanced by a careful weighing of the risks involved, has its place in research involving human subjects. This is also the case with regard to research involving donated gametes.

Additional questions arise about how to ensure that those who consider providing gametes for research make a choice that is voluntary and informed. Particular concerns arise about the possibility that they will be placed under undue pressure in order to entice them to donate and that women who are economically vulnerable will be exploited. These questions are not addressed here, as our focus is on the basic ethical issue of whether allowing gamete donation for research is ethically warranted, rather than on how to ensure that such donation is carried out within appropriate ethical bounds.

Developing Embryos through Research Cloning for Therapy

A major technical difficulty looms over the prospects of using currently available stem cells for therapy: the derivatives of these stem cells, if transferred to patients, would likely be rejected by their bodies as foreign and targeted for destruction.[23] Although recent research suggests that human embryonic stem cells and their derivatives are much less susceptible to immune rejection than adult stem cells, it confirms that such cells and derivatives may trigger a rejection response in some patients.[24] To overcome this problem, stem cell scientists are turning to the possibility of using non-reproductive cloning to develop human embryos from which they would derive stem cells that would be immunologically and genetically matched to specific patients. This use of such cloning would reduce the likelihood of immune rejection and avoid the need for adjunct immunosuppressive therapies.

Such non-reproductive cloning is termed "research cloning" here, rather than "therapeutic cloning," as some call it, since this procedure has not yet reached a stage of development at which it could be employed in the treatment of patients. It is also termed "research cloning" to indicate that the embryos developed by this method will not be used for procreative purposes but for research and eventual therapy. "Research cloning," in contrast to "reproductive cloning," is carried out in the laboratory in order to generate stem cells that can be

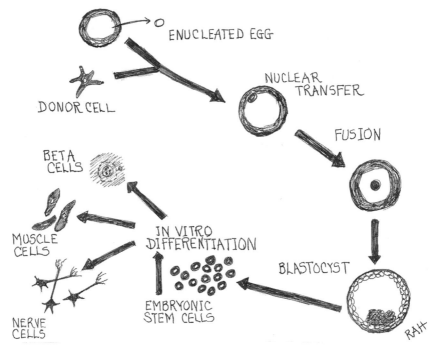

Figure 2.1. Research cloning (or somatic cell nuclear transfer). A nucleus from a patient is injected into a donated human egg whose nucleus has been removed. This construct is then activated electrically, chemically, or in other ways to form a blastocyst.

cultured to use for tissue replacement in therapy. The embryos developed in this process would not be transferred to any woman's uterus.[25] Finally, this method is termed "research cloning" instead of "somatic cell nuclear transfer for research" because the former nontechnical term is more meaningful to those who are not scientists.

Just what is research cloning? It involves removing the nucleus of a donated human egg, with all its genetic material, and replacing it with the nucleus of an adult somatic (body) cell from an individual patient. This results in an egg that contains the complete complement of the donor cell's nuclear genetic material. Medical investigators then use an electric impulse or chemicals to cause the somatic cell nucleus and egg to fuse together, resulting in a human embryo. (See figure 2.1.)

If researchers were to learn how to carry out this sort of cloning for therapeutic purposes, they would take a somatic cell from a specific patient, remove its nucleus, and transfer that nucleus to a donated human egg whose nucleus has been removed. They would clone that egg and at about five days of growth when it reaches the blastocyst stage derive stem cells from it. Next they would direct offshoots of these cells to differentiate into the cell type needed to treat the patient who initially provided the body cell and would then transfer these differentiated cells to that patient.[26] Because these cells would be almost genetically identical to the cells of the patient (except for their mitochondrial DNA, which is found in the material surrounding the nucleus of the egg), it is extremely unlikely that they would be rejected. Thus, research cloning would provide an additional source of human embryonic stem cells that does not involve the use of fertilized human eggs.[27]

For example, investigators engaging in research cloning would remove a skin cell or other body cell from a patient in need of additional heart muscle, insert it into a human egg from which the nucleus had been removed, and stimulate that egg to develop into an embryo. They would then derive stem cells from the inner cell mass of this embryo and establish embryonic stem cell lines from derivatives of these cells. Next they would take one of these lines and direct it to differentiate into heart muscle cells that they would transplant back into the patient. These heart muscle cells would have the same genes and immunological makeup as those of the patient and therefore would not trigger rejection.[28] Remaining heart muscle cells could be stored to have available as replacement cells, so that treatment of the patient could be repeated if necessary.[29]

To treat patients with gene-based diseases, research cloning could also be combined with gene transfer. Embryonic stem cells would be derived by means of research cloning, using the somatic cells of the patient with a genetic disorder, and derivatives of these cells would then be subjected to gene transfer or modification, differentiated, and transplanted back to that patient. The feasibility of this method has been demonstrated in an animal model using mice with a genetic disorder that has a human counterpart.[30] Such research cloning, it is hoped, could enable scientists to identify the origins of such conditions as Parkinson's disease and Alzheimer's disease.[31]

Thus, research cloning offers a way to learn what paths certain diseases take as they make headway in the human body. For example, it could enable scientists to identify the origins of such gene-based diseases as amyotrophic lateral sclerosis (Lou Gehrig's disease) and β- thalassemia and provide new information to use in treating patients with these conditions.[32] Furthermore, research cloning offers a way to develop more accurate models of various human diseases in order to test drugs and to explore the early stages of embryonic development in order to learn how and why embryonic and adult stem cells differentiate into more specialized cells.[33]

Current Status of Research Cloning

Several groups have shown that cloned embryonic stem cells can be derived from mouse cells and that these cells can be differentiated into several different kinds of somatic cells.[34] However, they have found it a more difficult feat to derive cloned embryonic stem cells using cells that are human.

Two accounts of human cloning for research and therapy were published by Woo Suk Hwang and his colleagues at Seoul National University in South Korea, one in 2004[35] and one in 2005.[36] Commentators initially observed that these studies amounted to a great leap forward in the development of research cloning.[37] However, these reports from the South Korean scientists proved false.[38] In 2006, they were retracted by the journal in which they were published.[39] Right now, stem cell investigators Evan Snyder and Jeanne Loring observe, "we do not know whether the procedure [i.e., research cloning] works at all, though we still suspect that the hurdles are more technological than biologic."[40]

Other centers have attempted to carry out research cloning in humans. A small biotech firm, Advanced Cell Technology, created a stir when it announced in 2001 that it had cloned several human embryos for transplantation into humans.[41] However, it is arguable that the resulting six-cell clusters, which died almost immediately, could not have been embryos because they did not lead to the development of a human being. In 2005, researchers at Newcastle University in the United Kingdom, led by Alison Murdoch, announced that they had cloned a human embryo.[42] That embryo, however, also ceased growing, although it lived for several days.

Investigators are attempting to discern why this cessation of growth occurs when research cloning is attempted and how to remedy it. Rudolph Jaenisch and his colleagues at Massachusetts Institute of Technology have found that two crucial genes essential to embryonic development fail to function in cloned blastocysts; they suggest that this might explain the problem.[43] If these genes were activated, this would enable the cloned blastocyst to continue to develop, they maintain.[44] Stem cell investigators are pursuing this and other avenues in hopes of finding a reliable method of research cloning.

Scientific and Practical Concerns Raised by Research Cloning

There has been some disagreement about whether research cloning is likely to provide a major new therapeutic route in stem cell research. Some contend that genetic irregularities found in mammalian embryos developed for reproductive cloning would also appear in human embryos cloned for research and therapy, rendering them unsuitable for use in patients. The President's Council on Bioethics, for instance, observed that the reproductive cloning procedure "resulted in high rates of death, deformity, and disability in the animals that come to birth following SCNT [somatic cell nuclear transfer]" and that research cloning would do the same.[45] In support of this observation, the council cited a study by Rudolf Jaenisch and colleagues indicating that about 4 percent of the genes in newborn mice that had been developed by means of reproductive cloning functioned abnormally.[46]

However, later studies by these same investigators, Hochedlinger and Jaenisch, found that the cells of blastocysts that were developed through research cloning showed no signs of the epigenetic abnormalities (abnormalities that affect a cell and that may indirectly affect the expression of its genome) that appear in animals cloned for reproductive purposes.[47] They explain the reason for this:

> The derivation of embryonic stem cells from cloned blastocysts may be the result of selection for a few successfully reprogrammed cells within a cloned embryo. In contrast, the development of a cloned embryo after implantation most likely does not allow for the in vivo selection of a few functional cells, thus causing developmental failure of the clone or phenotypic abnormalities.[48]

In short, they indicate that research cloning is more efficient than reproductive cloning because it selects for working, rather than abnormal, cells. They therefore maintain that embryonic stem cell lines derived from cloned embryos have the same therapeutic potential as those derived from IVF fertilized embryos.[49] They conclude that the concern that cloned embryonic stem cells would not be safe to use in patients because they would be peppered with genetic aberrations can be set aside.

Another difficulty with research cloning that has been posed by some scientists is that there would not be sufficient time to treat patients who have an acute injury, such as a heart attack, with derivatives of cloned embryonic stem cells, for these patients would require immediate treatment and cloning is not a speedy process. It would take days to obtain a somatic cell from these patients, as well as a human egg from a donor, and then to fuse them and grow stem cells from the resulting cloned embryos in order to differentiate them and transfer them to these patients.[50] Patients with an acute coronary condition could not wait that long to be treated. To make research cloning feasible for therapeutic uses in the acute care situation, it would be necessary to have multiple fresh donated human eggs at hand. This is not likely to happen since women could not provide eggs for research cloning on short notice. It would not be possible to develop a bank of frozen human eggs to call on in carrying out this sort of cloning since safe techniques for egg freezing are not yet assured. Alternatives to using human eggs in research cloning, such as reprogramming ordinary human body cells to function in ways akin to the cytoplasm of human eggs, are possible.

However, a final difficulty is that no matter what materials are used, individualized treatments using research cloning would be very expensive and would be available only to a few who could afford them. For such reasons, the use of research cloning in therapeutic stem cell research is not likely to become widespread in the near future.

Whether It Is Wrong to Clone Embryos for Research and Therapy

The question of whether it is ethically acceptable to create embryos for research and therapy also arises with respect to research cloning, for the procedure is generally taken to involve the development of a human embryo. Here, too, some recoil at the destruction of human embryos that takes place when embryonic stem cells are removed from human embryos. However, others hold the view stated earlier that it is ethically sound to use these cloned embryos in the service of developing medical therapies to treat seriously ill persons. (See chapter 3 for further discussion.)

Some, however, respond to this question by maintaining that the entity that results from research cloning is not an embryo at all. Paul McHugh of the President's Council on Bioethics, for instance, maintains that it is a "clonote," rather than an embryo, since, if transferred to a woman's uterus, it would die due to the severe epigenetic abnormalities that it bears.[51] In his view, whether the entity that develops as a result of cloning is an embryo depends on whether it could give rise to an individual human being. Since clonotes cannot do so, he concludes that they are not embryos and that it is ethically acceptable to use them to develop stem cells for research. However, if one views the early embryo as an individual human being, there seems to be no way that would be acceptable to carry out a definitive study to determine whether McHugh is correct, since manipulations of the clonote might well damage or even destroy it before it could exhibit whether it could produce a human being and therefore, ipso facto, be an embryo.

Others argue that to initiate research cloning would start us down a slippery slope toward human reproductive cloning. At the bottom of this slope, they argue, lie damaged fetuses and children with lethal conditions. Because of such probable outcomes of reproductive cloning, it has been roundly rejected by scientists, legislators, and others around the world. Yet some fear that if research cloning were allowed, reproductive cloning would not be far behind.

Alexander Morgan Capron, for instance, argues that "practically, if any laboratory is free to create human embryos through SCNT [somatic cell nuclear transfer], the result will be cloned babies or, at the very least, serious attempts to create them."[52] Since both reproductive cloning and research cloning start off in the same way, he maintains, there is a likelihood that at least some embryos cloned for research and therapy would be surreptitiously transferred to the bodies of women for gestation and birth.

Some members of the President's Council on Bioethics envision similar untoward scenarios and argue that this would present an agonizing dilemma for those who maintain that the human embryo is an individual human being:

> The only way to prevent [the production of cloned children] from happening would be to prohibit, by law, the implantation of cloned embryos for the purpose of producing children. To do so, however, the government would find itself in the unsavory position of designating a class of embryos that it would be a felony not to destroy. It would require, not just permit, the destruction of cloned embryos—which seems to us the very opposite of showing such cloned embryos "special respect."[53]

Both Capron and the President's Council therefore recommend that a moratorium should be imposed on research cloning, albeit for somewhat different reasons.

Any technology can be misused. That alone does not provide sufficient reason for banning it. Many life-saving medical measures, such as ventilators and dialysis machines, could be misused by those with evil motives intent on ending the lives of certain patients, and yet we do not bar these machines from hospitals on that account. As is the case for such lifesaving medical technologies, safeguards can be built into oversight mechanisms for research cloning in order to avoid the possibility that scientists might use purloined embryos developed for research cloning for reproductive purposes instead.

Currently, medical scientists who attempted to gain fame by stealing cloned embryos and using them to produce children would face major practical, professional, and legal difficulties. Such an act would call for the cooperation of a number of different specialists, as well as a completely equipped fertility clinic. These are unlikely to be available. A host of medical scientists have been made aware by notices from the Food and Drug Administration (FDA) that it has asserted jurisdiction over any attempts to clone a human being and that it would not permit reproductive cloning to proceed.[54] Clearly, to participate in such a practice would destroy a rogue scientist's professional life and open that individual to several different legal causes of action. Consequently, a scenario in which a medical professional were to abscond with embryos developed for research cloning and transfer them to a woman's body seems remote.

Finally, it is highly unlikely that those seeking to have a child who are willing to risk reproductive cloning would choose to use anonymous embryos stolen from research cloning laboratories. If they sought to have a child by means of cloning, rather than IVF, they most likely would do so in order to create a child who was a replica of a specific person or who could donate material to save the life of an already living child. Both of these scenarios would require a cloned embryo with a specific physical constitution rather than one whose future constitution was unknown.

All in all, the fear that allowing research cloning to proceed would inevitably lead to illicit reproductive cloning does not seem warranted and does not in itself provide sufficient ethical justification for prohibiting the use of this method.

Risks to Women Who Donate Eggs for Research Cloning

If research cloning were eventually to move into clinical use, this would create an immense and intense demand for thousands of human eggs from women. As noted in the discussion of egg retrieval, the process of egg donation is associated with risks and discomforts, and these are more difficult to justify when the women involved receive no personal health benefit and only distant altruistic satisfaction from such donation. Concerns about whether women would be adequately informed about these risks and whether undue pressure might be put on them to donate eggs to meet the increased demand are relevant in the context of research cloning. We have argued above that prospective egg donors who are fully informed of the risks of egg donation and who voluntarily and altruistically choose to proceed with such donation for research cloning should not be precluded from doing so.

Possible Alternatives to Research Cloning

Since research cloning raises a variety of scientific, ethical, and practical questions, some have suggested other ways of avoiding the problem of stem cell transplant rejection, the difficulty that led to the development of this technique in the first place.

One alternative would be to build up a collection of "universal" stem cell lines that would be immunologically compatible with most patients. This would be accomplished by genetically modifying a cluster of stem cell lines so that they would not trigger immune rejection in most patients. However, it has not yet been demonstrated in animals that it is possible to develop such stem cell lines; further research would be needed to assess the feasibility of this proposal in both animals and humans.[55] In addition, not all of the numerous genotypes needed for treatment of a multitude of patients would be encompassed by such universal stem cell lines. Both of these problems make the development of universal stem cell lines seem less feasible than research cloning for patient use.

Another alternative to research cloning is to build up stem cell banks that house hundreds of embryonic stem cell lines. Each line in this bank would represent a spectrum of immune profiles. Patients would receive cells from this bank that were immunologically compatible and that had been triggered to grow into the specific type of differentiated cells that they needed for therapy. The United Kingdom has established a stem cell bank that stores, characterizes, and distributes stem cells from embryonic, fetal, and adult issues and distributes them to researchers worldwide.[56] It has been hypothesized that the stem cell lines in this bank will represent a variety of genetic types that could serve the therapeutic needs of patients with many different immune profiles. Eventually, this bank plans to distribute stem cells for therapeutic uses.

However, a panel convened at Johns Hopkins University maintains that it would not be feasible to construct a stem cell bank that could hold a sufficient number of stem cell lines to provide matches for the millions of needy patients with different genotypes.[57] A plausible strategy, the majority of the panel members maintain, is to create a stem cell bank that contains the number of stem cell lines that are matched to the genes needed to cover the same percentage of persons in each of the major ethnic and ancestral groups. Such a strategy would avoid discrimination against those who are not Caucasian, these panel members believe. This could be accomplished by soliciting egg and sperm donors with the genes needed for this purpose and creating embryos with their gametes. Although such a bank would not meet the therapeutic needs of as many patients as possible, it would accommodate many in a fair manner.

This proposal faces several problems. Establishing such a bank would be a tremendous feat, for it would require defining ethnic and cultural groups, making complicated calculations about their genetic composition, and then finding and testing large numbers of willing potential gamete donors; this would be a monumental task. Many potential donors might be unwilling to volunteer to donate their gametes because if it were learned through genetic testing that they bore genes associated with genetic disorders and the results of their tests became available to their employers and insurers, this might subject them to discrimination in insurance and health care. Moreover, this method would cover fewer patients than a bank designed to include stem cell lines that possess the most commonly found genes in the general population. Thus, it sacrifices breadth of coverage for ethnic representation. Finally, this proposal, which would involve the creation of embryos for therapy, would not avoid the ethical concerns about the destruction of embryos that those who object to such destruction have raised. The proposal to establish this bank provides no discussion of these concerns. Consequently, those advocating the establishment of such a bank would have to address significant ethical and practical questions in greater detail before it could be put into place.[58]

Proponents of research cloning assert that the method they espouse is simpler than such proposed alternatives to it that have been proposed, for it would allow individual patients to receive stem cells that have been genetically customized to match their own tissue. They maintain that, despite current and future scientific unknowns, this technique offers a valuable approach that is scientifically, technically, and practically superior to many of the other proposed techniques for addressing major scientific and therapeutic issues associated with stem cell use. As long as steps are taken to prohibit the use of the resulting cloned embryos for reproductive purposes, either by law or by agency regulation, they believe that the danger of the misuse of these embryos would be almost nil. They recognize that research cloning would require thousands of eggs from women and that these would be extremely difficult to obtain, and they indicate that they are looking into ways to address this serious problem. (See chapter 8 for further discussion.)

Developing Embryos through Parthenogenesis for Research and Therapy

A technique known as parthenogenesis (from the Greek, "virgin birth") provides another possible source of human embryonic stem cells. In modern biology, parthenogenesis refers to a form of reproduction in which an egg develops into a new individual of its kind without having been fertilized by sperm. It occurs naturally under certain conditions among some invertebrates such as bees and ants, and some vertebrates, such as reptiles and snakes. However, parthenogenesis does not occur in mammals—including humans—in nature.

Parthenogenesis can be induced in the laboratory by stimulating an unfertilized mammalian egg with chemical or electrical signals in order to induce it to divide and grow like an early embryo.[59] Normally, a fertilized egg receives a set of chromosomes from the female and another from the male. However, in parthenogenesis the mammalian egg cell duplicates the set of female chromosomes (no sperm are involved) and then develops as though it had been fertilized. Because the resulting parthenote is missing a set of male chromosomes, it fails to develop an extraembryonic membrane and dies. Those who recommend attempting the use of this technique in humans to develop human embryonic stem cells argue that it offers a way of creating greater numbers of these cells than IVF or research cloning and is a simpler process than these other two.

In 2000, scientists at Advanced Cell Technology (ACT) announced that they had created human parthenotes by means of parthenogenesis.[60] They reported that they had activated twenty-two human eggs and that several of these had developed beyond the eight-cell stage to the point of cleavage before they died. No pluripotent stem cells could be harvested from these parthenotes, however, since they had not yet developed an inner cell mass that could yield stem cells. If the results of this report were reaffirmed at some future point, this would be the first known study in which human parthenogenesis was used successfully in the laboratory.

The significance of this study is open to opposing interpretations. Some would maintain that the resulting parthenotes were not human embryos because the research provided no evidence that they were capable of developing into human organisms.[61] Therefore, they would argue that the use of parthenogenesis is not subject to ethical objections from those who decry the destruction of human embryos in stem cell research. Others would maintain, in contrast, that these parthenotes constituted human embryos from the start but were compromised by the subsequent processes of parthenogenesis and could not survive because of this.[62] The former stance would seem to have the better of the argument, for these parthenotes never had the male chromosomes that would have enabled them to survive. It is not that such chromosomes were removed from them, thereby incapacitating them, but that they were never present. Because of this, these parthenotes were unable to develop and therefore did not qualify as human embryos.

The same investigators at Advanced Cell Technology, along with several scientists from other institutions, reported that they had isolated the first stem cell lines from primate parthenotes in early 2002.[63] They indicated that they had treated twenty-eight monkey eggs with chemicals to prevent these eggs from ejecting half their chromosomes (as they do in sexual reproduction) and to signal them to start dividing. Four of the resulting monkey parthenotes developed to the blastocyst stage, at which point the researchers derived a pluripotent stem cell line from one of them. They were able to culture a variety of monkey cell types from this stem cell line, including brain, cardiac, and muscle cells. This was the first report in which primate parthenotes were used to produce stem cells. Scientists disagree about whether this study indicates that pluripotent stem cells could be derived from human parthenotes as well.[64]

In 2003, David Wininger and his colleagues at Stemron of Maryland published a report indicating that they had grown human parthenotes to the blastocyst stage, at which point they derived stem cells from one of them.[65] The study marks the first time that human stem cells were derived from human parthenotes.[66] Here, too, since the parthenotes did not develop into human organisms but instead died, it cannot be said that they were embryos. However, this study does suggest that it is possible to obtain pluripotent human stem cells from human parthenotes.

In 2004, a team from Tokyo University announced the creation, birth, and survival into adulthood of a mouse developed by means of what they termed "parthenogenesis."[67] Tomohiro Kono and his colleagues altered the expression of a key gene in immature eggs of fetal mice in order to cause the genetic material of each egg to behave as though it had a male contribution; at this stage of development, the researchers maintain that the paternal genomic imprinting in fetal mice was lost. These eggs were then fused with mature eggs from female mice to create a total of 457 mouse pathenotes. Of these, 371 were transferred to twenty-six female mice, of which twenty-four became pregnant. Two mice were born as a result. One, named Kayuga after a princess in a Japanese folk story who was born from a bamboo stump, lived to adulthood and mated with a male, producing offspring. However, Kayuga apparently had many abnormal genes.[68] The other mouse was killed in order to conduct an examination of its genetic imprinting.

This study, its authors maintain, marks the first confirmed use of parthenogenesis to create a mammalian embryo that went on to develop into a living organism. The authors' thesis is that the lack of paternal genomic imprinting is the stumbling block to mammalian parthenogenesis and that this can be overcome by the alteration of certain genes in the mammalian egg. It should be noted that this study produced hordes of dead mouse parthenotes and that its extrapolation to humans would therefore be premature and dangerous.

This report suggested to some that human parthenotes could be developed by means of the same sort of genetic manipulations of human fetal eggs and that human stem cells could be derived from them. However, if this were possible—and this is unclear—the use of this method to provide a source of human pluripotent stem cells would not avoid the ethical issues raised by opponents of embryonic stem cell research. They would view any resulting human parthenotes as human embryos, since they could develop and become living human individuals, and would consider their destruction during the extraction of pluripotent stem cells as equivalent to killing an individual human being.

It is arguable that this study did not involve parthenogenesis in the classical sense of that term. In true parthenogenesis, the chromosomes of the egg are duplicated and no male contribution is involved. In this study, however, it is feasible to argue that the immature eggs used derived from mouse fetuses had not completely lost their male imprinting. Consequently, there could still have been some part of the genome that retained the male imprint in those immature eggs that was sufficient to support the development of the resulting mice. Therefore, according to this explanation, this study would not meet the hallmarks of true parthenogenesis and the mammalian parthenote would not constitute a mammalian embryo. This alternate interpretation is currently under discussion.[69]

Some reports have come from the United Kingdom indicating that human parthenogenesis has been carried out in that country. In 2004, a team led by Karl Swann of the University of Wales injected an enzyme produced by sperm into human eggs, causing them to divide as though they had been fertilized.[70] This technique changed the calcium ion structure of the egg but did not introduce male genetic material into it. The resulting human parthenotes, however, did not develop to a stage at which stem cells could be derived from them. In 2005, a team at the Roslin Institute in Scotland announced at a scientific meeting that it had used electrical stimulation to cause six human eggs out of 300 to develop into early-stage parthenotes.[71] Although these parthenotes matured to the blastocyst stage, the lead scientist in this study, Paul de Sousa, indicated that the team had not been successful in attempts at deriving human embryonic stem cells from these parthenotes.

Several scientific and practical difficulties have been raised about the use of parthenogenesis in stem cell research. Some maintain that cells in parthenotes may carry errors in the way that their genes are switched on and off, since they do not have the usual complement of paternally imprinted genes, and that human embryonic stem cells produced from them might consequently be too abnormal for use in therapy.[72] Another serious concern is that because human parthenotes would be dependent for their development on human eggs, this method would be limited in its impact, for human embryonic stem cells derived from these parthenotes would only be matched immunologically with the women who had donated those eggs and would therefore not be suitable for treating other women or any men. A final difficulty is one raised in discussions of several other proposed sources of pluripotent stem cells—this method would pose risks to the hordes of egg donors who would be needed if enough stem cells were to be developed to meet the needs of patients who might benefit from stem cell therapies. (See chapter 8 for further discussion.)

Harvesting Embryonic Stem Cells from Dead Embryos for Research and Therapy

To gain a larger supply of embryonic stem cells, Donald W. Landry and Howard A. Zucker of Columbia University have proposed harvesting these cells from dead embryos.[73] Much as it is ethically acceptable to retrieve organs from humans who have been declared "brain dead," they argue, so it is in accordance with the demands of ethics to retrieve embryonic stem cells from embryos that have been declared dead.

They note that a high percentage (perhaps two-thirds) of frozen human embryos that have been developed for IVF treatments stop dividing at the four-to-eight cell stage within twenty-four hours after they are thawed. These embryos are considered unsuitable for transfer to a woman's body to attempt fertilization. Yet some of these embryos have normal cells. Landry and Zucker propose that if, after an additional twenty-four-hour period, such embryos do not divide, they should be declared "organismically dead" and their embryonic stem cells should be extracted. A research team from Newcastle, United Kingdom reported in 2006 that it had carried out a study in accord with Landry and Zucker's hypothesis, for the group derived human embryonic stem cells from an "arrested" human embryo at the blastocyst stage.[74] The researchers waited from twenty-four to forty-eight hours after thirteen embryos had stopped dividing to declare that they were not viable and then grew some cells from five of them. They developed a fully characterized human embryonic stem cell line from one of these embryos. This study, the researchers maintain, shows that "arrested" embryos can provide a source of human embryonic stem cells.

A major difficulty that this study and the Landry-Zucker proposal raises is that it is not clear whether an "arrested" embryo is dead. If stem cells were removed from an "arrested" embryo and these cells subsequently began to divide when placed in a laboratory dish for research, this would call into question the accuracy of the decision that they were not viable In order to declare them absolutely dead, some critics indicate, investigators would have to wait so long that their cells could no longer be used in stem cell research. In short, it does not appear feasible to declare an embryo dead until it is too late to extract stem cells from its inner cell mass.

Landry and Zucker have responded to this objection by maintaining that embryos could be declared dead even if some of their cells were viable.[75] Scientists could determine that these embryos had lost "integrated function" as organisms, since they displayed no coordinated cell division, and could declare them dead on this basis, they respond. Just how to determine that an embryo with six to eight cells has lost "integrated function," however, seems an impossible task to some. For instance, Robert Lanza, a scientist with Advanced Cell Technology, states:

> You can't take an EEG to determine if there's loss of brain function. I've seen numerous embryos stop dividing, fooling the embryologist into thinking they're no longer viable; then, after a significant "resting" period, they go on to generate intact blastocysts. Unfortunately, the only sure way to know if an embryo is dead is if the cells are dead.[76]

Landry and Zucker, undaunted, indicate that it is possible to develop tests to ascertain whether the arrest of cell division of these embryos is irreversible. Michael Gazzaniga a member of the President's Council on Bioethics, agrees that it is feasible to declare these embryos dead but states that first criteria for embryonic death that are more specific and selective than those that Landry and Zucker provide must be developed.[77] George Q. Daley, a stem cell investigator at Harvard University, does not believe that this would resolve the questions that this proposal raises, for scientists would be concerned about whether these embryos were abnormal and, if so, whether research using cells derived from them might lead to erroneous conclusions.[78] He anticipates that attempts to generate pluripotent cells from dead embryos would be much less efficient than generating them from spare embryos remaining after the completion of IVF treatments.

Perhaps the most forceful challenge to this proposal is that if it were adopted in preference to current methods of obtaining embryonic stem cells, this would have the peculiar result that stem cells would be extracted from dead embryos while living embryos with usable stem cells would be discarded. This seems pointless to some. For instance, Janet Rowley, a member of the President's Council on Bioethics, observes:

Because they do not know in advance which embryos will not divide and which will, some portion of embryos (about half) will continue to divide and will be healthy embryos. What happens to these healthy embryos? The proposal says healthy embryos in excess of those to be implanted will be allowed to die while scientists struggle to recoup a few living cells from the dead embryos! This seems to me to be the height of folly.[79]

Rowley and others ask why would scientists choose to use cells derived from dead embryos when they could use existing cell lines or derive new ones from IVF embryos?

This proposal, while a serious attempt to avoid the destruction of embryos in stem cell research, raises so many questions of its own about its scientific feasibility and ethical necessity that it seems unlikely to provide a sound alternative to current methods of obtaining embryonic stem cell lines.

Biopsying Single Cells (Blastomeres) from Embryos for Research and Therapy

Yet another alternative proposed method for deriving human embry onic stem cells termed "single-cell embryo biopsy" involves removing a single cell (blastomere) from an embryo at the eight-to-ten–cell stage and deriving embryonic stem cell lines from it. Robert Lanza and colleagues at Advanced Cell Technology maintain that they have established proof of the principle that human embryonic stem cells can be generated from human embryos in this way without harming them.[80] In 2006, they carried out a "single-cell embryo biopsy" proce- dure in sixteen donated thawed human embryos at the eight-cell (blas- tomere) stage and derived 91 cells from them. Of these 91 cells, two developed into human embryonic stem cell lines that grew continuously in the laboratory for eight months. The researchers claim on the basis of this study that the remaining seven cells in a human embryo can grow into normal human beings with roughly the same rate of success as embryos that have not gone through the biopsy procedure. Lanza's team ended up destroying the embryos that were studied in order to make the most of the few embryos available but declared that in principle this technique can provide human embryonic stem cell lines without the destruction of embryos.

This procedure would be used in tandem with preimplantation genetic diagnosis (PGD), Lanza indicates.[81] PGD is a test for screening embryos developed by means of IVF for serious genetic and chromo- somal conditions. It involves removing one cell from an eight-cell embryo in order to assess its composition. If the cell removed bears signs of genetic or chromosomal anomalies, it and the embryo from which it was taken are usually discarded. However, if the cell removed carries no known markers for such disorders, the remaining seven cells are transferred to a woman's body in hopes of initiating a pregnancy. Lanza maintains that a second cell could be removed from the embryo that is being tested during PGD and provided for stem cell research. Thus, in theory, this technique could be used to diagnose an embryo, as well as to derive human embryonic stem cells. Since PGD offers evidence that removal of a single cell rarely damages the remaining embryo, he argues, removing an additional cell for stem cell research presents little likelihood of harm to the embryo.

More than 1,000 embryos have been tested by means of PGD without untoward effects on the children born of the embryos selected for transfer, according to one article.[82] Yet other writings urge caution about this proposed use of PGD because little nationwide data from independent laboratories has been published on the procedure's long-term success rates, error rates, and potential risks.[83] Moreover, it seems unlikely that couples whose IVF embryos are undergoing PGD would agree to the use of this procedure, for it would entail exposing IVF embryos that they have long sought to additional risks beyond those posed by PGD. Davor Solter of the Max-Planck Institute of Immuno-biology in Freiburg, Germany, observes that the probable need to freeze these embryos while stem cells were obtained from them would add to these risks, as would the need to keep them frozen until the results of that stem cell derivation were known.[84]

Another significant ethical concern that this method raises is that the single cell removed from the embryo might itself be totipotent—that is, capable of giving rise to an individual human being, much as a single blastomere removed from a rabbit or sheep embryo at the eight-cell stage can develop into a viable rabbit or sheep.[85] However, this is a matter of considerable debate. A study of whether a single blastomere is capable of producing a human being could not be undertaken since it would require transferring a blastomere to a woman's uterus in order to test its developmental potential, and this would be rejected as an unethical experiment, since it might result in the development of a child.

In short, the project of extracting single cells from embryos in order to develop embryonic stem cells raises serious scientific and ethical concerns. Critics maintain that the researchers carrying out "single-cell biopsy" have not demonstrated the safety or practicality of this procedure, since only two of 91 extracted cells in the Lanza study successfully developed into human embryonic stem cell lines. These concerns put into question whether this technique would provide an improvement over current methods of obtaining stem cells from embryos for research and therapy, especially in the eyes of those who view early embryos as individual living human beings.

Developing Embryo-like Entities through Altered Nuclear Transfer for Research and Therapy

William Hurlbut, a member of the President's Council on Bioethics, has developed another strategy for obtaining pluripotent stem cells that would use research cloning—with a twist. Basically, the procedure that he has proposed, which he terms "altered nuclear transfer," would start by altering a human somatic (body) cell so that it lacks one or more of the genes that embryos need in order to develop. Researchers would then insert the nucleus of this somatic cell into a human egg whose own nucleus had been removed and clone it, producing a mass of cells from which pluripotent stem cells could be extracted.[86] Hurlbut argues that this would not result in the creation of a human embryo (which he regards as an individual living human being), for the entity that resulted would not develop the sort of integrated organization that characterizes human embryos. Instead, it would result in an aberrant human cell cluster that could not survive more than a week or so. Since it would not constitute a human embryo, he maintains, this method would be ethically unobjectionable to those who reject the destruction of human embryos in stem cell research.

Hurlbut came up with the idea for "altered nuclear transfer" after he had learned that mouse embryos that carry a mutation in their *Cdx2* gene die at the five-day blastocyst stage because they fail to form a trophectoderm, the segment of the early embryo from which the placenta develops.[87] He reasoned that researchers could genetically manipulate the nucleus of a somatic cell by "knocking out" one or more of its genes, such as the *Cdx2* gene, that are necessary for normal embryonic development and then injecting this nucleus into an enucleated human egg. This egg would be activated in a process that imitates that used in research cloning to produce what Hurlbut calls a "limited biological entity."[88]

Initially, this cluster of cells would grow normally and produce additional cells that could be removed from its inner cell mass and cultured into pluripotent stem cells. However, Hurlbut explains, it would not have the potential to produce an individual human being and would inevitably die when some crucial embryonic component failed to emerge because of the earlier genetic modification. The gene that had been "knocked out" of the somatic cell at the beginning of this process could be inserted into the stem cells derived from this entity so that these stem cells would function normally and could be used to treat patients. Hurlbut contends that this method of altered nuclear transfer would avoid ethical controversy because it does not involve the destruction of embryos. What is destroyed in this procedure is only an amorphous mass of human cells.[89]

This proposal is no longer merely theoretical. Alexander Meissner and Rudolf Jaenisch have carried out the altered nuclear transfer procedure proposed by Hurlbut with certain modifications.[90] They silenced the *Cdx2* gene in the DNA of a mouse somatic cell and then injected this altered nucleus into a mouse egg whose own nucleus had been removed. Next they stimulated this egg to grow, creating an entity from which they derived mouse embryonic stem cells. Their final step was to reactivate the gene in these stem cells that had been silenced earlier in the newly constituted altered nuclear transfer entity. They found that this procedure efficiently generated pluripotent embryonic mouse stem cells. Indeed, this method had certain advantages over the "knock out" method proposed by Hurlbut, for it simply required the activation, rather than the reinsertion, of the gene that had been silenced in the initial somatic cell in the resulting mouse stem cells.

However, Solter argues that we do not know whether the *Cdx2* gene has the same function in humans as in mice and we could only learn this by studying human embryos—which could cause their destruction, the very result that this method was designed to avoid.[91] He maintains further that to be sure that every entity produced through altered nuclear transfer was incapable of normal human development, such entities would have to be tested; this would inevitably destroy a certain number of them. "Even if only 1 in 1000 or 1 in 1 million alternative-nuclear-transfer embryos possesses the capacity for normal development, the raison d'être of the approach collapses," Solter indicates.[92] Producing and destroying even one viable human embryo would defeat the very purpose of engaging in this method of creating embryonic stem cells in the first place. Consequently, this method would not satisfy those who object to the destruction of human embryos in stem cell research, Solter asserts.

Jaenisch maintains that that it would be a straightforward matter to verify the expression level of the *Cdx2* gene in humans by growing entities created by altered nuclear transfer in culture dishes and then testing their cells. He states that "although such surrogate assays cannot give 100 percent certainty in predicting the effect of CDX2 deficiency on human placentation, a positive in vitro result would provide sufficient confidence that a CDX2 knockout would abrogate the reproductive cloning potential of human blastocysts derived by altered nuclear transfer."[93] No medical procedure, he observes, gives a certainty of success of one in a million. Moreover, such large numbers of altered nuclear transfer entities would not be needed to reach a well-supported conclusion. Solter, in turn, points out that those who believe that it is wrong to destroy embryos in stem cell research would require just that—a certainty of success of one in a million.[94] If even only one of the entities produced by altered nuclear transfer were to have the capacity to develop into a human being, he argues, and it were used in altered nuclear transfer, these critics of embryo destruction would view this procedure as ethically unacceptable.

Some among those who object to the use of embryos for stem cell research have raised related metaphysical concerns about whether the entity produced by altered nuclear transfer might well turn out to be an embryo. For instance, Richard M. Doerflinger of the National Conference of Catholic Bishops, in discussing the procedure proposed by Hurlbut with the President's Council on Bioethics, stated:

> I for one am not convinced it fulfills my criterion for saying the resulting entity is never an embryo. Surely, it is not enough to say the genetic defect preventing organismal development was introduced into the genome from the very beginning. Any adult who develops Huntington's disease at the age of 40 had the genetic defect ab initio. But it also matters what development has taken place in the meantime. If that gene is expressed only after the 16-to-32–cell stage, it seems to me this would be an embryo that undergoes normal development as a human organism to a certain point and then dies.[95]

If the genetic alteration made to the somatic cell did not come into play until after the limited biological entity was created, that entity could be considered a human embryo that had been deliberately programmed to die. If so, then this proposal would not resolve the ethical issue at stake for Doerflinger and others who object to embryo destruction in stem cell research.

A group of stem cell investigators, thinking along similar lines, observed that "an alternative interpretation [to one that holds that the limited biological entities without the Cdx2 gene are not embryos] would be that the embryos that lack Cdx2 develop normally until Cdx2 function is required, at which point they die."[96] That is, the entities created by altered nuclear transfer could be viewed as embryos that were deliberately disabled so that they would die. These scientists went on to declare, in response to Hurlbut's proposal, that "we see no basis for concluding that the action of Cdx2 (or indeed any other gene) represents a transition point at which a human embryo acquires moral status."[97]

For the reasons presented here, the technique of altered nuclear transfer has received a mixed reception. It raises serious ethical and scientific questions of its own and does not appear to some commentators to overcome the ethical difficulties that it was designed to address. The primary issue in contention is whether the limited biological entity produced by altered nuclear transfer is a human embryo whose programmed development has been deliberately damaged, or is something else. Some—both those who view the early human embryo as an individual human being and those who do not—find this proposed strategy attractive and worth pursuing in animals. However, others who view the human embryo as sacrosanct, the President's Council on Bioethics reports, "find it aesthetically repulsive and ethically suspect to be *creating* such neither-living-nor-nonliving, near-human artifacts, a practice they regard as ethically no improvement over *destroying* early embryos."[98] Finally, some who do not view the early human embryo as an individual human being, reject this method as a distraction from the central issue of whether it is morally justifiable to use early stage human embryos in "the search to understand human biology and cure serious diseases."[99]

Developing Embryo-like Entities through Dedifferentiation for Research and Therapy

Yet another proposed alternative method proposed, known as "dedifferentiation," involves taking an adult cell and running its development backward to produce cells with the capabilities of embryonic stem cells. (See figure 2.2.) This method, those working on it indicate, would involve the creation of embryonic stem cells without using human embryos.

Harvard investigators Kevin Eggan, Chad Cowan, and their colleagues realized that something in the cytoplasm of an embryonic stem cell can turn an ordinary cell of the body into a genetically matched embryonic stem cell.[100] They aim to use this knowledge to control gene expression in a somatic cell and reprogram it so that it would develop into an embryonic stem cell. This stem cell would have the same genes as the somatic cell but would have a different pattern of gene expression. If they could accomplish this, they would bypass the need to use human eggs and would produce no human embryos.

To achieve this end, they fused already existing human embryonic stem cells with human skin cells, reprogramming the genes in the nuclei of the skin cells and transforming them into embryonic stem cells. That is, each somatic cell with the genes of the person from whom it was derived reverted to an embryonic stem cell. Eggan indicated that the fused cells had an almost identical gene expression profile to that of

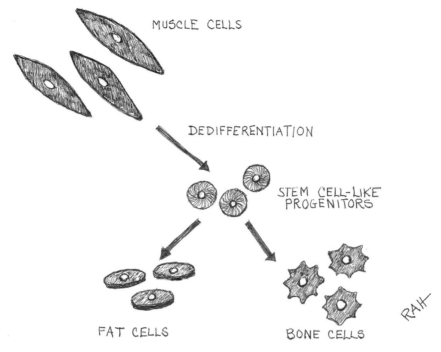

Figure 2.2. Dedifferentiation. Specialized body cells are taken back to a stem cell state and then redifferentiated into cells of another specialized type.

normal embryonic stem cells and behaved like such cells.[101] The study opens the door to the possibility that this dedifferentiation technique could be used to develop human embryonic stem cells that are genetically matched to specific patients. Any tissue grown from a patient's own somatic cells could be transplanted into that patient to treat disease without the danger of rejection.[102]

This method of dedifferentiation presents a significant technical problem, however. The fused cells produced in this experiment had two complete sets of genes, one from the somatic cell and another from the embryonic stem cell; this is double the normal number of sets. The extra DNA would have to be removed from the resulting embryonic stem cells before they could be transplanted into patients. These researchers have not yet figured out how to do this. For this and other reasons, they have indicated that this procedure is still in the early stages of research and does not yet provide a form of therapy. They have made clear that it is not a replacement for currently available techniques.[103]

Whether it is scientifically feasible to pursue dedifferentiation with an eye to developing therapies for patients with serious diseases is still an open question.[104] George Daley states: "Although this strategy is worth pursuing, it is extremely high-risk, and may take years to perfect, and may never work as well as nuclear transfer [research cloning], which we know we can practice today."[105]

The President's Council on Bioethics, while viewing dedifferentiation as a promising technique, has expressed a concern that dedifferentiation might be "pursued beyond (mere) pluripotency to the point of yielding a totipotent cell [a cell that could become any cell of the body]—in effect, a cloned human zygote."[106] Michael Gazzaniga of the President's Council on Bioethics also seemed to indicate that dedifferentiation might lead to the creation of a totipotent cell when he observed:

> I find this proposal strained at best. Winding the clock back on a developed somatic cell and to stop it at a critical point is supposed to be void of ethical issues while letting a cell grow forward to just before the same point as with SCNT [somatic cell nuclear transfer] is not ethical? This is the potentiality argument in reverse. In one version the film of life is running forward and in the other it is running in reverse. In both scenarios humans are making decisions about life and its origins.[107]

Bonnie Steinbock has also raised this issue, suggesting that if dedifferentiation were carried back to a point where it resulted in a totipotent cell, this would amount to the development of a human embryo.[108]

In short, this method, while considered to have scientific merit by several well-qualified scientific commentators, raises an ethical question for some others about whether it would involve the generation of human embryos. Since this is the very result researchers are seeking to avoid, the technique of dedifferentiation would end up in the same ethical thickets from which it was hoped it could provide deliverance, if this concern were on point. However, a dedifferentiated fibroblast cell will not become a fertilized egg. Such a cell has no cytoplasm and is 1,000 times smaller than a human egg. It is a cell, not an embryo. It would differentiate back to the embryonic stem cell stage and remain there without becoming an embryo. Consequently, the concern voiced by some that the technique of dedifferentiation would result in a human totipotent cell that was, in effect, a human embryo is misplaced.

This method has the advantage that it would not have to rely on the use of human eggs or material from embryonic stem cell lines. These features make it especially attractive to those who oppose the creation of such lines. Moreover, the fusion technique is not difficult and could be used to replicate multitudes of cells. One reporter notes, "For instance, researchers could produce hybrid cells that contain DNA from an individual with a disease and could study those cells to identify what's gong wrong."[109] However, this technique is not yet ready for therapeutic use in humans since considerably more needs to be learned about how it works and whether the cells produced in this way are normal.[110]

Comparison of Current Methods for Deriving Embryonic Stem Cells with Suggested New Modes

At this point in time, it is not clear whether some of the proposed methods of developing additional stem cell lines to supplement those currently available are scientifically feasible. Research cloning, for instance, is said to be theoretically possible but difficult to make a reality. Altered nuclear transfer has been shown to work in mice, but it is not clear whether it would be efficacious in humans. Dedifferentiation of adult stem cells, which appears to be the most promising technique, would take considerable time, perhaps another decade, some scientists believe, before enough would be known about cellular dedifferentiation to bypass some of the steps required today to pursue this technique.[111] Therefore, it, too, does not present an immediately available alternative method for developing human pluripotent stem cells.

No one of these sources of human pluripotent stem cells has been embraced by all involved in the debate about their development and feasibility. Stem cell scientists, in general, are inclined to continue using current sources that they know can provide embryonic stem cells— primarily embryos created by means of IVF. They also hope to develop research cloning, for, in general, they tend to view this as a significant technique for producing "custom-built" stem cells for studying the processes of human disease. Some of the other suggested alternative sources of embryonic stem cells strike many stem cell scientists as what Michael Gazzaniga terms "high-risk options that only have an outside chance of success and raise their own complex set of ethical questions."[112] Thus, there is currently no scientific stampede to develop any one of these alternative techniques over those that are currently in use.

Those with special concerns about protecting early human embryos from destruction have reservations about many of the old and the newly proposed sources and techniques for deriving pluripotent stem cells. They appear to view the dedifferentiation of adult stem cells as the most ethically acceptable of the lot, for it does not begin with the destruction of embryos. However, some among them are concerned that it could be difficult to control this process so that it ends just before an embryo appears in view, rather than at the point of embryo development.

This concern, I have argued, is based on a misunderstanding of the nature of the entity that results from the process of dedifferentiation.

Most of those interested in developing current and new sources of pluripotent stem cells recognize that several of these would require obtaining large numbers of eggs from women. Currently women are sought as egg donors primarily for reproductive, rather than research, purposes. Finding them in the reproductive context is not an easy matter. It is difficult to fathom how multitudes of such donors could be induced to donate eggs for research without putting coercive pressure on them or providing them with undue inducements. This prospect raises difficult ethical and policy questions revolving around the need to protect women who donate eggs for stem cell research from misinformation and misuse in a way that is consistent with good research ethics.

The burning question behind many of the proposals for developing embryonic stem cells is whether the early human embryo has such moral significance that it should not be destroyed in stem cell research. If that embryo has the same moral import as an individual human being, then those strategies for stem cell development that do not place the early embryo at risk should continue to be investigated. However, if the early human embryo does not have the same moral significance as an individual human being, this would make the use of several proposed alternative techniques ethically unnecessary. In chapter 3, I turn to the question of the moral significance of the early embryo in secular thought. In that chapter, I present a theory of the moral significance of the early human embryo that I call upon in subsequent discussions of oversight and regulation.

3

The Moral Significance of Early Human Embryos in Secular Thought

The dream of scientists and many patients of using human embryonic stem cells to treat the seriously ill has been interrupted by the alarmed voices of those who see human embryos as vulnerable living humans. These objectors do not reject stem cell research in itself, for they recognize that it may offer new forms of treatment and insights into human development. Instead, they reject human embryonic stem cell research because it necessarily involves the destruction of early human embryos. To destroy human embryos, these objectors declare, is to destroy individual living human beings and is therefore wrong.

Others, however, take different views of the moral significance of early human embryos. These range from the view that they do not have the potential to produce individual humans until after fourteen days of growth to the position that they are insignificant groups of human cells. Although these other commentators start from different positions, they reach the same conclusion: early human embryos at five to six days of growth are not individual human beings, and their use in embryonic stem cell research can be morally justifiable.

The debate about whether early embryos have the same moral significance as living human beings and are owed the same protections has become more heated since human embryonic stem cells were first cultivated in 1998. In part, this is because this question has increasingly been confused with the central moral question that arises in the abortion debate: How should we morally weigh the life, health, and well-being of a pregnant woman against the life of a fetus she is carrying? This latter question, however, is irrelevant in the context of stem cell research, for early embryos, rather than fetuses, are at issue, and these early embryos are outside the bodies of women. Consequently, these early embryos place no woman's life, health, or well-being at risk. For this reason, responses to the question whether it would be right to carry out an abortion do not necessarily fit responses to the question whether it would be right to carry out embryonic stem cell research. As Gilbert Meilaender points out, "No doubt it is, in our society, impossible to contemplate this question [whether early human embryos have the same moral significance as living human beings] without feeling sucked back into the abortion debate," but it "is a separate question."[1]

Are early human embryos individual human beings? Do they have special moral significance, meaning that they are the sorts of entities that should receive moral attention and consideration?[2] Do we owe them the many protections that we provide to living human beings? Is it morally acceptable to destroy them by extracting stem cells from their inner cell mass in the course of stem cell research?

Passions run particularly high about these questions, for they get to the core of just who we are and how we ought to treat those perceived by some as vulnerable fellow human beings. If we are to have a reasonable discussion about these questions with one another, rather than a heated mud-slinging match, we must make an effort to understand why others believe what they do and not dismiss their views out of hand as irrational or even evil.

Therefore, in this chapter, I explore five main views about whether early human embryos are individual human beings and what sort of moral significance they bear. These are (1) the time of fertilization view, (2) the fourteen-day or later view, (3) the potentiality view, (4) the group of human cells view, and (5) the person view. I consider whether it is morally justifiable to use early human embryos at five to six days after fertilization in research that involves their destruction in terms of each of these views and ultimately argue for the adoption of the fourteen-day or later view. I go on to maintain that because our view of the moral significance of early human embryos has broadened in light of recent findings about their possible role not just in reproduction but also in regenerative research, and because saving the lives and health of those already living, like bringing children into the world, is a worthy goal, it can be morally justifiable to use early human embryos (developed outside the body of a woman) for research that bears promise of treating serious disease.

We have more complete scientific knowledge today about the development of human embryos within and without the bodies of women than was available to past generations. Even so, scholars and commentators interpret the findings of recent developmental biology and embryology in different ways. This is because the metaphysical and ethical issues surrounding early human embryos are among the most complex and controversial that we face. The solutions that we bring to them, therefore, will not be simple and straightforward. Bearing this in mind, I now turn to consider the five major views that have been presented about the moral significance of early human embryos.

Five Views of the Moral Significance of Early Human Embryos

Of these five main ways in which people view what sort of moral consideration we owe to early human embryos, the first four—(1) the time of fertilization view, (2) the fourteen-day or later view, (3) the potentiality view, and (4) the group of human cells view—start from the assumption that individual human beings are owed great moral consideration and then attempt to fix the time at which these humans come into being. The fifth view takes a different approach. It rejects the notion that humans are morally significant and that it is important to establish when individual humans begin and instead starts from the assumption that "persons" are owed great moral consideration. It then goes on to explain when personhood begins and to assess whether early human embryos constitute "persons" and are therefore owed such consideration.

This means that to understand these five views we must consider what they say about the metaphysical significance of early human embryos—that is, how they explain what sort of beings they are and when they come into existence. The answers given in each case will lead us to give an account of the moral significance of early human embryos and what sort of moral consideration we owe them—that is, what sorts of moral attention and consideration we ought to extend to them.

Time of Fertilization View

Each of us is here today as a result of the merger of the egg of a woman and the sperm of a man. This merger is extremely significant from our current perspective as individual humans, for if that egg and that sperm had not joined, we would not be here. To some, it seems self-evident that since everyone alive began in this way, all fertilized eggs must be individual human beings. Robert George, a member of the President's Council on Bioethics, for instance, maintains:

> The being that is now you or I is the same being that was once an adolescent, and before that a toddler, and before that an infant, and

before that a fetus, and before that an embryo. To have destroyed the
being that is you or me at any of these stages would have been to destroy
you or me.[3]

To destroy an early human embryo in the course of carrying out stem
cell research, on this view, is to destroy an individual human being like
you or me, and such an act is profoundly morally wrong. This is the
view that informs the stem cell research policy adopted by President
Bush in 2001.

Metaphysical Justification of the Time of
Fertilization View

Some who hold this view assert that the unique genotype that is
established in the early embryo at the time of fertilization determines
its organization and the future direction of its development. John
Noonan, for instance, declares that "at conception the new being
receives the genetic code. It is this information which determines his
characteristics, which is the biological carrier of the possibility of
human wisdom, which makes him a self-evolving being. A being with
a human genetic code is a man."[4] That is, the fertilized egg is genetically
programmed from its very beginning so that all of its subsequent cell
divisions and the ways in which it differentiates and becomes an individual human organism are settled, according to Noonan. The early
human embryo is one and the same individual human being from the
start.

Those members of the President's Council on Bioethics who adopt
the time of fertilization view argue further:

> The fertilized egg is a human organism in its germinal stage. It is not just
> a "clump of cells" but an integrated, self-developing whole, capable (if all
> goes well) of the continued organic development characteristic of human
> beings. To be sure, the embryo does not yet have, except in potential, the
> full range of characteristics that distinguish the human species from
> others, but one need not have those characteristics in evidence in order
> to belong to the species.... The embryo is in fact fully "one of us": a
> human life in process, an equal member of the species *Homo sapiens* in
> the embryonic stage of his or her natural development.[5]

The early human embryo that figures in embryonic stem cell research,
in their view, is an individual, living, biologically human being. To
understand their position more fully, it is important to grasp the basics
of the very early biological development of the fertilized egg. Only then
can we grasp its metaphysical implications.

When sperm and egg fuse, the sperm, with its twenty-three chromosomes, enters the cytoplasm surrounding the nucleus of the egg. Within

the next eighteen to twenty-six hours, the second polar body (a small sphere with twenty-three chromosomes), is ejected from the egg, leaving it with twenty-three chromosomes. The chromosomes of the egg and the sperm now merge within the nucleus of the egg to complete fertilization. The resulting cell, which has forty-six chromosomes, half from the egg and half from the sperm, is termed a "zygote." The paternal set of chromosomes does not become activated until several days later when, after several divisions or cleavages into smaller cells called "blastomeres," the genome present at the completion of fertilization switches on and affects subsequent embryonic development.[6]

Advocates of the time of fertilization view maintain that the genetic code of the early embryo is set at the time when sperm and egg form a zygote. The rest of its growth, they explain, involves working out what occurs genetically at the time of fertilization. Therefore, they conclude, the zygote constitutes a unique individual human from fertilization onward.

Some supporters of the time of fertilization view observed in 1999 and 2002 that research in the mouse at that time reinforced the theory that the zygote directs the development of the cells that spring from it.[7] They pointed to the work of several investigators who maintained that the mouse zygote exhibits polarity, meaning that it has an up-down or left-right axis from the start.[8] Since such studies apparently displayed that the human zygote has an anterior-posterior orientation that continues during its subsequent divisions into several cells, they held, the human embryo takes on an individual identity at the time of fertilization. This identity determines its overall body plan and future development. In adopting this theory, they challenged the scientific consensus reached in the 1970s that the early embryo does not exhibit a distinct polarity until five or six days after fertilization when the zygote has been succeeded by the blastocyst, a slightly oblong ball of a few dozen cells.

Thus, on the time of fertilization view, the zygote or fertilized egg is an individual entity whose newly constituted genome directs the multiplication of its cells, the direction of its development, and the differentiation of its tissues. It organizes itself into an embryo, fetus, infant, child, and adult without ceasing to be the one and same living being.[9]

Moral Implications of the Time of Fertilization View

Because the human fertilized egg is an individual human being, according to the time of fertilization view, it necessarily follows that it has the same moral significance as you or me and that it is owed all the moral protections that we give to living individual humans. Once sperm and egg fuse, the resulting human being is owed protection from destruction from that point onward, they hold. This means that it is wrong to destroy that embryo in the process of deriving the precursors of human embryonic stem cells from its inner cell mass. Much as we would not kill one human being in order to save another, they argue, we should not kill the early human embryo in carrying out stem cell research—even if this might enable us to save many other human beings through the resulting therapies. Some among them liken embryos remaining at in vitro fertilization (IVF) clinics that would be otherwise be discarded to dying children and maintain that just as we make extra efforts to save living children from death, we should do the same for these frozen embryos.[10] We can do this by offering them for adoption by couples who want to have children, they believe.

Critique of the Time of Fertilization View

The time of fertilization view raises important questions about the appropriate interpretation of recent embryological findings, such as just when early embryos develop a distinct axis, as well as a number of metaphysical questions, such as those that center on the issue of numerical identity. Answers to these questions—esoteric as they may seem—will have import for the soundness of the view of the moral significance of early human embryos that is held by advocates of this view. I therefore turn to consider the scientific and metaphysical issues and problems that the time of fertilization view raises. These have largely been explored by advocates of the fourteen-day or later view.

In critiquing the time of fertilization view, they argue that if instead of looking back from our current position as living human beings, we look forward from the point at which sperm and egg merge, it does not seem obvious that all fertilized eggs must be individual human beings. There are several reasons for this. For one, recent findings in human embryology and reproductive medicine have cast doubt over the contention that the genotype of the zygote or fertilized egg contains specific instructions that enable it to control its own development. C. A. Bedate and R. C. Cefalo, for instance, state that "the formation of the embryo depends on a series of events that will have to occur during the course of ontogenesis, some of which are outside the control of the genetic program."[11] Several other scientists are in accord with this view. They observe that the activation of the genes in each cell into which the zygote divides is influenced by such factors as the cell's location, its previous history, cell-to-cell contacts, and cytoplasmic, electric, and biochemical signals.[12] This leads them to maintain that the way in which the early embryo grows depends largely on its interactions with neighboring cells and other environmental cues, and that the genotype of the zygote does not determine the organization and development of the early embryo once and for all. This conclusion runs contrary to that reached by advocates of the time of fertilization view.

Supporters of the fourteen-day or later view argue further that twins, triplets, and higher multiples share the same set of genes and yet are separate individuals. Consequently, the genetic constitution of the zygote does not establish that it is an individual human being, they claim. Moreover, two different blastomeres with different genes can, on occasion, fuse to form one chimeric blastocyst.[13] Yet this blastocyst has two sets of genes, even though it is one individual, which suggests that genes alone do not determine individual identity. They point out further that human sperm, eggs, and many tumors are genetically unique and yet are not individual human beings.[14] Therefore, they conclude, having cells with a specific genetic code is not sufficient to identify early embryos as separate individual humans.

These critics of the time of fertilization view also note that scientists who have studied the development of zygotes have found that sometimes more than one sperm penetrates an egg, creating a fertilized egg that will never develop.[15] This indicates, they assert, that not all fertilized eggs constitute individual human beings. At other times, zygotes stop developing and are absorbed into the placenta.[16] These zygotes, too, cannot be living individual human beings. In addition, recent evidence reveals that a stunning percentage of early embryos—in the range of 75–80 percent—die early in pregnancies,[17] many because of genetic anomalies.[18] Harold J. Morowitz and James S. Trefil state:

> Slightly fewer than a third of all conceptions lead to a fetus that has a chance of developing. In other words, if you were to choose [an embryo] at random and follow it through the first week of development, the chances are less than one in three that it would still be there at full term even though there has been no human intervention.... It is simply not true that most [embryos], if undisturbed, will produce a human being. The probability that a conception will result in a live birth is actually quite low. Note that since we have assumed that all conceptions lead to cell division, we have almost surely overestimated the true success rate.[19]

Therefore, it is difficult to accept that early embryos, which die in such massive numbers, are individual human beings, those who adopt the fourteen-day or later view argue, for most do not result in humans. Indeed, we do not act as though these embryos are such beings. We have not launched worldwide public health efforts to save them, as we have done for individual human beings who are dying of malnutrition or AIDS, and we have not urged people to stop engaging in sexual intercourse on grounds that to continue to do so would result in the development of a large number of human beings (embryos) that will inevitably die.

Even those zygotes that are structurally and functionally normal and begin to develop cannot be said to be individual human beings, supporters of the fourteen-day or later approach argue, for they do not function as stable organized entities. They point out that the first two cells into which the fertilized egg divides function as distinct cells, rather than two-celled individuals. Each of these cells is totipotent, meaning that when one cell is separated from the rest (up to the eight-cell stage) and provided with a hospitable environment, it can become a separate individual.[20] The fact that early embryos can split into twins or higher multiples until fourteen or fifteen days after fertilization[21] indicates that the period of early embryonic development up to about fourteen days after sperm and egg meet is a time of great fluidity. This means, they conclude, that the zygote is not a fixed and distinct individual human entity.

Advocates of the fourteen-day or later view return to the possibility that identical twins can develop from a single fertilized egg to argue that if the fertilized egg is already an individual human being that directs its own development, it is difficult to explain how one human being can divide into two or more.[22] For instance, Peter van Inwagen muses as follows: "Suppose I was once a mass of adhering cells that was still capable of splitting into two masses, each of which would have developed into an organism that was genetically exactly like me. Suppose, then, that this had happened. What would have become of me?"[23] Would he have been sacrificed to these subsequent individuals? Or would he somehow have contained them? Since one being cannot be identical to two, the original fertilized egg cannot be said to be identical to each twin. Yet we have no basis for identifying that fertilized egg with either twin in preference to the other, for they are identical in their characteristics and neither is temporally prior to the other. This leaves us with no rational basis on which to describe the fertilized egg as an earlier stage of either one of the twins.[24] The only conclusion that remains is that the fertilized egg is not identical to either of the twins that has emerged. Yet this is no explanation at all. The possibility of twinning, consequently, means that we cannot say that the fertilized egg is identical with a specific individual. This does not depend on whether twinning is rare or frequent; it depends on the possibility of twinning— and we know that this possibility exists. Therefore, the phenomenon of twinning presents a serious problem for the time of fertilization view.

Further, those holding the fourteen-day or later view challenge the claim of supporters of the time of fertilization view, noted above, that scientific evidence suggests that the zygote exhibits polarity and has an orientation to develop in a specific direction from its very beginning. Time of fertilization advocates maintain that this evidence proves that the fertilized egg is, after all, a single human individual. Those holding the fourteen day or later view, however, point out that researchers have subsequently found evidence that supports the older scientific view that the polarity, or directional orientation, of early mammalian embryos does not appear until they reach the blastocyst stage at five or six days after fertilization.[25] These researchers could find no distinct axis that tilts mouse zygotes in a certain developmental direction until that stage. Moreover, this tilting, they maintain, comes about through a process that includes chance occurrences, rather than one occurrence that is directed from the moment that a fertilized egg first appears.[26] According to N. Motosugi and colleagues, for instance, "the mammalian embryo gradually acquires axes of asymmetry . . . , initially through a random process or using available, but not essential, cues."[27] Their and other studies in embryology support the scientific view that the zygote does not display some sort of directional orientation from the start, contrary to the claim of those holding the time of fertilization view.

The arguments between those holding these two different views continue to this day. For instance, those who take the time of fertilization position acknowledge that identical twinning is still possible during the development of the early embryo and that this presents a problem for their view, since it puts into doubt whether the zygote is a single individual. Yet Alfonso Gómez-Lobo, a member of the President's Council on Bioethics and an advocate of the time of fertilization approach, responds to this problem as follows: "A stick in my hand is potentially two sticks: I could break it in half. But this does not entail that as long as I do not break it my stick is not one stick."[28] Similarly, he argues, when twinning occurs, the individual that is the zygote continues while a second one appears. The singleness of the cell formed at fertilization need not be denied, he maintains. And so the arguments go back and forth. At some point it is necessary to step back from them in order to understand just what it is that advocates of the fourteen-day or later view maintain apart from their critique of the time of fertilization view and to assess the adequacy of the fourteen-day or later view.

Fourteen-Day or Later View

According to those who adopt the fourteen-day or later view, the development of the early human embryo rests on a cascade of events that leads to the formation of a distinct individual with differentiated parts at about day fourteen. This individual retains its identity as the same entity through its subsequent stages of development. This means, supporters of the fourteen-day or later view argue, that the early embryo at the fifth or sixth day after fertilization, the stage at which embryonic stem cells are removed from it for embryonic stem cell research, is not an individual human being.

Metaphysical Justification of the Fourteen-Day or Later View

They hold, in contrast with advocates of the time of fertilization view, that the zygote or fertilized egg becomes a biologically stable organized individual at the point in its development when certain significant changes occur at about day fourteen.[29] At this time, the cells piling up on the embryonic plate form the primitive streak, a thickening plate of cells among the assembled cluster of cells, from which the brain, the nervous system, and the organs of the body grow; the first neural groove now appears, indicating the beginnings of the nervous system; and the cells of the early embryo begin to differentiate into specialized tissues and systems—neural, cardiovascular, and so on.[30] These sorts of changes marked by the appearance of the primitive streak occur at approximately day fourteen.

Several developments at this point are especially significant. The first is that the cells of the early embryo begin to function either as part of the embryo proper or as extraembryonic supporting materials that will be discarded later. The second is that it is irrevocably settled by this time that an embryo proper that is distinct from the membranes that nourish it is present. A third is that twinning can no longer occur after this point. These findings support the view that the cells of the early embryo form a distinct individual human entity at about the fourteenth day after fertilization. Such evidence, along with the multiple arguments set out above in response to the time of fertilization view, has led supporters of the fourteen-day or later view to reach their position.

On the fourteen-day or later view, the appearance of the primitive streak at about day fourteen after fertilization marks the point at which the embryo, in the form of the embryo proper (the embryo itself), separates off from the embryonic supporting material, starts to develop specialized tissues and systems, and becomes a distinct and separate individual. Some among those who accept the fourteen-day point as metaphysically significant adopt a more developmental approach than this suggests: they maintain that the individual is not fully formed as such at the fourteen-day point but that it continues to develop and becomes a complete individual at some later point in this process. However, they disagree among themselves about just when this later point has been reached. Some say that it is when brain waves first occur in the fetus, others when it is viable and could be kept alive outside the uterus, and others at still later points. The range of views about this is wide, and each of these views is supported by sophisticated philosophical arguments. However, the proponents of all of them agree that the early human embryo at five to six days after fertilization, the time relevant to embryonic stem cell research, is not an individual human being.

Moral Implications of the Fourteen-Day or Later View

What sort of moral consideration, if any, do we owe to this early human embryo? Do we have a duty to protect it from destruction? Or is it morally justifiable to use this early embryo in stem cell research?

The fourteen-day or later view provides a large umbrella that covers a range of subviews about just when the embryo formed at the fourteenth day after fertilization is owed protection from destruction. Some say that it is from day fourteen onward, since it is at that time that it constitutes a living human individual. Others say that the human embryo is in process at day fourteen and that it increases in moral weight as it develops until it reaches a point at which it is owed the same moral consideration as a living human being. This point corresponds to the metaphysical point or period of development at which it is said to be an individual human entity. However, discussion of these views of the moral significance of fetuses and infants at points after the fourteenth day from fertilization is beyond the scope of the issue at stake here, the moral significance of human embryos at the fifth or sixth day after fertilization.[31]

Many who hold a version of the fourteen-day or later view argue that although we do not owe the early human embryo before day fourteen all the moral protections that we accord to living individual humans, we owe it a certain kind of moral consideration and respect. The 1994 Human Embryo Research Panel of the National Institutes of Health, for instance, maintained in its report that the emergence of the primitive streak at fourteen days after fertilization represents "a major milestone in embryonic development." It went on to state that "although the preimplantation embryo warrants serious moral consideration as a developing form of human life, it does not have the same moral status as an infant or child."[32] Because the early human embryo has a certain moral weight, we owe it serious moral consideration. Yet, the panel maintained, this "does not rule out well justified research" on the early human embryo.[33]

This view reappeared in the cloning report of the President's Council on Bioethics. Members who favored research cloning declared that the early human embryo "has a moral status somewhere between that of ordinary human cells and that of a full human person," and declared that

> the embryo in its earliest stages (certainly in the first fourteen days) is not the moral equivalent of a human person but that it commands significantly more respect than other human cells. We also hold that the embryo can be used for life-saving or potentially life-saving research while still being accorded the "special respect" it deserves.[34]

We can both respect early human embryos and yet use them "for serious, not frivolous reasons."[35]

John Robertson also adopts the notion that the early human embryo is owed special respect. He maintains that it is "a potent symbol of human life" and that the ways in which we treat it reflect and even define the value that we place on human life generally. However, "symbols do not make moral claims on us in the same way that persons and living entities with interests do," he adds. We need to choose "what level of costs in lost research are acceptable to maintain a symbolic commitment to human life."[36]

Daniel Callahan finds the view that the early embryo is owed "special respect" both sensible and yet puzzling. He confesses to a "nagging uneasiness" about such respect, as it is "an odd form of esteem—at once high-minded and lethal." Indeed, it seems to him that special respect was given by the Human Embryo Research Panel to the research that uses human embryos, rather than to the embryos themselves! The human embryo seemed to have no value at all to members of that panel, he argues.[37] Members of the President's Council on Bioethics who adopt the time of fertilization view go even further and maintain that the view of some of their colleagues that early embryos are owed special respect is incoherent and self-contradictory. They cannot fathom how those holding it can claim both that human embryos deserve special respect and yet endorse research that requires their destruction.[38]

Their colleagues who adopt the special respect view respond by pointing out that various religions condone the killing of animals for food and yet express respect for those animals.[39] This, too, is the case with the early human embryo, they argue; we can condone the destruction of the early embryo for life-giving research without losing sight of the respect that we owe it. Michael Meyer and Lawrence Nelson note more specifically that in certain Native American cultures when animals are killed for food those who have destroyed them are expected to express respect for such animals by apologizing to them after their death for having had to do so.[40] Therefore, the notion that one can respect an entity and yet destroy it under justifiable circumstances is not incoherent, according to these advocates of the special respect view.

Those who hold this view, however, need to establish a standard by which to assess when it is morally justifiable to destroy early human embryos in research and when it is not. Robertson maintains that special respect for early human embryos means that they should be created and discarded in research only if this would aid in "the development of useful knowledge."[41] He does not define what he means by "useful knowledge" more closely. The report of the Human Embryo Research Panel was somewhat more detailed. It maintained that the use of embryos in research is allowable under two conditions: the research should be of a sort that "by its very nature cannot otherwise be validly conducted"—that is, the use of embryos is a last resort—and in order to validate a study "that is potentially of outstanding scientific and therapeutic value."[42] The panel went on to recommend that researchers carefully limit the number of embryos they use and not allow them to develop longer than a specific research protocol requires, but in no event beyond fourteen days after fertilization. This view, while underwriting guidelines for carrying out research involving human embryos, does not elaborate on what sorts of research would justify destroying human embryos.

Bonnie Steinbock is more specific about this. She would allow early embryos to be used and destroyed in "important research, for example, in reproductive medicine, genetics, or cancer and other diseases, as these are endeavors with the potential for enormous human benefit."[43] She cautions that it would be wrong to use these embryos in trivial research or to treat them frivolously, for they are owed a degree of respect. Robert P. Lanza and colleagues add that "in this context, respect means that that research must be justified in terms of its scientific validity and likely therapeutic benefit. It also means that the number of embryos used should be minimized consistent with the need for the scientific validity of the study."[44] This standard would rule out the use of early human embryos for, say, routine testing for toxins but would justify their use in research directed toward, say, the treatment of Parkinson's disease.

In summary, some who adopt the fourteen-day or later view (including some who emphasize the "later" interpretation of it) take the concept of "special respect" for early human embryos at day five or six after fertilization as a way of saying that although these embryos are not individual humans and have no characteristics on the basis of which we would say they are owed protection from destruction, we should treat them with respect because they represent a connection with human life. This means that we do not have a moral license to destroy them arbitrarily—but it does not mean that we should never allow them to be destroyed in research. In some instances, their significance as symbols of human life can be acknowledged and yet they can be used in research that is aimed at treating and perhaps curing those who are more than symbols of human life—living human beings.

Critique of the Fourteen-Day or Later View

Advocates of the time of fertilization view reject these arguments. They find the twinning argument—that no discrete individual is formed until approximately the fourteenth day after fertilization—unpersuasive. For instance, those on the President's Council who adopt the time of fertilization view argue that "if one locus of moral status can become two, its moral standing does not thereby diminish but rather increases. . . . The fact that where 'John' alone once was there are now both 'John' and 'Jim' does not call into question the presence of 'John' at the outset."[45]

This response, however, misses the point. No one presenting the fourteen-day or later view asserts that the appearance of Jim diminishes the moral standing of John. Instead, the issue is one of numerical identity. If John is a single individual from the time of fertilization on, where did he go when he became two individuals? Did he become one of the twins? If so, which one? If not, what happened to him when Jim appeared? Each twin is a distinct individual and therefore each cannot be identical with the earlier fertilized egg. The answer given above by Gómez-Lobo that the appearance of twins is like the appearance of two sticks after one stick has been broken will not do, for John is an early embryo, rather than an inert stick, and would be destroyed, rather than transformed into two different individuals, if broken in two. The metaphor does not work.

These members of the President's Council also question the moral significance of the primitive streak, stating that "changes that occur at fourteen days are merely the visibly evident culmination of more subtle changes that have taken place earlier and that are driving the organism toward maturity." They go on to maintain that nothing that occurs after the embryo's individual genetic identity is established serves to exhibit that it has developed "novel human individuality."[46] However, this amounts to a simple reassertion of their original position, rather than a response to the significant evidence derived from embryology set out by those presenting the fourteen-day view that calls that position into question.

The notion of special respect presented by some who are proponents of some version of the fourteen-day or later view (who in certain instances emphasize the "later" aspect of this view) is also open to criticism, for it is difficult to discern just when this special respect is owed to early human embryos. It is extended to them because they serve a symbolic function in our society, not because of any attributes of theirs, they maintain. Thus, it can be retracted or outweighed when greater goods that would be served by the destruction of these human embryos come along. Indeed, as long as early embryos are not treated with contempt or derision, it appears that almost anything can be done with them, even though they are still said to be owed "special respect" as symbols of human life. This notion is therefore perplexing and needs further discussion if it is to be used in support of the claim that early human embryos are owed some sort and degree of moral consideration.

It is difficult at this point in our analysis to resist the conclusion that the metaphysical and embryological arguments in support of the fourteen-day or later view are better supported and more convincing than those presented in favor of the time of fertilization view. The problems that supporters of the time of fertilization view have found with some of the arguments for the fourteen-day or later view appear to be based on misunderstandings of the latter view. In addition, they fail to respond adequately to other arguments against their position that have been developed by those who adopt the fourteen-day or later view. Several significant scientific and metaphysical problems that the time of fertilization view itself raises remain at issue, however. The fourteen-day or later view also needs to address further the question of why early human embryos are owed "special respect" in the research context, where, unlike in the procreative context, they do not symbolize "continuing human life."

Potentiality View

Some philosophers and theologians challenge both the time of fertilization and the fourteen-day or later views, arguing that even though the zygote or fertilized egg is not an individual human being, it is a potential human being and will, in the normal course of events, grow into an actual one. It develops gradually from conception through the various stages of prenatal development until it emerges completely actualized. Consequently, those presenting this potentiality view argue that the fertilized egg and the embryo and fetus that develop from it are owed protection from destruction from the time of conception onward.

Metaphysical Justification of the Potentiality View

According to this view, the human embryo has the potential to become a human being at fertilization. On one version of it, "we know that a new human individual organism with the internal potential to develop into an adult, given nurture, comes into existence as a result of the process of fertilization at conception."[47] That is, the fertilized egg has within itself in the normal course of events a certain power to develop into a post-birth human being.

To understand this view more fully, we must delve into certain fascinating philosophical questions about the meaning of "potentiality." When supporters of those this view talk about the potentiality of the fertilized egg in terms of what occurs in "the normal course of events," they do not mean by this what happens to it statistically. That is, they do not count up how many zygotes develop in a certain way and then draw conclusions about their potential in the normal course of events from this. To accept the understanding of potentiality that such counting implies would mean, for example, that in a society where disease led to the death of 95 percent of all children, children would not be potential adults, since statistically they would never develop into adults.[48] This seems wrong. The fact that a child would face a significant chance of death in such a society does not cancel out the fact that it is capable—or has the potential—of becoming an adult in the normal course of events. Thus, the notion of the potential as the statistically normal misses the point. Those presenting the potentiality argument mean by the "normal course of events" that the relevant processes will unfold in virtue of the child's biological constitution, not by virtue of certain exigencies in that child's environment.

Some deny this and assert that an entity's potential is whatever might possibly happen to it. John Harris, for instance, maintains that ascribing potential to a being involves making a provisional prediction about its future. He asserts that "to say that the fertilised egg is a potential human being is just to say that if certain things happen to it (like implantation) and certain other things do not (like spontaneous abortion) it will eventually become a human being."[49]

However, if a being's potential is whatever might happen to it, then its potential is immense. A fertilized egg, on this notion of "potential," would be not only a potential human being but also a potential form of glue, were it dumped into a bubbling vat in order to fuse its ingredients for this purpose, or a potential culinary delicacy, were it ground up and served as an hors d'oeuvres at a party. This concept of the potential is so broad and undiscriminating that it loses its core meaning. A fertilized egg's potential is limited by the way that it is formed biologically. This is not to deny that there is a certain amount of plasticity in the developmental process; an entity's potential to develop into a certain sort of being might be realized by more than a single developmental path.[50]

Moreover, to say an entity is a potential human being does not mean that it will become an actual human being if it encounters no resistance during its development. An acorn is a potential oak tree, even if has no chance of growing into one because someone burns it up when using it as fuel. A fertilized egg, according to those who set out the potentiality view, is still a potential human being, even if it does not have a supportive environment and will die. When it does not receive nutrition and other necessities, it retains its potential, but that potential will not be realized.

In short, the potentiality view maintains that the fertilized egg or zygote, in virtue of its biological constitution, has the potential in the normal course of events to develop into a post-birth individual human. Because of its potential to become a living human individual, it is owed protection from destruction, proponents of this view hold.

Moral Implications of the Potentiality View

On the potentiality view, the fertilized egg is morally significant because it is potentially the very same being as the later human being that emerges from the process of prenatal development—and that human being is morally significant. That is, advocates of this view accord moral significance to the zygote because it has the power, within the normal course of events, to become one and the same being as the later morally significant individual human being. It would be wrong deliberately to use it in research that would destroy it, in their view, for that would prevent it from realizing this potential in the normal course of events.

Critique of the Potentiality View

This view raises intriguing questions about the moral significance of the potentiality of the fertilized egg. One such question is whether a potential being is as significant morally as the actual being that it might become. Some would argue that the potential is not yet actual and that what counts morally is the being that actually exists, not the potential being. Therefore, they would hold, the fertilized egg does not have the same moral significance as the post-birth human individual, and it is consequently permissible to destroy that fertilized egg. However, advocates of the potentiality view response would maintain that the fertilized egg, even though potential, is the same individual as the later human being and that the moral significance of the latter is retroactive and moves backward to the former. Therefore, they would say, it is not permissible to destroy fertilized eggs. A further question: arises: Should the potential of an entity always be realized, as proponents of the potentiality view imply? It seems that it need not be. There is no moral requirement, for instance, to save acorns, with their potential to develop into oak trees, from destruction or to bring to fruition the potential of a chick egg to become a chicken. However, those who hold the potentiality view would respond that potential of the fertilized egg is morally more significant than that of an acorn or a chick egg, for the human who will, in the normal course of events, develop from the fertilized egg will have great moral significance, whereas the oak tree and the chicken will not.

Advocates of the potentiality view, however, seem to falter in these responses. They need to provide an argument for the claim that a potential entity that would have moral significance if it were brought into being, must be brought into being. The properties that develop when the potential of the fertilized egg is actualized are relevant to how we should treat it, once actualized, but those properties do not exist in the fertilized egg. Therefore, we do not necessarily owe it the same sort of moral consideration that we owe to the later actualized entity. Moreover, even if an actual human being would have greater moral significance than an actual acorn or an actual chicken, that does not provide an argument for maintaining that the potential human being must be actualized.

Many—but not all—of those who present the potentiality view have not addressed these rather complex sorts of philosophical questions. They have simply asserted that the fertilized egg and the later individual human that might develop are one and the same individual and that because the latter has moral significance, the former must also and must therefore be preserved in being and protected from destruction. Yet this begs the question. Is it the case that the fertilized egg is potentially the very same being as the early embryo and the later individual human being? To respond, it is necessary draw a distinction between two kinds of potential that have been sorted out by Stephen Buckle.[51] One is the potential to *become* a distinct being in the future, and the other is the potential to *produce* a certain state of affairs in the future; but they differ in important respects. Both kinds of potential refer to a capacity or power in an object or group of objects.

Buckle defines the potential to become as follows:

> The potential to *become* is the power possessed by an entity to undergo changes which are changes *to itself*, that is, to undergo growth or, better still, *development*. The potential to *become* can thus be called developmental potential. The process of actualizing the potential to become preserves some form of individual identity.[52]

The potential to become attaches only to those distinct individuals that preserve their identity over time. That is, the individual at the beginning of the process of becoming that this notion of potentiality encompasses must be the very same numerical individual at the end of it. The sort of identity involved here is not personal or qualitative identity but what Derek Parfit has termed (and philosophers generally call) numerical identity.[53]

The potential to produce, in contrast, is the capacity to cause something else. It does not require that the being at the start and the end of the process of production must be numerically the same. Further, the potential to produce is not restricted to single entities; it also can be ascribed to entities composed of several discrete components that jointly lack unifying features and organization. Such entities, in combination, can have the potential to produce.

For instance, a mixture of oxygen and hydrogen has the potential to produce water, but these two elements have no overarching organization that renders them a single entity. Together, they do not become water, but together they produce something else, water. Similarly, human sperm and egg that are placed in a laboratory dish containing nutritive ingredients have the potential to produce something else, a fertilized egg. However, these two gametes have no joint unifying features that make then a single entity. Therefore, they do not have the potential to become the fertilized egg, but instead the potential to produce the fertilized egg. We can only speak of entities as having the potential to become where they are unified simple or complex wholes.

Proponents of the potentiality view presume the potentiality to become, rather than the potentiality to produce, for they hold that the early human embryo has the potential to become the very same later human individual. They maintain that "the fertilized egg is a potential human subject if *it* will eventually become a human subject, not merely because it will cause, or help to cause, a human subject to come to exist."[54]

This view raises a significant difficulty. The fertilized egg will not eventually become a human subject because it is *not the same entity* as the embryo proper or the human individual at the other end of the developmental process. Buckle explains this as follows:

> The changes that the fertilised egg undergoes are not changes through which it develops into, or itself *becomes*, the embryo proper. Rather, it undergoes a process of differentiation in which the various cells developed in the earliest stages after fertilization take on a range of different functions, only one of which is the development of the embryo proper; and no one group of specialized cells can be singled out as the same individual as the fertilized egg.[55]

The embryo proper that forms around the primitive streak, as noted in the discussion of the fourteen-day or later view, is not the entire collection of cells that develop from the fertilized egg but a small subset of them. It is this set of cells that is the embryo proper from which the individual human being develops. The other cells form extraembryonic material that supports it. Consequently, the fertilized egg does not stand at the beginning of the process of development of the embryo proper, for it does not become the embryo proper. Instead, it produces or causes the embryo proper. It is not itself numerically identical with the embryo proper. Yet the potentiality argument maintains that the fertilized egg and the embryo proper are the very same individual and that the fertilized egg becomes the embryo proper and the individual human being that can develop from that embryo proper. This conclusion is mistaken. Therefore, the potentiality view does not establish that the fertilized egg is a potential human being.

This failure of the potentiality argument has important implications for the question whether the time of fertilization or the fourteen-day or later view should prevail. I have argued that those who support the time of fertilization view have not provided convincing responses to the metaphysical arguments of those who hold the fourteen-day or later view. Instead, they have basically reasserted their earlier justifications for their position. Now it is clear that the potentiality view also has significant weaknesses and does not stand up to analysis. Therefore, the fourteen-day or later view emerges as the best supported of the three major views analyzed thus far.

Group of Human Cells View

Some argue that the early embryo at five to six days after fertilization amounts to a group of cells clustered together that do not constitute specific differentiated cells or tissues. These cells do not have the internal complexity and integrated functioning that we find in human organisms and therefore are not entitled to any special moral consideration, in their view. This is the group of human cells view.

Metaphysical Justification of the Group of Human Cells View

Members of the President's Council on Bioethics who set out this view indicate that they view the early human embryo as biological tissue rather than human life. The early-stage human embryo, they hold, has no characteristics that "spell the difference between biological tissue and a human life worthy of respect and rights."[56] It is a collection of primitive and undifferentiated cells that have not been formed into specific cells and tissues of the human body.

They rehearse several of the arguments given by those who hold the fourteen-day or later view to support their conclusion that this collection of cells is not a unique individual that functions in the integrated way in which a human organism functions. Thus, they point out that, until the primitive streak forms, the developing embryo may split into twins and two blastocysts may fuse to form a single one. Such embryological findings and their reasonable interpretation, they contend, confirm their view that the early human embryo is not a unique integrated individual but a collection of cells.

They also take into account the potentiality view but argue against it, maintaining that "the potential to become something (or someone) is hardly the same as being something (or someone), any more than a pile of building materials is the same as a house."[57] Any potential that the early human embryo may have to develop into an individual human being, they assert, can only be realized by its implantation within the uterus of a woman—and most early embryos developed coitally fail to implant. They conclude that this indicates that whatever potential to develop into a living human being the early embryo may have is very limited.

Moral Implications of the Group of Human Cells View

Supporters of the group of human cells view find no moral difference between the issues raised by the use of early human embryos in stem cell research and those raised by the use of any other sort of biomedical research materials. They can discern no sound reasons for treating early embryos as though they require special moral attention. Because the early embryo does not have any trace of a nervous system and therefore "no capacity for suffering or conscious experience in any form," it does not, in their view, represent "a human life worthy of respect and rights."[58]

They base their main moral argument in support of using materials from early human embryos in stem cell research on an analogy with the use of human organs in transplantation. If it is right to use one collection of tissues, a human organ, to treat those who are seriously ill, they argue, then it is right to use another collection of tissues, an early human embryo, in research that might lead to promising new therapies. Since the early embryo, like a human liver or kidney used in transplantation, lacks a brain and the capacity for consciousness, they maintain, it is equally acceptable morally to use cells derived from it in stem cell research and treatment.[59]

Those who adopt this view argue that a moral boundary can be drawn to limit the use of embryos for research. They would set it at fourteen days of development when human embryos are no longer clumps of cells but start to show signs of developing into distinct individuals with the beginnings of a nervous system. In short, they accord "no special moral status to the early-stage . . . embryos."[60]

Critique of the Group of Human Cells View

Those who present the group of human cells view tend to move between two notions of the moral significance of early human embryos. One is that these embryos amount to a collection of 100 to 200 undifferentiated human cells that have even less moral significance than the differentiated human cells, tissues, and organs found in the human body. The other is that these embryos are on a moral par with such differentiated cells, tissues, and organs. They expressly adopt the first notion and yet, as the analogy that they draw between the use of early embryos in stem cell research and the use of organs for transplantation reveals, they sometimes seem to adopt the second. They do not resolve this inconsistency.

It arises because advocates of the group of human cells view misconceive the notion of potentiality, as some on the President's Council of Bioethics point out. A pile of miscellaneous raw materials has no definite potential and might become anything at all, these critics observe. This is not the case with the early human embryo, which has some sort of potential (which they do not define) to form a human being. The question at issue is whether this group of cells constitutes an integrated biological whole with the potential to develop into an individual human being. Those who hold the group of human cells view imply that it does not, since it is not an integrated organic entity. Yet advocates of the group of human cells view do not specifically grapple with the possibility that this collection of cells might go on to become one or more human beings.[61] Therefore, they underestimate the moral seriousness of the question of whether to engage in research that involves the destruction of such cells.

The group of human cells view leaves open important questions about the metaphysical and moral significance of the early human embryo that need to be addressed if it is to provide a credible position. It does not acknowledge that the early human embryo could go on to produce the embryo proper which, in turn, could become a living human individual. Because of such lacunae, it does not offer a well-supported view that could provide the basis for deciding whether it would be morally acceptable to use early human embryos in stem cell research. This means that the fourteen-day or later view still stands as the primary candidate for providing a metaphysically and morally sound approach to this question.

Person View

Some would claim that the first four views presented here are "species-ist," for each assumes that being a member of the species *Homo sapiens* is in itself a criterion of moral significance. That is, the arguments set out above seek to understand when the lives of human beings begin because they attribute moral significance to all members of the human species. Each of these arguments goes down the wrong track, according to these critics, for being a member of the human species is irrelevant to the question of what protections we owe to early human embryos. What matters morally, they maintain, is whether a being possesses certain properties that render it a person, not whether it is a member of a certain species.

Metaphysical and Moral Justification of the Person View

Peter Singer is one of the primary spokespersons for this view. He urges us to accept that being a person is distinct from being human and insists that the primary condition that must be met to be owed protection from destruction is being a person.[62] By a "person," he means a being who exhibits a certain cluster of characteristics, of which rationality and self-consciousness are the most prominent. Singer maintains that the gorilla Koko, for instance, is a person because

> [she] communicates in sign language, using a vocabulary of over 1000 words ... has achieved scores between 85 and 95 on the Stanford-Binet Intelligence Test ... demonstrates a clear self-awareness by engaging in self-directed behaviours in front of a mirror ... lies to avoid the consequences of her misbehavior ... engages in imaginary play ... remembers and can talk about events in her life.[63]

Humans who carry out various forms of reasoning and display self-awareness are also persons. However, not all humans are persons, Singer claims. Although newborn infants are humans, they are neither rational nor self-conscious and therefore do not count as persons. Human embryos and fetuses also are not persons. Indeed,

on any fair comparison of morally relevant characteristics, like rationality, self-consciousness, awareness, autonomy, pleasure and pain, and so
on, the calf, the pig and the much derided chicken come out well ahead of
the fetus at any stage of pregnancy—while if we make the comparison
with a fetus of less than three months, a fish would show more signs of
consciousness.[64]

Consequently, when considering whether it is wrong to abort fetuses
less than three month of age—who clearly are not persons—he argues
that "abortion terminates an existence that is of no intrinsic value at
all" and is therefore morally acceptable. Presumably he would apply
the same argument to the early embryo at five to six days after fertilization; Singer would maintain that the destruction of such an embryo
in stem cell research also "terminates an existence that is of no intrinsic
value."[65]

Critique of the Person View

Singer's argument depends, in part, on the view that being human and
being a person are two separate and distinct notions. Yet in considering
his explanation of what it means to be a person, we come to realize
that it is not distinct from our understanding of what it means to be
human but, to the contrary, depends on that understanding. Koko, for
instance, has characteristics and capacities that we associate with being
human in the ordinary, everyday, not the biological, sense of being
human. That is why she has a claim to humane treatment. Singer
cannot escape writing about her in terms that are typical of those we
use in describing humans. This is because the notion of being a person
is derived from that of being human.

   When we say that an individual is human in the ordinary, everyday
sense, we mean that this individual has not only the physical characteristics of organisms that belong to the species *Homo sapiens* but also
certain personal characteristics and capacities, such as those for sen-
tience; perceiving things; having a concept of self; having abilities to
reason, generalize, and learn from past experience; having capacities to
love and to feel sympathy and empathy; having the empathy to recognize and value the interests of others; and many other capacities. We
have no fixed notion of how many and what sorts of these features and
capacities an individual must display to be said to be human.[66]

   What we mean by a person is remarkably similar. Indeed, if we
substitute the term "person" for "human" in the above description of
the spectrum of features and capacities of humans, we will come up
with the same description.[67] The very notion of being a person that
Singer has developed requires an individual to have characteristics that

we understand only in terms of what it means to be human. A being with personal characteristics that are quite different from those of humans would not be a person.

Imagine an alien who does not closely resemble a human in its physical aspects, for it is a living organism with no nose, ears, or legs and rolls along rather than walks. Further, it is devoid of all emotions. It does not love anything, fear anything, hate anything, or care about anything. It calmly and wantonly kills and reproduces without joy, sorrow, or reason. It does not seek any ends and does not evaluate ends rationally, for ends really do not matter to it. Whatever happens just happens. Since it doesn't care about anything, it cannot be motivated to act in order to achieve certain ends rather than others.

Would this alien count as a person in Singer's eyes? Is it rational or self-conscious? What makes these questions difficult to answer is that the kind of rationality and self-consciousness that the alien exhibits is vastly different from that of humans. Consequently, we cannot tell whether it is the sort of self-conscious rational being that Singer considers a person. The very notion of being a person that he has developed requires that an individual have certain characteristics that we understand only in terms of what it means to be human.

What is at issue when we ask whether it would be wrong to destroy an early human embryo in stem cell research is not whether this embryo exhibits a whole cluster of adult human characteristics and capacities and is therefore a person. It is unreasonable to expect this of human embryos during the prenatal stages of human development, as Singer does, in order to be justified in claiming that they should not be destroyed, just as it would be unreasonable to expect this of prenatal "great apes, . . . whales, dolphins, elephants, monkeys, dogs, pigs and other animals [who, according to Singer,] may eventually also be shown to be aware of their own existence over time and capable of reasoning."[68] If the standard of already existing personhood, as defined by Singer, were the only criterion available for deciding whether a being would live or be destroyed, few human embryos would survive, nor would many prenatal great apes, whales, dolphins, and so on!

The person view must be rejected, therefore, not only because it misleadingly substitutes the notion of "person" for "human," but also because it unreasonably requires that human embryos must exhibit certain capacities and characteristics at every point in their development in order to be protected from destruction. That is, this view must be rejected because it sidesteps the question of whether the early human embryo is an individual human being.

Emergence of the Fourteen-Day
or Later View

I have considered, in turn, four different views about whether early human embryos are individual humans and one that focuses and on whether they are persons. The first, the time of fertilization view (1) creates too many unanswered embryological and metaphysical questions about when individual human beings begin to develop as such and, consequently, leaves us with puzzles about the moral significance of early human embryos. Next, the potentiality view (3), among other problems, mistakenly ascribes to early embryos the potential to become, rather than the potential to produce, and therefore mistakenly identifies the fertilized egg with the later individual human being. The group of cells view (4) falters not only because it pursues two mutually conflicting notions of the moral significance of early human embryos, but also because it, too, misconceives the meaning of the notion of potentiality and therefore fails to develop defensible moral conclusions. Finally, the person view (5) sidesteps the question of whether early human embryos are individual human beings because it overlooks its reliance on the very notion of the human as foundational. Moreover, it leads to an unreasonable expectation that early human embryos at day five or six after fertilization must exhibit personal characteristics typical of adult humans if they are to be free from the threat of destruction.

The view that appears to be open to greater support, both metaphysically and morally, than the other four is the fourteen-day or later view (2). It offers a reasoned interpretation of recent embryological findings and several well-supported arguments that lead to the conclusion that the early embryo at five or six days after fertilization is not an individual entity. However, the notion that this early embryo is owed "special respect" will need further elaboration if the fourteen-day or later approach is to justify the use of early human embryos in stem cell research. This additional elaboration will be presented and developed below in the course of discussing the ethical implications of creating embryos for research.

The Moral Significance of Early Human Embryos in
Stem Cell Research

Must we create early human embryos only for procreative purposes? Or is it also morally acceptable to develop them for research? These questions arise in several different contexts. When stem cell research is at issue, these contexts include those in which embryos would be created for research by means of IVF using donated gametes or through cloning using donated eggs and somatic cells.

Clearly, commentators who maintain that early human embryos are individual human beings will object to their creation for use in research that involves their destruction. However, some who veer away from that view also reject the creation of embryos for use in research that leads to their destruction.[69] And some who appear to hold the fourteen-day or later view also consider it wrong to engage in research that involves destroying embryos.[70] The basic argument of these critics of the creation of embryos for research is that doing so ignores the part that early human embryos play in reproduction and therefore wrongly treats them as dispensable research material to be used for the benefit of others. Maura Ryan, for instance, asks:

> If we do not recognize the human embryo as potential human life, as laying some claim on us morally that distinguishes it from a tree, as having a significance independent of our bestowal, what prevents us from producing as many embryos as we need for research just as we grow trees for furniture . . . ?[71]

The human embryo, she maintains, has "a moral standing that, even if not equivalent to full personhood, distinguishes it from things and non-human forms of life."[72] She does not elaborate on the basis on which she attributes exclusively reproductive significance ("the potential for human life") to human embryos.

Others argue that reproduction is not the only good end that early human embryos can serve and that the moral significance of these embryos is not solely procreative. Scientific research aimed at important goals, such as treating serious disease and avoiding birth anomalies, is also directed toward a good end and research using early embryos can rightly seek that end. Michael Sandel, of the President's Council on Bioethics, for instance, argues that

> if the creation and sacrifice of embryos in IVF is morally acceptable, why isn't the creation and sacrifice of embryos for stem cell research also acceptable? After all, both pursue worthy ends, and curing diseases such as Parkinson's is at least as important as enabling infertile couples to have genetically related children. . . . Stem cell research on IVF spares and on embryos for research (whether naturally or cloned) are morally on a par.[73]

The moral significance of early embryos in the research context differs from their significance in the procreative context, since they have different roles in each. This does not mean that these embryos are devoid of all moral significance in the research setting. In the context of stem cell research, the moral significance of embryos is *not reproductive* but *preservative* and *regenerative*; that is, in that context, embryos serve to restore and renew human life rather than to start it on the way into this world. In such instances, human embryos take on moral significance because of their possible contribution to the restoration of human life.

Here we get to the nub of the issue. Historically, we became aware of the existence of human embryos and their role in procreation only recently. We came to associate them exclusively with that end because that was the only end that we were aware that they could serve. When we came to realize that we could develop human embryos in vitro in order to further the procreative quest of those who are infertile, we continued to assume that reproduction was the sole possible end for which human embryos could be created outside the uterus of a woman.

But more recently, we have come to realize that human embryos can play a regenerative role and that there is no iron law of nature or morality that says that embryos created in vitro must only be used for procreation. We are not morally required to insert every human embryo that has been developed by means of IVF into the uterus of a woman so that it can realize its potential to produce an embryo proper. We accept that it is morally sound to refrain from introducing a great many embryos into a woman's body at one time because to do so would jeopardize her life and health and that of any resulting children. And, with that realization, we have come to recognize that embryos remaining outside the bodies of women can not only be used to develop new human beings but can serve another worthy end—to preserve and regenerate the lives of those living human beings who suffer from disease or injury. Recognition of this additional regenerative end that early human embryos can serve does not constitute "an assault on the character of procreation,"[74] for procreation is not denigrated by the creation of embryos for research. Procreation retains its value as a good end. However, research directed toward the care and treatment of those with serious diseases is an equally good end, and early human embryos can play a morally sound and important regenerative role in reaching toward that end.

Early human embryos created in vitro that will be used in stem cell research have moral significance because of their potential preservative and regenerative role. Because of such moral significance, they ought not be treated arbitrarily or frivolously when stem cell research is considered just in the same way that they ought not be treated arbitrarily or frivolously when procreation is at issue because of their moral significance. However, to maintain that in the research context, early human embryos in vitro have symbolic value as "continuing human life," as some commentators have maintained, is to make what philosophers call a "category mistake," for it confuses the procreative with the regenerative context. In the regenerative research context, early human embryos have moral significance because they might restore and renew the lives of those already living. Because of this we should not use such embryos frivolously or arbitrarily. Instead, we should carefully screen all proposed human embryonic stem cell research to ensure that it promises to provide important knowledge related to treating and healing living human beings, is carefully designed, and can only be conducted with cells derived from such embryos.

Thus, it can be ethically sound to use cells derived from early human in vitro embryos in significant scientific research that is directed toward treating and even saving the lives of living human beings. Such research does not diminish the moral significance of human embryos as possible vehicles for procreation but recognizes this, even as it also recognizes the moral significance of human embryos as possible vehicles to another good end: countering disease and forms of ill health and disability that affect those who are living. Early human embryos, therefore, have moral significance and are owed special respect not just because they symbolize the coming into being of human life in the procreative sense, but also because they symbolize the renewal of human life in the restorative and regenerative sense. When this broadened view of the moral significance of early human embryos is adopted and joined with the fourteen day or later view, that view provides justification for the careful, well-considered creation and use of human embryos in stem cell research.

Of the various views of the metaphysical and moral significance of early human embryos that have been considered here, the fourteen-day or later view emerges as the most supportable. The time of fertilization, potentiality, group of cells, and person views, as argued above, all succumb to inherent metaphysical and moral difficulties. In contrast, the fourteen-day or later view presents a strong biological and metaphysical case for the conclusion that a distinct individual human entity begins to develop at day fourteen after fertilization when gastrulation is underway and the primitive streak begins to form and to organize the cells of the developing embryo proper. The fourteen day or later view can explain satisfactorily the moral significance of the early embryo at day five or six after fertilization in terms of the restorative and preservative role that stem cells derived from it can play in renewing the stuff of human life.

4

The Moral Significance of Early Human Embryos in Religious Thought

In a pluralistic democratic society such as that in the United States, no exploration of the moral significance of early human embryos would be complete it if were to consider only secular views of this matter. The views of those who adhere to religious traditions within that polity also need to be taken into account if we are to gain a more complete picture of the reasoning of many citizens about contentious issues as we develop public policy. That is especially the case today, when the views of active and influential religious adherents about whether stem cells derived from human embryos should be used in research have been playing a prominent role in public policy decisions about this research.

Some who object to the use of early human embryos in stem cell research embrace religious traditions that teach that early embryos are individual human beings who are owed the same sorts of protections as living persons. Such early embryos, like all human beings, reflect the image of the divine, they believe. Consequently, to destroy such early human embryos in the course of stem cell research, in their view, is to throw the gift of life back into the face of the divine.

Those who follow certain other religious traditions do not regard early human embryos as human beings that have the same moral significance as already born human beings but instead hold varying views about this. Some among them maintain that once early embryos reach the fourteen-day mark, they become individual entities that are owed either all the protections of living human beings or increasing protections as they develop after that mark. Others maintain that it is when these embryos develop some feature, such as brain waves or the capacity to survive on their own, that they become protectable human beings.

These religious adherents come together in agreeing that early embryos need not be used exclusively for procreation but can also serve a role in forms of research that offer the hope of healing for those who are sick and suffering. To use early embryos in stem cell research directed toward such therapeutic ends, they maintain, carries out the mandate of stewardship and compassion given us by the divine.

Religious Voices in the Public Square

Some among the religious groups and individuals that have articulated their views about the moral significance of early embryos and stem cell research in the public square in the United States have created a considerable stir, for, moved by the rightness of their cause, they have thrown verbal thunderbolts at those with whom they disagree. This has led some who are not religious—who at times have used extreme language of their own—to question whether religious voices ought to be heard in the public square at all in a secular pluralistic society. Religious believers, these commentators insist, should keep their convictions within the walls of their houses of worship.

Some who argue that religious beliefs should not be voiced in public discussions of policy matters assume that such beliefs, regardless of kind, are difficult to defend rationally. Robert Audi, for instance, states that religious adherents should not express their religious views in the public square unless they have "adequate" secular reasons for them— that is, reasons whose truth is sufficient to justify them.[1] He assumes that this would lead to silence in the overwhelming majority of cases in which religious speakers appear on the public scene.

Until religious spokespersons have their say, however, it is not possible to tell whether they have adequate secular reasons for their beliefs. Even if Audi were to broaden his view of what it means to have an adequate reason—a move that seems necessary in view of the variability of standards for assessing the sufficiency of reasons—so that reasons are adequate when they appear to those presenting them to adhere to certain canons of rationality, that would still leave us with a vital question: Why must citizens with reasons for their religious views that they consider defensible be prohibited from stating them in the public square, especially when secular thinkers with reasons that might strike Audi as inadequate are allowed to speak out? To presume from the start that religious reasons can never be adequate is to beg the question.[2]

It is important to grasp the varying rationales behind the views of citizens who follow different religious traditions, for their beliefs inevitably affect the way in which they broach important moral and public policy matters. And it is important to comprehend why people make the claims that they do in order to address their concerns as participants in a democratic polity. James Childress observes that "religious communities, several with ancient roots and long traditions of moral reflection, significantly shape the moral positions taken by many U.S. citizens on new technological developments. Hence, it is important to understand how these communities...argue for their positions as well as the conclusions they reach."[3]

Some of the beliefs of several religious traditions, particularly of the Christian and Jewish traditions, have been translated into secular form and become part of our heritage as a democratic republic, Courtney Campbell points out.[4] For example, when religious believers speak out about treating humans as ends in themselves, about the potential for the abuse of power by those in legislative and regulatory positions, or about the need to provide medical treatment in fair and just ways to those who are marginalized, they bring to public attention core values that have shaped and continue to shape our republic.

It not only religious persons who use distinctively religious understandings to illuminate contentious points of policy. One of the most famous arguments concerning abortion, that presented by Judith Jarvis Thomson, a thinker prominent in secular philosophical commentary, calls on an understanding of the biblical parable of the Good Samaritan (Luke 10:30–35).[5] She asks her readers to grasp the moral point of this parable told in a religious context and then transfer that understanding to a secular public context. Explicitly religious spokespersons, such as the nineteenth-century abolitionists, the early-twentieth-century social gospelers, and the 1960s civil rights marchers, also stimulated secular thinkers to develop new insights into pressing issues of public concern using religious writings, metaphors, and images.

Moreover, religious representatives may present perspectives that are not familiar to many who participate in or follow discussion in the public square. The very distinctiveness of their religious views may spur others to examine and question their own views. As a result, these listeners may sharpen their views and make changes in them that they now realize, having heard the religious view presented, are warranted. Jeremy Waldron notes that some religious spokespersons may express ideas "that bear no relation to existing conventions or commonly held opinions, but which nevertheless gain a foothold as soon as they are considered and discussed by persons with open minds."[6]

An even more basic reason to hear out those who speak out of religious conviction in a democratic republic, Michael J. Perry observes, is that one's basic moral/religious convictions are (partly) self-constitutive and are therefore a principal ground—indeed, the principal ground—of political deliberation and choice. To bracket such convictions is therefore to bracket—to annihilate—essential aspects of one's very self. To participate in politics and law . . . with such convictions bracketed is not to participate as the self one is but as some one—or, rather, some thing—else.[7]

That is, to deny religious speakers a place in the public square is to deny them the opportunity fully to enter into public debate as distinct individuals with beliefs that define who they are, an opportunity that is important to our form of democratic polity.

The many contributions of religious voices to public discussion and the importance of religious beliefs to self-identity provide strong reasons in a democratic republic not to exclude religious viewpoints from the public square—as well as strong reasons not to accept what religious believers say unthinkingly.[8] To be accepted or excluded, however, are not the only possible fates that speakers from various religious traditions face. They can also be ignored.

This has been the case for a wide variety of spokespersons for religious groups in the United States in recent years. It is no secret that one religious viewpoint has had the ear of those in charge of administering federal public policy in the United States until recently and that those with this viewpoint have been extremely influential in the development of stem cell research policy.[9] It is also no secret that many other religious thinkers in the United States who hold different views about the moral considerations raised by stem cell research have been largely overlooked by leaders in the Congress and the White House until recently. Indeed, the presidential bioethics body established by the Bush administration to examine stem cell research science, ethics, and policy heard from Christian commentators and no other specifically religious speakers in the course of developing its report about this research.[10] In contrast, an earlier presidential bioethics commission, the National Bioethics Advisory Commission (NBAC), heard from a wide spectrum of religious representatives and scholars about the views of their traditions regarding stem cell research.[11] This provided NBAC's members with a broader understanding of the moral issues involved in the pursuit of embryonic stem cell research, a member of this body subsequently indicated.[12]

Public debate can become tainted when only one religious viewpoint is welcomed in public decision making. To shun alternative voices conveys the message that citizens must first accept a particular approved set of religious premises in order to be heard. This, in turn, raises questions about fundamental fairness and respectful treatment, which are among the central moral values embraced within a pluralistic democratic republic. The views of a variety of religious believers need to be heard and addressed responsibly if we are to have the sort of rich and broad open debate necessary to carry on a thriving democratic form of governance.[13]

With this in mind, I proceed in this chapter to explore the convictions of several religious traditions that have found a home in the United States about the moral consideration owed to early human embryos, a significant moral issue raised by the prospect of pursuing embryonic stem cell research. Special attention is given to the Western Christian religious tradition because the political reality is that this tradition has carried great weight in the development of recent embryonic stem cell research policy in the United States. Yet the theological and moral reality is that the version of the Western Christian tradition put forward by those religious representatives who have influenced current stem cell research policy reflects just one strand within that tradition. The presentation of a more complete picture of the Christian tradition is in order.

Other religious traditions also embrace significant values and concerns that, if heard, might well enrich and sharpen current public debate about embryonic stem cell research. The sheer extent of religious diversity in this country, however, means that it is not possible to present the views of all religious groups found within the United States about the moral consideration that we owe to early human embryos. Therefore, I focus here on the beliefs of several of the major religious traditions, in addition to those of the Western Christian tradition.

Christian Tradition

Some Christian denominations hold that the human embryo should be treated as a living human being from the time of conception. Several other Christian religious groups, however, maintain that an individual human being does not come into existence at fertilization but instead develops from a later starting point. All of these Christian denominations begin from the same religious sources and yet end up with starkly opposing views of when human embryos become individual human beings who are owed protection from destruction. How and why has this come about?

All Christian denominations look to the Bible for basic religious truths. Many also turn to the historical Christian tradition, which incorporates the teachings of the early church fathers and councils, as well as later moral and theological commentaries. Almost all of these denominations also acknowledge, to varying degrees, the importance of reason and experience in understanding religious standpoints. Some add to these sources of religious beliefs the teachings of church leaders who are considered to have special access to divine truth. The weight of these different resources varies from denomination to denomination. I consider the basic approaches to the Bible and the Christian tradition that have been adopted by several of the mainstream Christian denominations, taking into account the relative weight that they give to reason and experience, when considering the question of the moral significance of early human embryos.

The Bible

Christian commentators view the Bible as a holy book with richly varied sorts of passages, including historical descriptions of events, stories, commandments and moral instructions, parables, and poetry. They take the functions of these different kinds of passages into account when they refer to specific scriptural writings to support their conclusions. Yet Christian scholars do not necessarily all do this in the same way. They may emphasize different aspects of certain passages that they find relevant and consequently develop varying understandings of these texts.

Genesis 1:26

The creation story in Genesis 1:26, which declares that human beings were created in "the image of God," has been read by some to display that the divine imprint has been set on human embryos and that because of this they should be treated as human beings from the moment of conception. This passage, according to certain commentators, reveals that all humans, no matter what their stage of life, reflect the image of God.[14]

However, others point out that the creation story features two adults, Adam and Eve, who are fully formed; it makes no mention of human embryos.[15] They note further that the concept of the "image of God" is often understood to refer either to the capacity of humans to enter into a relationship with God or to the created character of humans as rational, creative, and moral beings.[16] Thus, this concept applies to already living human beings and neither excludes nor includes early embryos within its compass. It simply does not address them.

To read this passage as indicating that early embryos are individual human beings assumes what needs to be proved, some claim,[17] since whether early human embryos bear God's image and, if so, in what sense, are the very questions at issue. A response to them cannot be held at the start but must come at the end of an inquiry. In view of such considerations, this passage neither supports nor opposes the view that early human embryos constitute human beings from the moment of conception. It simply does not address this question.

Jeremiah 1:5

Another passage that has been taken to establish that early human embryos are individual human beings is Jeremiah 1:5, which reads: "Before you were in the womb I knew you, before you were born I set you apart; I appointed you as prophet to the nations." Since God knew Jeremiah even before he was conceived, God must surely have known him once he entered the womb, on one reading. This means that Jeremiah had to be an individual human being at the time that he was conceived. Therefore, all human embryos must be individual human beings at the time that they are conceived, according to this interpretation.

However, if we take this passage as providing information about precisely when individual human beings begin to exist, and it teaches that God knew Jeremiah before he appeared in the womb, Jeremiah would have had to exist in some preexistent realm before he entered this one.[18] Yet the Christian tradition and other monotheistic religions reject this view. It therefore seems a misreading of this passage to take it to declare just when individual human beings come into existence.

Instead, it is a poetical passage that tells about God's knowledge of and care for Jeremiah and all humankind. It does not declare definitively the very time at which all human beings began to exist. Similar texts that have been taken to indicate that the embryo is a living human being, such as Isaiah 49:1, Galatians 1:15, and Ephesians 1:3–4, also express wonder about God's plans but do not state that the early embryo is an individual human being starting at the moment of conception. They do not address this question.

Psalm 139:13–16a

This psalm reads, in part,

> For it was you who formed my inward parts;
> you knit me together in my mother's womb. . . .
> my frame was not hidden from you,
> when I was being made in secret,
> intricately woven in the depths of the earth.
> Your eyes beheld my unformed substance.
> In your book were written all the days that were formed for me,
> when none of them as yet existed.

This passage refers to the growth of a human from something formless to fullness and completeness. Some see it as displaying that David was an individual human being from the moment of his conception, since God knit him together in the womb and knew him there.[19] Consequently, they maintain, all other early embryos must also constitute individual human beings from the time of their conception.[20]

Others find that although this passage declares that God is intimately involved in the development of each individual human being, it does not state just when that development begins.[21] Instead, its whole thrust is to use poetic imagery to celebrate God's relationship with God's chosen people. Thus, its point is not to establish the moment of conception but to affirm that the Israelites cannot see life apart from their relationship with God. This and similar texts, such as Job 31:15, tell of God's presence, reliability, and providential care but do not specify when human life begins.[22]

That thoughtful scholars and readers could reach such varying interpretations of such scriptural passages was one of the factors that led a group of conservative Christian theological commentators to conclude that biblical texts alone cannot resolve the questions of whether early human embryos are individual human beings and when we owe protection to them.[23] Conservative Christian scholar Gilbert Meilaender observes, "We cannot, I think, claim that the Bible itself establishes the point at which an individual life begins, although it surely directs our attention to the value of fetal life."[24]

Western Christian Historical Tradition

Many Christian religious bodies also consider understandings of the moral significance of the early embryo that have arisen within the historical Western Christian tradition. That tradition is often represented in public debate as invariably holding that the early human embryo is a living individual human being. Yet the Western Christian tradition long held that the early human embryo is not an individual human being. It also maintained for a considerable period of time, as we shall see, that it is wrong to destroy early human embryos, not because this amounts to homicide or the killing of a human being, but because this interferes with the process of procreation.[25]

Exodus, Aristotle, and the Early Church

The scriptural starting point for the view of the moral significance of the early embryo that developed within the Christian tradition is found in Exodus 21:22–25. This is the only passage in the Hebrew Bible and the New Testament that specifically relates to the growth and loss of embryos. Theologians within the early church who were considering the sort of protection owed to the embryo and the fetus therefore relied on this passage. It reads in the translation from the Hebrew as follows: "If men strive, and wound a pregnant woman so that her fruit be expelled, but no harm befall [her], then shall he be fined as her husband shall assess, and the matter placed before the judges. But if harm befall [her], then shalt thou give life for life."[26]

This passage maintains that the husband (who is considered to be in charge of the woman) is owed compensation from the assailant for hurting the woman. If she is killed, the life of the assailant must be forfeited. Thus, the penalties meted out by the law of Exodus relate to the harm caused to the woman, not to the embryo or fetus. To bring about the loss of the embryo or fetus is not seen as the moral equivalent of killing a human being, according to this passage. The rabbis who have interpreted it, reports Immanuel Jakobovits, who was for many years the leading rabbi of Great Britain, have concluded that it indicates that the embryo or fetus is not owed the same protections as a living human being.[27]

When Exodus was translated from Hebrew into Greek in the third century B.C.E. in what is known as the Septuagint version, the text that resulted was somewhat different. The relevant passage in Exodus now reads: "And if two men strive and smite a woman with child, and her child be born imperfectly formed, he shall be forced to pay a penalty: as the woman's husband may lay upon him, he shall pay with a valuation. But if it be perfectly formed, he shall give life for life."[28]

The passage distinguishes between the "imperfectly formed" embryo or what came to be known as the "unformed" embryo and the "perfectly formed" or "formed" embryo. A fine had to be paid by the assailant as the penalty for the loss of the embryo, but he owed his life as the penalty for the death of the fetus. It is the gestational age of the embryo, rather than the injury caused to the woman, that is significant in this translation.

The scientific and metaphysical views of Aristotle, who undertook the first known study of developmental anatomy in the fourth century B.C.E., were behind this translation. In Aristotle's embryology, the embryo grows from an initial formless mass that has resulted from the union of semen with menstrual blood in a process that takes place in several stages. The embryo first develops a nutritive or vegetative soul that enables nourishment, then a sensitive or animal soul that enables the development of organs required for sensation, and finally a rational or intellectual soul that enables the power to reason and completes the human form. That is, the early embryo is unformed until the rational soul shapes the matter in the womb.[29] Aristotle did not view the rational soul as an immaterial spirit but, rather, as the animating principle that forms and actualizes the embryo, making it a human being with particular contours and characteristics. The Septuagint translation of the Exodus passage reflects this Aristotelian view.

Early Christian theologians, influenced by Aristotle, embraced the distinction between the unformed embryo, which was not yet human and the formed human embryo, which was. Aristotle had concluded from his developmental studies of animals that the formation or animation of the embryo took place forty days after fertilization for the male and ninety days after fertilization for the female.[30] Many key theologians in the developing Christian moral tradition adopted this view and maintained that the embryo was not formed and so indisputably human until it reached these gender-related points. Destruction of an unformed embryo did not constitute homicide, since it did not involve the killing of a being with a human soul.[31]

Subsequent Western Christian Thought

Aristotle's view of the nature and development of the human embryo was adopted by several early Christian theologians. Tertullian, who lived at the turn of the third century, was opposed to abortion but appeared at some points to maintain the distinction between the formed and unformed embryo. For instance, he wrote, "The embryo therefore becomes a human being in the womb from the moment that its form is completed."[32] An early fourth-century church father, Gregory of Nyssa, more clearly adopted the Aristotelian approach when he declared that the unformed embryo is "something other than a human being."[33]

Augustine, a theologian of the late fourth and early fifth centuries who had an immense influence on Western Christianity, accepted the distinction between the formed and unformed embryo. He termed the unformed embryo a "living, shapeless thing" and observed that "it could not be said that there was a living soul in that body."[34] "Who," he asked, "is not rather disposed to think that unformed fetuses perish like seeds which have not been fructified?"[35] Even so, Augustine considered it wrong to destroy the unformed embryo, not because this amounted to homicide but because to do so served the same purpose as contraception or sterilization—to avoid procreation. He considered these practices to be sinful in that they broke the link between sex and procreation and therefore denied what he viewed as the primary end of the sexual act. Sexual desire, Augustine held, had emerged only after the Fall as God's crowning punishment for Adam and Eve's disobedience and was not the proper motivation for sexual intercourse.

This remnant of his earlier Manicheanism led him to reject sexual union as an end in itself and to view all sex as illicit unless excused by the intent to procreate.[36] Although it was wrong to destroy the unformed embryo because this frustrated procreation, it was even more sinful to destroy the later formed embryo in Augustine's eyes, for this amounted to killing a human being.

There were dissenters. Several early church theologians rejected this view and held that the soul was immediately infused into the body at conception. For instance, Basil the Great in the fourth century, refused to accept what he termed "the fine distinction" between the unformed and formed embryo.[37] This view, however, was not the predominant position within the Christian tradition.

During the Middle Ages, Western Christian thinkers retained this distinction.[38] Thomas Aquinas, a thirteenth-century theologian and a leading Christian thinker, taught that the embryo does not have a human, rational soul from the start but the kind of soul responsible for growth and development common to all forms of life. However, when the embryo grows to a stage at which it resembles human form, the human soul enters, transforming it into an individual human being, he maintained. Consequently, Aquinas refused to view the destruction of the early embryo as tantamount to homicide.[39] Even so, like Augustine, he regarded any act that causes the death of the unformed embryo to be a serious moral lapse on a par with the use of contraception because it interferes with the procreative purpose of sexuality.

Over the centuries of Western Christian thought, the distinction between the unformed and the formed embryo or fetus was accepted by such varied theologians as Jerome, Augustine, Gratian, Lombard, Aquinas, and Sanchez.[40] The destruction of the unformed embryo was considered wrong because this frustrates the process of procreation, not because this is a form of homicide. However, according to Roman Catholic theologian John Connery, the destruction of the formed embryo was viewed more gravely as "anticipated homicide, or interpretive homicide, or homicide in intent, because it involved the destruction of a future man. It was always closely related to homicide."[41] The distinction expressed in this view was entrenched in canon law in the Catholic West until the nineteenth century.

Protestant Reformers

No one view of the moral significance of the early embryo can be traced across the works of the Protestant reformers. They rejected the sort of Aristotelian scholastic reasoning that prevailed in the Roman Catholic Church of their time and aimed to return to early church teachings and those beliefs explicitly found in the Bible. Yet they could not escape the developed Western Christian tradition entirely, as it had provided the framework for the theological and moral thinking in which they had been schooled. For instance, Melanchton, a significant sixteenth-century follower of Luther, retained the traditional view that the soul is infused into the fetus at forty days after fertilization and that early embryos, therefore, are not living human beings.[42]

It is more difficult to ascertain the views of Luther himself about the moral consideration owed to early embryos, as he did not write systematic theological and moral treatises. Indeed, he rejected the authority of reason as "the fountain and head of all mischiefs."[43] Christian theology, he argued, could be repaired only by breaking free from Aristotle. David Steinmetz reports that "when Luther asked 'What, then, is a human being?' he answered that a human being is not a rational soul individuated by a body, as Aquinas might have put it, but a creature who trusts either the true God or an idol."[44] Yet it is clear that Luther considered it wrong to destroy the fetus by means of abortion. He wrote: "How great, therefore, the wickedness of human nature is! How many girls there are who prevent conception and kill and expel tender fetuses, although procreation is the work of God."[45] However, he did not indicate whether he made any moral distinction between the fetus and the early embryo or between preventing conception and causing an abortion.

Calvin was more apt to take theological considerations into account. He, too, rejected abortion of the fetus, commenting that "the unborn, though enclosed in the womb of its mother, is already a human being, and it is almost a monstrous crime to rob it of the life which it has not yet begun to enjoy."[46] At times, he seemed to distinguish the early embryo from the fetus, as when he wrote in a commentary on Psalm 139 that "the embryo when first conceived in the womb has no form."[47] Yet elsewhere he rejected the Aristotelian account of the timing of the ensoulment of the fetus, maintaining instead that the soul is infused into the embryo at conception.[48]

Thus those who adopted various forms of Protestantism did not embrace a single view of the moral significance of the early embryo. They had no theological or practical reason at that time to delve into what they viewed as fine distinctions between the early embryo and the later fetus, although they made it clear that they believed it wrong to destroy the later fetus.

Effect of the Scientific Revolution

Ancient and medieval Christian scholars knew little about human sperm and even less about human eggs and did not have an understanding of how the process of fertilization occurs. Consequently, their views about the morality of causing the deaths of embryos rested on precarious scientific grounds. However, interest in the empirical study of nature grew in the sixteenth and seventeenth centuries. For instance, Leonardo da Vinci provided illustrations of fetuses and the dissected uterus of a pregnant woman in a 1521 notebook of sketches.[49] Scientists and thinkers of the time were examining living and dead humans in order to learn just how they functioned. The information provided by such drawings and other findings about the embryo led scientific investigators to question Aristotle's biology.

Two rival theories of fertilization were developed in the seventeenth century that hearkened back to ancient theories but dressed them in the new science.[50] The first, derived from Aristotle, was the epigenetic view, a developmental theory that held that new structures emerge in the embryo that were not present from its beginning. Naturalists who examined embryos growing in animals pointed out that all of the organs had not yet formed. They therefore postulated that an individual being must gradually emerge, guided by vital teleological forces that are not strictly material. The second theory, known as the preformation view, developed as a negative response to the epigenetic view. It sought to account for life in terms of matter in motion and concluded that the organs must already be present in a preformed figure found within the egg or sperm. Embryonic development, according to this theory, required the growth of existing structures rather than the formation of new ones.

When William Harvey carried out a series of experiments in 1633 focused on the reproduction of deer during the mating season, he could not find a fluid mixture surrounded by a membrane inside the uteruses of does.[51] If Aristotle's view that the semen gives shape and animation to menstrual fluid in order to form the embryo were correct, he should have found this sort of mass. This and several other experiments led scientists to reject Aristotle's epigenetic view and to embrace the preformation theory.

The invention of the microscope allowed scientists of the seventeenth century to gain more detailed information about gametes and embryos. Since all the organs of the adult were believed to be prefigured in one of the gametes, it is not surprising that when Anton van Leeuwenhoek viewed sperm directly through his microscope in 1678, he claimed to see a tiny human being, the homunculus, beneath the lens. (See figure 4.1.) This "finding" supported the major preformationist view that the male sperm contains a small. well-formed human being whose nourishment and growth is sparked by material from the woman.[52]

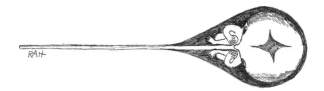

Figure 4.1. Homunculus. A tiny human folded up inside the spermatozoa (after Nicolas Hartsoeker in the seventeenth century) was believed to be activated during reproduction. Other authorities maintained that the homunculus was hidden within the human egg.

Scientists, philosophers, and theologians in the eighteenth century continued to support the preformation theory, by and large, although they adopted differing theses about just how the embryo got started on its developmental journey.[53] This left little room for any distinction between formed and unformed embryos. In 1827, Karl Ernst von Baer discovered the human oocyte, and scientists began to attribute a more prominent role to the female element in fertilization.[54] They reasoned that if gametes from both men and women played a part in the creation of children and these gametes united at conception, an individual human being must somehow be present at conception, albeit not in a specific gamete. As a result, the epigenetic theory was abandoned.

Many Christian theologians now began to give greater credence to the notion of immediate human ensoulment at conception. This view was supported by the affirmation of the dogma of the Immaculate Conception of the Blessed Virgin Mary by Pope Pius IX as an article of faith in 1854. Since, according to this doctrine, Mary was without sin from her conception, it was reasoned, she must have been ensouled at the time of conception, rather than ninety days later. In 1869, the same pope announced, in view of the implications of this dogma and the recently modified preformationist embryology, that the punishment for destroying either an unformed or a formed embryo would now be the same—excommunication.[55] The distinction between unformed and formed embryos was dropped from the canon law of the Roman Catholic Church which, up to this time, had imposed excommunication only for the abortion of a formed fetus. John Noonan states that "if a moment had to be chosen for ensoulment, no convincing argument now appeared to support Aristotle or to put ensoulment at a later stage of life than fertilization."[56] The distinction between "unformed" and "formed" embryo no longer had the significance that it had held for the earlier historical Christian tradition.

Current Views of the Moral Significance of Early Human Embryos within the Christian Tradition

Yet this distinction has been resurrected, albeit in modified form, in recent Christian thought. Embryological findings have led some Christian thinkers within the Roman Catholic tradition to question the moral significance that theologians and the magisterium (teaching authority) gave to the fertilized egg starting in the nineteenth century.[57] For instance, noted theologian Bernard Häring wrote in 1973 that before the fourteenth day of embryonic development "there has not yet emerged a human person . . . individualization seems not yet to have reached that point which is indispensable to personhood. In our philosophical tradition, it is a common presupposition that only a human life possessing irreversible individuality can be a person."[58] The Roman Catholic Congregation for the Doctrine of the Faith observed in its *Declaration on Procured Abortion* in 1974 that "this declaration expressly leaves aside the question of the moment when the spiritual soul is infused. There is not unanimous tradition on this point and authors are as yet in disagreement."[59]

In 1987, however, the Congregation for the Doctrine of the Faith responded to the question "How could a human individual not be a human person?" in *Donum Vitae* (Respect for Human Life):

> The human being must be respected—as a person—from the very first instant of his existence. . . . Thus the fruit of human generation, from the first moment of its existence, that is to say from the moment the zygote has formed, demands the unconditional respect that is morally due to the human being in his bodily and spiritual totality. The human being is to be respected and treated as a person from the moment of conception.[60]

In 2006, Pope Benedict XVI also enunciated this view, telling those at a Vatican conference that there should be no moral distinction between the embryo before and after implantation, although he acknowledged that there is no explicit teaching on the first days of life in scripture.[61]

Roman Catholic scholar Margaret Farley pointed out in her testimony to NBAC that "there is no single voice from within the Catholic community on such questions."[62] She stated:

> A growing number of Catholic moral theologians, for example, do not consider the human embryo in its earliest stages (prior to the development of the primitive streak or to implantation) to constitute an individualized human entity with the settled inherent potential to become a human person.[63]

The Roman Catholic tradition is engaged in an ongoing process of discernment, she explained, that remains faithful to its theological and ethical convictions and takes account of the best scientific evidence. Thus, in her view, whether to consider the early human embryo a living human being is still under discussion within the Roman Catholic Church.

According to Father Demetrios Demopoulos, the Eastern Orthodox tradition holds that the early embryo is a potential human person and is therefore owed protection from destruction in stem cell research. He stated in testimony to NBAC:

> Whether created *in situ* or *in vitro*, a zygote is committed to a developmental course that will, with God's grace, ultimately lead to a human person. The embryo and the adult are both potential human persons, although in different stages of development. As a result, Orthodox Christians affirm the sanctity of human life at all stages of development.[64]

Protestant bodies have not adopted one view of the moral significance of early embryos but tend to take opposite approaches to this issue.[65] The Southern Baptist Convention, for instance, agrees with those Roman Catholics who believe that human embryos should be treated as human beings from the moment of conception.[66] However, the Southern Baptist denomination steps away from the Eastern Orthodox view somewhat in that it holds that the human embryo is an actual, rather than a potential, person.

Several other Protestant groups articulate a case against viewing the early human embryo as an individual human being. For instance, several scholars within the Anglican-Episcopal tradition agree with those in the Roman Catholic tradition who maintain that the early embryo is not capable of becoming a distinct individual until fourteen days after sperm and egg meet. At this time, they maintain, the human embryo may begin gradually to develop into a living human being if it is not damaged and surrounding conditions enable it to do so.[67]

A resolution of the 213th General Assembly of the Presbyterian Church (USA) of 2001 endorsed embryonic stem cell research that is directed toward compelling goals:

> We believe, as do most authorities that have addressed the issue, that human embryos do have the potential of personhood, and as such they deserve respect. That respect must be shown by requiring that the interests or goals to be accomplished by using human embryos be compelling and unreachable by other means. . . . Prohibition of the derivation of stem cells from embryos would elevate the showing of respect to human embryos above that of helping persons whose pain and suffering might be alleviated.[68]

The United Church of Christ also regards human embryos with great respect, consistent with their potential to develop into full personhood, but does not regard them as equivalent to persons.[69] Its Committee on Genetics therefore recommends that any research on early human embryos should not be carried out on such human embryos beyond the fourteenth day of development and that it should proceed before that stage only if it has well-justified objectives, shows proper respect for the early embryos, and does not allow them to be implanted after they have been involved in research.[70]

The biological story of the embryo will continue to emerge as our knowledge of developmental embryology increases. This, in turn, will have a significant effect on the theological views of the moral significance of the early human embryo of those within the Christian tradition, for any theological account of what we owe to this embryo will have to demonstrate an understanding of the scientific evidence available if it is to have credibility.

Moral Significance of the Early Embryo in Several Other Religious Traditions

The Talmud, the Koran, and several other holy scriptures do not specifically address the moral significance of the early embryo, although religious scholars have read various passages from these scriptures in ways that provide an indirect answer to this question. As do Christian scholars, learned thinkers in other religious traditions weigh and balance relevant passages from their holy book in order to develop a coherent and textually supportable view of when individual human beings come into existence. We review the teachings of four major religious traditions besides the Christian tradition—the Jewish, Islamic, Buddhist, and Hindu traditions—about this question and the implications of their responses for the pursuit of embryonic stem cell research.

Jewish Tradition

"Be fruitful and multiply," God urged newly created human beings (Genesis 1:28). This biblical command to procreate permeates the Jewish religious tradition. Having children, forming a family, and, more broadly a people who will prosper is essential to Jewish thought.[71] What are the implications of this procreative ethos for the moral significance of the early embryo?

No single voice or council speaks for the entire Jewish tradition.[72] Even so, Jewish scholars have generally held that until the fortieth day after conception embryos are, as stated in the Babylonian Talmud, "as if they were simply water."[73] Rabbi Moshe Dovid Tendler testified to NBAC that "there are two prerequisites for the moral status of the embryo as a human being: implantation and 40 days of gestational development. The proposition that humanhood begins at zygote formation, even *in vitro*, is without basis in biblical moral theology."[74] Rabbi Elliot Dorff affirmed this view in his statement to NBAC, maintaining that "genetic materials outside the uterus have no legal status in Jewish law, for they are not even a part of a human being until implanted in a woman's womb and even then, during the first 40 days of gestation, their status is 'as if they were water.' "[75] Leaders of several branches of Judaism in the United States also have declared that traditional Jewish thought "states that an embryo in vitro does not enjoy the full status of humanhood and its attendant protections."[76]

In specifically addressing the ethics of embryonic stem cell research, Rabbi Mark Washofsky observed:

> Medical research, after all, partakes of the *mitzvah* to preserve human life (*pikuach nefesh*), which our tradition teaches is the highest of all moral duties. Thus, the large supply of "excess" embryos that exist in fertility clinics constitutes a resource of life-saving potential, and Jewish tradition, which commands us to preserve life, allows and encourages us to utilize these embryos for the purposes of human stem cell research.[77]

Human embryos, within the Jewish tradition, may be discarded or used for reasonable, beneficial purposes. The primary question raised by their use in stem cell research is whether this might have lifesaving consequences for those who are among the living, according to these Jewish commentators. When this is the case, such research is commanded, according to the Jewish tradition.

Islamic Tradition

The Koran, the holy book of Islam, consists of the revelations that the prophet Muhammad received from the time of his call as the prophet in 610 until his death in 632. Muslims believe that the Koran was directly communicated by God and is therefore inerrant. Consequently, it serves as the source for ethical and theological beliefs within the Islamic tradition.

The section of the Koran that refers to the creation of human beings describes this as follows:

> And certainly We created man of an extract of clay, then We made him a small drop in a firm resting-place, then We made the drop a clot, then We made the clot a lump of flesh, then We made [in] the lump of flesh bones, then We clothed the bones with flesh. Then We caused it to grow into

another creation. So blessed be Allah, the best of creators. Then after that you will most surely die. Then surely on the day of resurrection you shall be raised. (Holy Koran 23:12–16)

The Creator starts with a drop from which the human being is gradually fashioned through a developmental process.[78] The Koran later declares that God "breathes His own spirit" into the human after he has formed the limbs and organs of the human (Holy Koran 41:9–10).

Some Muslim commentators suggest that when Allah says "Then We caused it to grow into another creation," this indicates that there is a distinct stage later in biological development at which perceivable human life forms.[79] This allows for a moral distinction between the early and later human embryo, even though the Koran does not provide a particular point at which this occurs. This is a contested point among Islamic scholars.[80]

The majority of Sunni and some Shi'i scholars hold that the human embryo is ensouled and becomes an individual human at 120 days (four lunar months, plus ten days) after conception.[81] Yet the majority of Shi'i and some Sunni scholars disagree and regard the embryo as ensouled at forty days.[82] Thus, the tradition that elaborates the embryology of the Koran, according to Abdulaziz Sachedina, is divided between those who describe the embryonic stage when human destiny is recorded by an angel sent by God as occurring either on the fortieth or forty-second night or else after 120 days.[83]

The significant point is that even though Islamic scholars disagree about the time of ensoulment, they all agree that it occurs later than five days after conception, the time when embryonic stem cells are derived from the early embryo. Sachedina therefore observes that "it is correct to suggest that a majority of the Sunni and Shi'ite jurists will have little problem in endorsing ethically regulated research on stem cells that promises potential therapeutic value, provided that the expected therapeutic benefits are not simply speculative."[84] Thus, in Islamic thought, it seems that research using embryonic stem cells is acceptable if it is undertaken with the purpose of providing treatment to those who are sick and suffering.

Buddhist Tradition

The first of the Five Precepts of Buddhism states that we should avoid killing or harming any living being. Compassion is a central virtue in the Buddhist tradition, and this implies an obligation to care for all life at any stage.

There is some debate among Buddhist scholars, however, about whether the human embryo is owed protection from the moment of fertilization. Damien Keown maintains that "most Buddhists regard fertilization as the point at which individual human life commences and believe that the embryo is entitled to moral respect from that time onwards." He adds, "in terms of the more conservative majority view, any destructive experimentation on embryos is considered a breach of the first precept against taking human life."[85]

In contrast, Michael G. Barnhart argues that the central Buddhist concept of consciousness, which he terms *vi~n~nana* is not a quasi-Aristotelian soul "that individuates and constitutes an ontological individual moving along the karmic ladder to eventual enlightenment." Such an interpretation of this concept, Barnhart finds, is difficult to reconcile with the rejection by Buddhism of the ego, or *atman*. An individual is transitional and in process. Buddhist texts, Barnhart maintains, provide no reason to take individual consciousness to be present at any particular point in the process of embryonic development. Therefore, "no Buddhist need equate a presentient fetus with a sentient human," he concludes.[86] The destruction of embryos in stem cell research, on his interpretation of Buddhism, would be allowed if, after weighing the full range of circumstances, it became clear that this would be a compassionate practice in the service of others.

Hindu Tradition

Rebirth is basic to Hindu thought. The soul passes through a cycle of births and deaths until it attains salvation (*Moksa*). The ultimate goal of those practicing Hinduism is to attain a state of enlightenment that releases the soul from the cycle of earthly reincarnations and allows it to become one with Brahma, the Creator. *Moksa* is realized when all one's *karmas*, or the effects of one's choices and actions from previous lives, are removed by the practice of ethical and spiritual living. One's *karma* determines whether one's soul achieves a higher or lower state of existence in its next life.

According to Vedic scripture, the classical Hindu religious texts, birth takes place when one passes from one life to the next. A traditional Hindu lawgiver, Manu, who lived in the second century B.C.E., taught that the soul takes form at conception and is progressively invested with all the elements necessary for human development.[87] Therefore, there is no time when the human embryo is not ensouled. The duty of nonviolence, *ahimsa*, requires Hindus to refrain from taking life in any form. Abortion of a fetus is regarded as a form of violence that results in bad *karma* and thwarts the soul's progress toward enlightenment.[88] Presumably, destruction of the human embryo would also result in bad *karma*. Yet there are exceptions to the rule against abortion that are dictated by the central Hindu virtue of compassion, and the same may be true of the use of early embryos in stem cell research.

Some alternative Hindu traditions put the beginning of personhood at three to five months gestation. Indeed, a minority tradition holds that incarnation does not occur until as late as the seventh month.[89] These views have affected contemporary Hindu beliefs, and today some Hindus accept as moral the use of early embryos in research that is directed toward therapeutic ends.

Relevance of These Religious Views to Public Policy Regarding Human Embryonic Stem Cell Research

This study of several major religious traditions and their adherents indicates that they evaluate the morality of using early human embryos in stem cell research in different ways that are not obviously reconcilable. Yet it is important in a pluralistic democratic society to hear their views so that others may understand what is of significance to them, respond respectfully, and attempt to find common ground among them and with them, even when that may seem unlikely.[90] Those in positions of power who decide against listening to a variety of religious voices in public discussion and instead set the direction of debate in favor of a single religious tradition diminish public respect for those other religious views. In effect, they decide a priori that these other religious voices have nothing of value to contribute and thereby arbitrarily limit the scope and depth of public debate. Deliberately ignoring religious voices that do not express certain Christian convictions in the public square defeats the very purpose of having such a square in the first place. As Aristotle declared, the very existence of the polis depends on the human power of speech, the ability of individuals to set forth their understandings of "the just and the unjust."[91]

Significant questions of public policy are not necessarily irresolvable because different religious traditions have varying and sometimes opposing beliefs about them. It is essential in a democratic republic to seek out a reasoned basis for deliberative discussion across religious and secular boundaries—that is, to seek principles of mediation between different and even opposing views in the public square, rather than to exclude some in a sort of a priori despair about reaching common ground.[92] In a pluralistic democratic society, ideas need to be set out in an open public forum to be tested and accepted, rejected and reworked, all with the ultimate purpose of developing well-reasoned and warranted public policy. Of course, this requires that religious spokespersons present their views in a responsible, non-coercive manner, explaining and giving reasons for them in ways that are not dogmatic and that do not undermine the democratic process and participatory politics.[93] It is essential to encourage an open and challenging form of debate in a polity such as ours, in which nothing is taken for granted and nothing is rejected without justification, including religious discourse, if we are to have the sort of broad and full discussion that is essential to democratic flourishing.

5

Creating Human-Nonhuman Chimeras in Stem Cell Research

Another significant debate about the ethics of stem cell research, besides that swirling around the moral significance of early human embryos, centers on whether human stem cells or their derivatives should be used to create chimeras—in this case, organisms that combine human and nonhuman cells. Stem cell investigators have been inserting human embryonic stem cells and specialized human stem cells into animals during the prenatal and postnatal stages of their development to learn how and why human stem cells function in a developing organism. Ultimately, they hope to discern how they might be used therapeutically in humans. Some of this research has met with resistance from some other scientists, ethicists, religious figures, and members of the public who are concerned that novel half-human, half-animal beings might emerge from such research.

Stem cell scientists involved in this chimeric research explain the need for it by pointing out that studies of different kinds of stem cells derived from mammals, such as mice, while providing detailed knowledge about how mammalian stem cells function, can only take them so far. At some point, they need to examine the distinctive ways in which human stem cells function. They can culture human stem cells in vitro (in a laboratory dish) and follow how they differentiate into skin, pancreatic, and many other sorts of cells, but it eventually becomes necessary for them to use the knowledge that they have gained from laboratory studies in a living environment. They cannot ethically carry out such studies in humans because the risks to such subjects are largely unknown. Therefore, stem cell scientists have initiated research that involves inserting different kinds of human stem cells into animals that are at various stages of growth to discover how these human cells function in developing organisms and to explore the ways in which they repair and replace diseased or injured tissues.

Critics of such research recall the ancient Greek myth of the Chimera, which was a "thing of immortal make, not human, lion-fronted and snake behind, a goat in the middle, and snorting out the breath of the terrible flame of bright fire."[1] (See figure 5.1.) This beast was terrorizing the land of Lycia, when Bellerophon was sent by the king to kill it. He flew above the Chimera astride the winged horse Pegasus and riddled it with arrows, ending its life. The Chimera, as well as such interspecies creatures as the part-human, part-bull Minotaur, inspired fear in the ancient Western world. Any creature that merged sharply different categories of being invited evil and chaos. A modern version of the chimera myth was played out in H. G. Wells's *The Island of Dr. Moreau,* where mysterious creatures who were part-human and part-animal gradually broke through their civilized veneer to rampage through their island home and destroy their maker. "There is a kind of travesty of humanity over here," the protagonist in this tale observed.[2]

Such stories still hang over proposals to insert human stem cells into nonhumans. It seems unnatural and repugnant to many to develop living creatures that are comprised of parts from several different species—particularly when one of those species is the human.

Is it wrong to create such chimeras? Some maintain that it is not, pointing out that we have been combining human and animal materials for years with no ill effects, medical or ethical. Others argue that it is wrong, voicing various concerns about the development of human-nonhuman chimeras that can be separated into four main ethical arguments: to do so is wrong because it (1) is unnatural, (2) crosses species

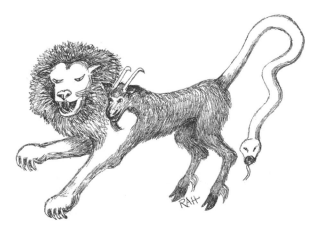

Figure 5.1. Chimera. The chimera was a fearsome creature that was depicted in Greek mythology with the head of a lion, the middle portion of a goat, and the tail of a snake.

boundaries, (3) is morally repugnant, and (4) violates human dignity. In this chapter, I explore the moral weight of each of these arguments and maintain that one—the human dignity argument—has special moral force. However, it does not rule out all human-nonhuman chimeric research. I then address what sorts of human-nonhuman chimeric research should be considered out of ethical bounds and what sorts should be taken as ethically sound. Finally, I develop some basic guidelines for conducting human-nonhuman chimeric research and for setting limits to it.

Development of Interspecies Chimeras in Scientific Research

The development of chimeras that combine cells from two different species is not unique to stem cell research. Scientists have been developing different sorts of chimeras for years. Some, for instance, have fused goat and sheep embryos, creating a creature known as the "Geep" because it looks something like a sheep but also has characteristics of a goat.[3] Others have transplanted regions of the brains of quails into the brains of chicken embryos, developing chicks that squawk like quails.[4] The aim of these experiments was not frivolous; it was to develop interspecies chimeric models to use in the study of cell migration. Still other scientific researchers have created mice with human immune systems, human skin tissue, and human-like kidneys in order to study a variety of serious diseases that afflict humans and to develop treatments for them based on the understandings that they gain from such research. These sorts of chimeric experiments have been greeted with interest, and even curiosity, but have not elicited any significant public outcry.

Investigators specializing in stem cell research also have carried out studies that have resulted in various human-nonhuman combinations. Several teams, for instance, have injected adult human blood and skin stem cells into mice in order to study how these human cells grow and proliferate in a living environment.[5] Others have transferred adult human bone marrow cells into fetal sheep, in hopes of eventually learning how to repair damaged livers and hearts in human beings.[6] Still others have injected human stem cells into fetal pigs to ascertain whether they might be able to grow human organs in animals.[7] Although these transfers of human stem cells to animals have received some attention, they have not triggered intense public debate about the ethics of pursuing human-nonhuman chimeric research.

In 2001, Vaclav Ourednik, Evan Snyder, and colleagues inserted human neural progenitor cells (stem cells that have begun to differentiate into brain cells) into the forebrain of fetal monkeys.[8] Their purpose was to study how such human neural cells emerge in a developing brain and what role these cells play in rescuing any dysfunctional neurons that reside there. They found that the human stem cells did not pool in one place but followed the same developmental path as the monkey cells surrounding them, generating neurons and glial cells that integrated into the monkey brain and were controlled by the brain of that primate.[9] This study did not raise ethical concerns among other scientists and the public, even though it involved the use of primates, which are closely related to humans. The lack of debate about it may have been due to the fact that it used human stem cells that had begun to differentiate, rather than unspecialized human stem cells with the potential to develop in many different sorts of cells.

Another stem cell research group led by Ronald S. Goldstein engaged in a study involving the insertion of human embryonic stem cells into early chick embryos in 2002.[10] The goal of this research was to test the ability of these unspecialized human cells to differentiate into a variety of types of cells within a prenatal nonhuman system. The human embryonic stem cells differentiated and integrated with the tissue of the host chicks in ways that were controlled by the hosts, this research team found. The group was apparently mindful of the need to avoid creating humanized chicks, for they were careful to prevent the human cells from interspersing among the developing tissues of the chicks and did not allow their eggs to hatch after the chicks were born. Despite these precautions, several scientists expressed disapproval of this study, maintaining that it had crossed a contentious ethical line.[11] They were concerned that the use of human embryonic stem cells had run the risk of creating chicks with human features.[12]

The debate about whether researchers should develop human-nonhuman chimeras became more heated in 2002 when some investigators at Stanford University indicated that they proposed to expand an earlier 2000 study in which they had inserted human fetal neural stem cells into the brains of newborn mice, producing mice with brains composed of some human segments.[13] The purpose of this study was to discern pathways that human stem cells might take during neural development. Ultimately, these researchers hoped to create networks of human neural cells that could be used therapeutically to reconstruct damaged brain tissue and restore brain function in patients with diseases that affect the brain, such as Alzheimer's and Parkinson's.[14]

The investigators found that the human fetal neural stem cells that had been inserted into the mice had migrated to various regions of their brains where they had intermingled with the resident mouse brain cells and matured into the type of cells characteristic of each region.[15] They concluded that chemical signals from the developing mouse brain, rather than the human neural cells, had controlled the responses of the mice. That is, the mice were still mice with brains that contained some human cells.

When Irving Weissman, the lead investigator in this research project, subsequently announced that he planned to conduct another study that would produce mice whose brains were populated entirely by human neural cells, some other scientists saw this proposed experiment as a risky one that would raise the ethical stakes. Media reports about it envisioned the birth of curious creatures that looked like mice but thought like human beings, and expressed alarm.[16] A group organized by the New York Academy of Sciences to formulate guidelines for stem cell research, in part in response to this and other human-nonhuman chimeric experiments, could not reach agreement about whether to endorse or oppose such research.[17]

In response to the concerns raised, Weissman indicated that the Stanford group would refrain from proceeding with this experiment until it had received a report from a university advisory committee.[18] That committee, in an unpublished report, recommended that the researchers take a cautious step-by-step approach to this research, building in stopping points as they proceeded. At each stopping point, if no signs of human brain structures and no human-like behaviors appeared in the mice, the researchers could go on to the next step. However, if such structures and behavior did begin to appear, no matter how preliminary, they were to stop this sequential process immediately, discuss its significance, and, in light of their conclusions, either go on with the study or stop it entirely.[19] The Stanford stem cell research group has since indicated that it has no immediate plans to develop a mouse with a brain composed entirely of human cells.[20]

A groundbreaking study that explored the development of human stem cells in a prenatal nonhuman system was published in 2005 by a research team headed by Fred Gage and Alysson Muotri at the Salk Institute in La Jolla, California. These investigators injected approximately 100,000 undifferentiated human embryonic stem cells into the brain ventricles of fetal mice.[21] (Mouse brains contain 75 to 90 million cells.) This was part of an effort to make realistic models of neurological disorders such as Parkinson's disease that researchers could study in order to develop treatments for such conditions. The group found that the unspecialized stem cells inserted into these fetal mice differentiated into human neurons that settled into the adult mouse forebrain and integrated with the mouse cells found there. The inserted human cells occupied .01 percent of the mouse brain, a trace amount, and did not affect the ways in which the mice functioned.[22] This study provided evidence that human embryonic stem cells can differentiate and become functioning human brain cells in a developing organism without restructuring the brain. It suggested that such human stem cells, if injected into humans, would mature into the cells that surround them, filling in where there has been injury or destruction.[23] Although this research raised considerable public interest, it did not create an ethical storm, as had some of the earlier human-nonhuman chimeric studies, perhaps because it had used relatively few human embryonic stem cells and provided assurance that the human stem cells had not "humanized" the mouse brain.

The underlying ethical concern that such chimeric research raises is that the resulting human-nonhuman chimeric hosts might retain sufficient numbers and kinds of human stem cells to develop as human beings in certain ways and yet retain certain distinctively nonhuman features that would interfere with the ways in which their human aspects functioned.[24] The more specific scenario at issue is that human stem cells inserted into an animal might cause it to develop a human brain or human germ (reproductive) cells. That is, the resulting human-nonhuman host, if it developed a human brain, might struggle to think and act like a human being and yet be deterred from doing so by some of its remaining nonhuman features. Or if this human-nonhuman chimera were to develop human sperm—in itself a highly unlikely happenstance—and were to mate with another chimera that had developed human eggs—an even more unlikely happenstance—they might produce human offspring (a happenstance that is almost nil). Those who object strenuously to the creation of human-nonhuman chimeras have these sorts of untoward scenarios in mind.

Arguments against Creating Human-Nonhuman Chimeras

In biological terms, the chimera is an organism that combines cells from two different species in such a way that each of its cells retains its original species identity.[25] The "Geep" mentioned above was a chimera, in that it combined cells from sheep and goat and each of its cells was either a sheep or a goat cell. A human-nonhuman chimera would have cells that are either human or animal; these cells would retain their own genetic identity. In contrast, when every single cell in an organism's body fuses cells from two different species, that organism is known as a "hybrid." The mule, for instance, is a hybrid in that each of its cells combines horse and donkey chromosomes.

I consider four arguments that can be drawn from the claims made by those protesting the development of any sorts of human-nonhuman chimeras. These are (1) the contrary to nature argument, (2) the species integrity argument, (3) the social taboo argument, and (4) the violation of human dignity argument. Some might maintain that all four could be merged in an attempt to form one coherent case against the creation of human-nonhuman chimeras. By considering these arguments separately, however, we can gain a better sense of the strengths and weaknesses of each before going on to develop an argument for adopting one, the human dignity argument, as the most supportable.

Contrary to Nature Argument

Some contemporary scholars and commentators decry the development of human-nonhuman chimeras on grounds that this would amount to a violation of the laws of nature. There is a natural ordering of living things that should not be contravened in scientific experimentation, they hold. The works of nature are to be understood and valued in teleological terms—that is, in terms of the goals toward which they are directed; those goals should not be nullified.[26] Those embracing this position maintain that living things have an inner tendency to reach their appropriate ends or purposes and do so by exercising certain characteristic biological functions. According to traditional Aristotelian natural law theorists, the very fact that a living entity pursues a certain end through certain biological processes is its own justification.[27] They hold that the order of nature has normative force. That is, a life that functions in accordance with its intrinsic principles of operation as it reaches toward its appropriate ends displays a kind of goodness.[28] Accordingly, for natural law theorists, it is a moral good for each kind of being to be aligned with its proper end and a moral wrong to alter its natural functioning in ways that distort or violate this end. This natural law approach was adopted by the Stoics and several leading medieval scholastic thinkers, such as Thomas Aquinas,[29] and has been developed more recently by several contemporary moral theorists.[30]

There is a sense of the continuity between humans and nonhumans in much of natural law thought.[31] Even so, natural law theorists maintain that natural human ends and ways of functioning to achieve those ends differ radically from those of, say, mice or monkeys.[32] The very nature of human beings, they maintain, sets moral limits on any scientific interventions that would modify or transform that nature and redirect it toward nonhuman ends—or that would transform humans into animals or animals into humans. To carry out such transformations would wrongfully violate the order of nature, on which our scientific, social, and moral orders are grounded.[33] Thus, the contrary to nature argument seeks to retain what it sees as the natural order of things by prohibiting the creation of human-nonhuman chimeras.

This argument rests on two questionable assumptions: that an organism's ways of functioning are teleologically directed toward a certain end or ends and that those ways of functioning should not be altered. The natural world, however, is subject to interpretive framing in light of philosophical, social, biological, and ethical understandings. This means that having a certain mode of functioning—say, being able to reproduce in a certain way—is not, in itself, ethically significant.[34] It is what we make of that mode of functioning and other human functions, the ends to which we put them, that has ethical import. Although the realities of nature put constraints on our ethical judgments about the ways in which we should intervene into the natural world and human functions, they do not require that we refrain from such interventions when they are directed toward ethically defensible goals. Furthermore, the natural world is in constant flux. Organisms do not remain static but evolve and change over long periods of time. Although we may appreciate and value the way that many aspects of the natural world unfold, this gives us no reason to think that there is a moral requirement built into nature that all things must remain in a fixed natural state.

When considered on its own terms, the contrary to nature argument fails to provide a way to distinguish between those interventions into nature that further natural ends and those that do not. For instance, it would be ethically unacceptable, on this argument, to make use of in vitro fertilization (IVF) because this practice alters and therefore subverts a natural human function, reproduction. Yet it is arguable that IVF provides a way of overcoming impediments to reproduction that nature has set in place for some among those who hope to have children and that its use would help them achieve that procreative end. The contrary to nature argument does not provide a clear explanation of when an intervention into the order of nature, such as in vitro fertilization, is justified and when it is not. It offers no bright line to help us to distinguish between ethical and unethical interventions but, instead, leaves us to speculate endlessly about the natural purposes of virtually all living entities.[35]

Therefore the objection that it is a violation of the natural order to create human-nonhuman chimeras must be set aside on grounds that this position equates, and thereby confuses, biological description with ethical norms. The contrary to nature argument does not provide sufficient explanation of when and why an intervention into the order of nature is wrong and therefore provides inadequate ethical justification for its conclusion that it is wrong to develop human-nonhuman chimeras.

Species Integrity Argument

There is something about crossing the boundaries between species that gives many pause. It seems wrong to them to merge cellular materials from humans with those of other species, for they believe that there are built-in moral barriers between the species that should not be crossed. No one view of why such crossings are wrong has emerged from critics of interspecies mingling. To understand their position, it is essential to understand the meaning of "species" if we are to understand what it means to cross boundaries between species.

The classical conception of species, which derives from Aristotle, was based on the presumption that to define a species involves making an objective determination about something given in nature. On this view, similar biological organisms are members of a natural kind or species, and each of these species has an essential and unchanging nature or essence that makes it the kind of being that it is.[36] That is, there is an underlying "natural state" in terms of which the resemblances between individuals of a species are explicable.[37] On this definition, species are internally homogenous and discontinuous with one another, and their boundaries are real and objective. To violate those boundaries is to destroy the very essence of the species and to invite chaos in the natural world. A species integrity argument based on this classical notion of species is a form of the contrary to nature argument, for it takes species to be built into the order of nature and holds that it is wrong to violate that order by crossing species boundaries.

In later centuries, biologists found this view of species unsatisfactory because it used arbitrary criteria, such as whether animals were domestic or wild, to group organisms into species.[38] Consequently, they developed alternative notions of species to accommodate their scientific interests. In their initial attempts, they ascribed significance to similarities in the visible appearances, functions, or behaviors of organisms and drew species boundaries between living beings on this basis.[39] The eighteenth-century father of biological taxonomy, Karl Linneaus, for instance, developed a graded hierarchy of species based on similarity of appearance. His system, which used more defined characteristics than Aristotle's to group organisms into a species, brought order to a previously disorganized discipline and led to the flowering of taxonomic research.[40]

However, in the nineteenth century, Darwin revolutionized the concept of species with his theory of evolution and led biologists to maintain that species are not static, timeless classes of organisms but evolving ways of categorizing them. Species necessarily change over time as they go through many separate events in which new ones are formed and labeled. Consistent with this view, Ernst Mayr developed a significant notion of species in the 1940s. He focused on the mode of reproduction as the most important criterion for defining species and argued that species are groups of interbreeding natural populations that are reproductively isolated from other reproductive groups.[41] His view ran into difficulties, however, because many asexually reproducing organisms, such as bacteria and the 5 percent of birds that interbreed, do not fit into such a classification system. Some biologists therefore sought still other criteria for defining species, often basing their alternative species categorizations largely on biologically interesting criteria that furthered their particular scientific concerns and approaches, rather than on some eternal essence.[42] As a result, as many as twenty-two different concepts of species have been developed by naturalists.[43]

However, categorizing entities into various biological species will not in itself justify the claim that it is wrong to obliterate the boundaries between species in stem cell research. Before one can declare that it is wrong to cross species boundaries it is necessary to select one from among this multitude of concepts of species and explain the moral unacceptability of crossing species boundaries in terms of it.

Jason Scott Robert and Françoise Baylis provide a critique of the view of species as fixed essences and maintain that there is no one authoritative definition of species. Even so, they argue that in everyday life we use a notion of fixed species and maintain that we have developed social conventions with significant moral import on this basis. More specifically, they hypothesize that we have developed conceptual boundaries between humans and nonhumans in the Western world that give humans a distinctive moral status. We do not grant animals such moral status, they suggest, but instead grant them moral significance only insofar as doing so meets human needs and interests. This leaves us with no way of understanding our moral obligations to novel beings such as human-nonhuman chimeras that do not fit into human or nonhuman species categories, on this argument. In order to avoid social and moral confusion and to retain the distinctive moral status that we ascribe to humans, they hold, it is necessary to keep the tightly guarded species boundaries between humans and nonhumans that are at the basis of our system of assigning moral status.[44] They therefore reject the creation of human-nonhuman chimeras, declaring in their conclusion that to protect the privileged place of human animals in the hierarchy of being, it is of value to protect (folk) essentialism about species identities and thus effectively trump scientific quibbles over species and over the species status of novel beings. The notion that species identity can be a fluid construct is rejected, and instead a belief in fixed species boundaries that ought not to be transgressed is advocated.[45]

Thus, according to this argument, the creation of novel beings that are part human and part nonhuman is sufficiently threatening to the social order that it should be prohibited.

Critics of Robert and Baylis point out that they provide no confirmation of the claim that crossing conventional fixed species boundaries would create social and moral chaos.[46] Indeed, this claim appears to be disconfirmed by a variety of scientific endeavors involving fixed species boundary crossings that have not led to moral confusion within society. We have created hybrids such as mules by mixing nonhumans of two different species and have inserted pig heart valves into humans and human livers into sheep without provoking moral confusion. No objections were voiced about research in which material from humans was combined with that of other species to develop a blood clotting factor for hemophilia, insulin for diabetes, and erythropoietin for anemia.[47] It is possible that we would take the creation of human-nonhuman chimeras in moral stride, as we have in these other instances. Indeed, Louis Charland suggests that we might well provide new ways of naming and defining species as we create such chimeras.[48] Although Robert and Baylis are surely correct in implying that as a matter of social convention we still adhere to the classical notion of species as unchangeable and eternal essences, such conventions are amenable to modification when there is good reason for this, such as to treat disease and improve health.

The species integrity argument in its older or newer forms, therefore, does not offer reliable criteria for ascertaining when the lines between species have been crossed. Moreover, even if it were to do so, it offers no accepted argument about why such crossings would be wrong. There are a number of significant instances cited above in which we have crossed species boundaries for good reasons without creating public unease or social chaos.

Social Taboo Argument

Undoubtedly, the initial reaction that many have to the very thought of creating human-nonhuman chimeras is one of repugnance or revulsion. Critics of the creation of human-nonhuman chimeras claim that this is not just an idiosyncratic individual reaction of a few but is grounded in conventions or taboos found across many cultures. Such taboos serve to promote social well-being and important community values. Leon Kass, for instance, claims that repugnance provides the basis for strictures in many societies against such practices as incest, bestiality, and cannibalism. Indeed, Kass argues that "repugnance may be the only voice left that speaks up to defend the central core of humanity."[49] He asserts that we have some rarely articulated and "perhaps not altogether articulable" sense that putting human stem cells and their derivatives into animals would evoke such repugnance among many in our society.[50]

The fact that certain practices elicit repugnance, on this view, is sufficient to indicate that they are wrong. Attempts can be made to support such reactions of revulsion with argument, Kass acknowledges, but he asks, "Would anybody's failure to give full rational justification for his or her revulsion at these practices make that revulsion ethically suspect?"[51] Sheer repugnance is foundational to this approach and is said to lead inexorably to the intuition that certain practices are ethically unacceptable.

Repugnance appears to be grounded in both emotions and moral intuitions. The force that each of these should be given in ethical decision making is a contested philosophical issue. Responding to certain situations with anger, outrage, or revenge can be appropriate. Surely we are ethically warranted in feeling outrage at the murder of innocent people or the rape of a child. What makes such outrage justifiable is not the emotion of outrage, however, but our reasons for responding in this way. Emotions can sometimes occur by chance and can be misplaced. Indeed, at times, they can obscure, rather than clarify, our ethical reflections. Consequently, we need to provide reasons for ethical judgments based on our emotional responses that provide coherent and supportable grounds for those judgments.[52]

Moral intuitions are also said to support responses of repugnance. Such intuitions traditionally have been viewed as stemming from an authoritative inner voice[53] and are said to have direct epistemological force; they are considered by some to require no further justification. Thus, we intuit that it is wrong to kill innocent and helpless people and right to assist a child about to be raped. Although intuitions undoubtedly have a role in ethical thinking, as these examples exhibit, they are not infallible; they can be mistaken. Moreover, intuitions are sometimes mutually conflicting; in such instances, both cannot be right. These sorts of difficulties work against the claim that we have an inborn moral sense that provides us with infallible moral intuitions about matters such as the creation of human-nonhuman chimeras.[54]

In short, intuitions and emotions, separately or jointly, do not provide a sufficient basis for making moral judgments; such judgments need to be supported by reasons. This means that social taboos based on repugnance alone cannot justify rejecting the creation of human-nonhuman chimeras in stem cell research.

Even so, it is important to acknowledge that such taboos play a significant part in preserving core social judgments and values within societies. They serve to bring order out of cosmological and social chaos by perpetuating traditions and ways of thinking.[55] The taboo against incest, for example, forces societies to expand, bringing in new members who can help them to survive and flourish. However, taboos have their downside, for the same taboos are not held universally across all cultures and, within a culture, they can outlive their social role and become liabilities.

The social taboos listed by Kass are not universally accepted. A paradigm taboo that he believes is universal, that against cannibalism, is not found in all cultures; cannibalism still exists today in some societies as a socially sanctioned practice. Taboos against crossing humans and nonhumans, in particular, have not been held universally. The ancient Egyptians, for instance, depicted some of their honored gods with animal heads or bodies, and Native Americans have revered sacred figures that combine human and nonhuman features. Moreover, some of the taboos that have been entertained within our society in the past have subsequently been discarded or are now in question.[56] Blood transfusions, organ donations, and interracial marriages have all been viewed as morally taboo at various points in our social history. Yet we have since reversed each of these taboos. Similarly, those ancient taboos that prohibit mixing different sorts of beings, particularly humans and nonhumans, appear to have diminished in force today, for we accept such practices as the insertion of pig heart valves into human beings without ethical qualms. Because social taboos are variable and come and go within societies, they alone cannot provide an adequate basis for making ethical assessments about whether to create human-nonhuman chimeras.

In discussing social taboos, Jeffrey Stout distinguishes the "repulsive" from the "abominable," or what has been termed here the "repugnant."[57] The repulsive mixes categories that are usually kept sharply separate but does so in ways that are not socially or cosmologically significant. The abominable or repugnant, in contrast, not only displays great anomalies but also poses a threat to the established cosmological and social order. Stout observes:

> An anomalous or ambiguous act is more likely to seem abominable where it seems to pose, or becomes symbolic of, a threat to the established cosmological or social order.... A great deal hangs, therefore, on

whether the anomaly in question is viewed as a mediator between realms or as a transgressor across boundaries that guard cosmic and social order. I shall henceforth confine the term abomination to transgressors (or transgressions) of this kind."[58]

Some acts, such as growing a human ear on the back of a mouse (in order to develop new outer ears for children without them),[59] do not have major cultural or global import in our society and would therefore undoubtedly be categorized by Stout as repulsive but not abominable or repugnant. In cultures that distinguish humans from animals even more sharply than ours, however, such an experiment would be viewed as abominable just because it obscured that distinction.

Thus, repugnance, on Stout's view, is not a primitive emotion at the foundation of such moral judgments as that it is wrong to create human-nonhuman chimeras. Instead, it arises from an antecedent commitment to social and cosmological categories relative to which such chimeras seem anomalous. This means that it is not the creation of these chimeras that needs to be defended but, instead, the social and cosmological system that grounds taboos against combining the human and the nonhuman.

Such taboos, which emerge from diverse historical and cultural contexts, are subject to alteration as the social system in which they arise alters. This sort of alteration is occurring today as the context in which mixing human materials with those of animals moves away from ancient fearsome and socially abhorrent chimeric creations of fantasy toward human-nonhuman combinations that are initiated to study the development of human stem cells and, ultimately, to treat those with disease.[60] There is an ethical imperative today to resist earlier taboos against developing human-nonhuman chimeras, since such taboos do not take into account the reasons that such chimeras might rightly be pursued within the different contexts in which we live today.[61] Thus, the simple assertion that human-nonhuman chimeras are taboo, unvarnished by a rationale or justification and grounded in a social context that no longer exists, does not provide an adequate basis for rejecting stem cell research in which human and nonhuman cells are combined.

Human Dignity Argument

Another concern raised by proposals to create human-nonhuman chimeras in stem cell research is that this would merge humans and nonhumans in ways that would denigrate or even eliminate the distinctive moral significance of each, with particular emphasis on its effect on humans. The contrary to nature, species integrity, and social taboo arguments presume that there is something about human beings that ought to be honored and protected from denial and diminishment. It is this on which the argument from human dignity focuses.

The notion of human dignity has been invoked in debates about a variety of issues, such as euthanasia and human cloning. Yet those presenting it have not tended to elaborate on what human dignity means, and it therefore tends to be enveloped in a cloud of confusion.[62] For instance, Kass has expressed concern about the threat to human dignity that he finds presented by such recent biotechnological innovations as reproductive cloning. However, he offers only a hint of what he means by human dignity, indicating that it has to do with "the worthiness of embodied human life, and the worth of our natural desires and passions, our natural origins and attachments, our sentiments and aversions, our loves and longings."[63] He does not explain what it is that gives embodied human life, our natural desires and passions, our loves and longings this worthiness and consequently leaves us with only a vague notion of what he means by human dignity.

Such formless notions of human dignity led Ruth Macklin, at one time, to argue that dignity is a superfluous concept that means no more than respect for human autonomy and the right to self-determination.[64] Although she is surely correct that the violation of human dignity involves the arbitrary infringement of human autonomy, human dignity means more than this. For instance, if a person autonomously chose to enter into slavery, that would denigrate human dignity, even though that individual made an autonomous choice to do so. The concepts of human autonomy and human dignity are not coextensive; they are distinct moral categories that overlap in certain respects. The former is a subset of the latter rather than inclusive of it.

John Harris also finds the way in which the notion of human dignity has been used too inexact and defines it as "not using individuals as a means to the purposes of others."[65] This, however, is a stricture that follows from the recognition of human dignity rather than an explanation of what it means.

Can the notion of human dignity be rehabilitated? It was Immanuel Kant who brought the concept of human dignity to the fore of Western thought.[66] His view of human dignity provided the foundation for his special understanding of the moral law.[67] He maintained that humans have an unconditioned and incomparable worth or dignity because they are moral agents whose actions can be imputed to them.[68] Their dignity is manifested in their capacities to set ends for themselves and to act to achieve those ends in the practical sphere. Because they have a rational nature and the ability to act on principles, Kant held, humans possess a distinctive dignity. Alan Gewirth, a recent thinker influenced by Kant, maintained that the primary ground on which human agents logically must be said to have dignity is that they have purposes that they can act to fulfill.[69] This generic purposiveness underlies the ascription of dignity to all human agents, he argued. Although Kant's and Gewirth's views capture an important aspect of human dignity—human cognitive abilities—they omit other significant factors that inform our common understanding of this concept.

Human dignity is a widely shared notion that signifies that humans typically display certain sorts of capacities that render them worthy of respect. It is not only that they have capacities for reasoning, choosing freely, and acting for moral reasons, as Kant argued, or for entertaining and acting on the basis of self-chosen purposes, as Gewirth held, that leads us to attribute a certain dignity to humans. It is also because humans can display such capacities as those for engaging in sophisticated forms of communication and language, participating in interweaving social relations, displaying sympathy and empathy in emotionally complex ways, and developing a secular or religious world view, that they are said to have human dignity. Human dignity is not the sort of concept for which we can provide a strict dictionary definition complete with necessary and sufficient conditions, much as we cannot provide strict definitions of human kindness, personhood, human rights, or a poem. Instead, when we talk about human dignity, we are considering a family or cluster of capacities, no one of which is necessary or sufficient for capturing what we mean by it.[70] An individual may have only a few among the capacities that we associate with human dignity or a great many and yet be said to have human dignity. Wittgenstein observed that certain terms "have no one thing in common which makes us use the same word for all . . . they are related to one another in many different ways."[71] Human dignity is one of those terms. We use it to mean a family of capacities, all of which are present in a paradigm case of human dignity but not all of which need be present in all cases of human dignity.

Having human dignity is conceptually distinct from behaving and bearing oneself in a dignified manner. Dignified comportment is a characteristic exhibited by some who respond to untoward circumstances in a noble and uplifting manner; such individuals display what Daryl Pullman has termed "personal dignity."[72] Having human dignity, in contrast, is, as Gewirth states, "a characteristic that belongs permanently . . . to every human as such";[73] it does not come and go depending on how one responds to circumstances. A person can behave in ways that are boorish and selfish and thereby diminish her "personal dignity" and yet retain her human dignity in that she is still owed certain sorts of responses and treatment by others.

To respect those with human dignity involves treating them in certain ways and refraining from treating them in others just because they have some among this family of capacities associated with human dignity. That dignity is degraded and demeaned when the cluster of relevant human capacities is deliberately and wrongfully diminished or eliminated in human beings. This occurs when they are subjected to such acts as murder, torture, enslavement, rape, or maiming.[74] These acts are wrong not only because they injure humans physically and psychologically but also because they deny them the exercise of many of the capacities distinctively associated with human dignity.

When it comes to the question of whether to develop human-nonhuman chimeras, proponents of an argument from human dignity would maintain the following: it would be wrong to encase within an animal's body those physical components of humans that are necessary for exercising the cluster of capacities associated with human dignity because this would eliminate or diminish those very capacities. The torturer or enslaver of human beings wrongs them, not only because he or she harms them but also because he or she denies them the option of exercising many of the capacities associated with human dignity. The creator of the human-nonhuman chimera would do even worse—he or she would obliterate or enfeeble those very capacities.

At the core of the concerns raised by the human dignity argument about developing human-nonhuman chimeras is the following: certain human bodily components that are closely connected to the capacities associated with human dignity might be transferred to human-nonhuman chimeric beings and in that setting would be severely restricted in their exercise or even destroyed. Such human dignity–related capacities are especially associated with the structure and activities of the human brain—whether one views the relationship between thought and the brain as one of materialistic identity, dualistic correlativity, or in some other way.[75] If investigators were to introduce substantial numbers of specialized human neural stem cells into a nonhuman and those human stem cells were to migrate to the resulting chimeric brain and control its functions, the host would, in effect, become a host of mixed species (in an ordinary under-standing of species) with a human brain that attempted to think and act like a human. The human dignity argument maintains that to carry out such a study would violate human dignity because it would render the resulting chimera incapable of exercising its distinctively human capacities, since its brain would be imprisoned in an animal-like body. To insert undifferentiated human embryonic stem cells into an animal embryo would raise similar questions. If these pluripotent human embryonic stem cells were to integrate with the brain of the developing embryonic animal and the resulting human-nonhuman chimera were to emerge with a human brain, this would violate human dignity for the same reasons.

Possible Criticisms of the Human Dignity Argument

Is the human dignity argument a form of the species integrity argument that I have already rejected? Helga Kuhse observes that "it would not be enough to say that human life has dignity because it takes the form of a featherless biped or because humans have opposing thumbs."[76] Surely she is right. (See discussion of speciesism in Chapter 3.) However, this is not a species-dependent argument that contends that because humans have certain physical features, they therefore have human dignity. It is a species-dependent argument in an extended sense in that it maintains that because humans have certain distinctive capacities, they have human dignity. Those human physical features that figure in the workings of the human brain and its peripheral support systems, in particular, are especially connected with the exercise of the capacities associated with human dignity, for they play a part in the various ways that humans think and feel.

Robert Streiffer asks whether "the transplantation of human stem cells or their derivatives into developing animals could, at least in principle, significantly enhance the research subject's moral status"—that is, could give an animal the moral status of "a normal human adult."[77] From the point of view of the animal, Streiffer observes, such status-enhancing chimeric research would be "absolutely unacceptable" because the animal, as a research subject, could not be guaranteed the protections that should be provided for those with the moral status of normal adult human beings. This is because we cannot know in advance of such studies which among them would be "status-enhancing." This epistemological uncertainty leads Streiffer to allow the insertion of differentiated human stem cells into animals but to ban the introduction of undifferentiated human stem cells into nonhuman primate blastocysts. This eliminates the risk of harm that such research would cause to animals if they were to emerge from it with the moral status of normal human adults.

Streiffer does not provide an explanation of what it means to have "the moral status of a normal human adult." On what basis would we determine that a sheep or a bonobo had been enhanced to the point where it had such moral status? This is not just an epistemological issue, but also a conceptual one. Streiffer rejects species-based and cognitive capacity standards of moral status but provides no other standard of such status. Moreover, his focus on avoiding the creation of an animal with the moral status of a normal human adult, however that is conceptualized, seems too narrow in that it fails to reflect concern about the possibility of developing a chimeric being with the moral status of a normal human child or a disabled human adult or child. Such outcomes would also surely raise ethical concerns, even though the resulting individuals presumably would not have the moral status of normal human adults. On the human dignity argument, the epistemological problem, while still present, is not intractable, for a chimeric individual would have to exhibit only some among the capacities associated with human dignity at any stage of development to render it outside of ethical bounds to create a human-nonhuman being.

Critics of the argument from human dignity might claim that since it maintains that having human dignity involves the possession of certain capacities, only those humans with such capacities, but not all humans, can be said to have dignity.[78] For example, these critics might argue, since newborn infants cannot exercise some of the capacities associated with human dignity, they therefore lack such dignity. This would mean that human dignity argument proponents would have to acknowledge that it would not be wrong to develop a human-nonhuman chimera with the capacities of a child, such commentators would claim.

This criticism would rest on a misunderstanding of the argument from human dignity. It does not insist that all who have human dignity must exhibit a fixed number of specific capacities. Instead, it contends that they need some of those capacities but that they need not fully exercise them. Thus, it uses an ordinary understanding of what human beings are and the distinctive capacities that they have now and might develop to point out that they are owed respect because of this. Although the newborn infant does not exhibit all of these capacities, we take him or her to have some of them and therefore to be owed treatment accorded to those with human dignity. The argument from human dignity also accords such dignity to disabled humans with limited capacities associated with human dignity because they might develop a fuller set of such capacities in the future due to greater maturity and to medical and social assistance. We do not want to chance mistakenly treating them as lacking in human dignity, thereby placing them outside the orbit of the protections accorded to those with such dignity.

The argument from human dignity might also be criticized as wrongly dismissing the value of animals and unfairly giving preference to human beings. It is the case that some advocates of human dignity have denigrated the worth of animals. However, that is not necessary to the logic of the human dignity argument. Animals of different species have varying and distinctive capabilities, some of which resemble those associated with human dignity in certain respects. For instance, Franz DeWaal, a noted primatologist, finds that several different kinds of primates exhibit attachment and empathy; internalization of prescriptive social rules; concepts of giving, trading, and revenge; and tendencies toward peacemaking and social maintenance.[79] Yet they do not display the complex behavior involved in making ethical choices from among many available alternatives and rejecting some of these on moral grounds, nor do they exhibit certain other human dignity–associated capacities. The range of capacities associated with human dignity, as far as we know at this time, belongs uniquely to humans. In short, it is the case that many animals, particularly primates, have certain capacities that require us to treat them with respect. However, animals have a different sort of dignity from that of humans. No denigration of animals or humans need follow from this.

In summary, the argument from human dignity does not fall into several of the difficulties that hover over the other arguments discussed above against the development of human-nonhuman chimeras in stem cell research. Furthermore, it provides an explanation of why it would be wrong to create certain sorts of human-nonhuman chimeras and yet does not condemn the creation of any and all human-nonhuman chimeras.

Setting Ethical Limits to Developing Human-Nonhuman Chimeras

The responses of scientists and the public to the possibility of developing human-nonhuman chimeras in stem cell research suggest that the degree of ethical unease to which many of us react to such research varies with (1) the sort of human stem cells under study, (2) whether they are differentiated (specialized) or undifferentiated (unspecialized), (3) where in the host animal they are inserted, (4) how closely related this animal is to humans, (5) when a prenatal animal is used as host, how far in its development that animal has progressed, and (6) what sort of outcome is expected.

We do not object to the transfer of most sorts of differentiated human stem cells into, say, the kidneys or hearts of mice, pigs, or monkeys, for this is not likely to result in the emergence of chimeric beings with the capacities to think, feel, and act like humans. However, when we entertain the possibility of transferring human neural stem cells or human germinal stem cells, or else undifferentiated human embryonic stem cells into prenatal nonhumans, raising the possibility that these cells might overwhelm their brains or their germline, we draw back, for we realize that such transfers might result in the production of human-nonhuman chimeras with distinctively human features and capacities. Many are especially concerned that chimeric beings that are neither fully human nor fully animal would emerge with human brains or human sperm and eggs.

To avoid these untoward possibilities it is necessary to place certain restrictions on the design of studies involving the transfer of human stem cells into prenatal animals. In particular, it requires placing certain limits on the transfer of differentiated human neural stem cells and undifferentiated human embryonic stem cells into prenatal nonhumans, for such human cells might spread throughout the bodies of these developing nonhumans. It also requires us to restrict the role that primates, which are more closely related to humans than other sorts of nonhumans, play in this form of stem cell research in order to avoid the creation of human-nonhuman chimeras with features and capacities extremely close to human. I begin the development of such limits on human-nonhuman chimeric research by first considering the impact that transplanting *specialized human neural stem cells* into nonhuman hosts could have on their brains in particular. I then address the possible effects of transferring *human embryonic stem cells* into nonhuman hosts in light of the possibility that those cells might differentiate and enter their brains or germline.

Limits to Transferring Human Neural Stem Cells into Prenatal Nonhuman Hosts

To date, none of the transfers of specialized human neural stem cells into nonhumans that have been carried out appear to have affected the brains of recipient nonhumans in ways that have resulted in the emergence of distinctively human capacities, features or functions in them. For instance, Ourednik and colleagues, as noted above,[80] transferred human neural progenitor cells (stem cells that have begun to differentiate into brain cells) into the forebrain of fetal monkeys and found that these human cells developed along the same pathways as the monkey cells surrounding them. The human neural cells became an integral part of the monkey brain and were controlled by it; consequently, no problematic human-monkey chimera resulted. The Weissman study discussed earlier[81] involved inserting human fetal neural stem cells into the brains of newborn mice. These human cells migrated to various regions of the mouse brain where they apparently integrated with mouse neural cells and matured into cells characteristic of the region of the brain in which they were located. This study suggested that the developing mouse brain, rather than the human neural cells, controlled the responses of the mice and that no mouse-human chimera of ethical concern had emerged.

Indeed, it seemed highly unlikely even before such studies were carried out, that if stem cell investigators were to insert specialized human neural stem cells into, say, a mouse embryo, and were to bring it to term, the mouse that emerged would have a human brain. This is because mouse skulls are not large enough to accommodate the human brain and because their brains do not have the size, complexity, and organizational structure to be transformed into human brains.[82] Human neural cells, which develop more slowly than those of mice, could not somehow seize control of themselves and speed up their development to accommodate the mouse brain.[83] Instead, studies suggest that the human cells would mimic the nonhuman host's structure and functions and would become "the practical equivalent of mouse cells."[84] Consequently, a human-mouse chimera with a human brain would not result from such a study.

Would the story be any different if a large primate embryo, such as a chimpanzee, bonobo, or gorilla (each of which is more closely related to humans than a mouse in genetic structure and physiological complexity and function), were injected with human neural stem cells? Might this embryo, if brought to term, result in a primate with a human brain? If so, would this primate think and act like a human?

The evidence available in the scientific literature about the ways in which the brains of primates function suggests that in the case of primates as well, human neural cells would not gain control of themselves and direct themselves to meet the needs of the developing primate brain. Instead, these human cells would function in the ways that the primate brain directed them. This is because human neuronal networks differ from those of primates in their developmental timing. If a network of human neural stem cells were somehow to take over the primate's brain, that human network would not develop at the same pace as that of the primate and would therefore fail to become a functional human neuronal network.[85] Thus, available evidence suggests that it seems highly unlikely that the transplantation of human neural stem cells into mouse or primate embryos would result in the development of nonhuman hosts with a human brain.

Karpowicz, van der Kooy, and I point out that it is important to recognize that this appears to be the case only when separate, dissociated, unorganized human neural stem cells are injected into nonhuman embryos. Inserting whole masses of associated human neural stem cells into nonhuman embryos might run the risk of human pattern development and formation in the brains of such nonhumans, particularly primates, possibly resulting in a human-nonhuman chimera with a human-like brain.[86]

Evidence for this claim is derived from the "Geep" and the "chick-quail" studies cited above. These involved the transfer of associated goat cell masses into sheep blastocysts[87] and whole regions of the quail brain into embryonic chicks.[88] During embryonic development, these experiments indicate, the replacement of the whole inner cell mass of an embryo or whole regions of the brain can result in a host with characteristics and capacities of the kind of entity from which the organized associated cells were derived. It is theoretically conceivable—albeit highly unlikely—that to transfer an embryonic human cortex into a chimpanzee, which is closely related to humans, would give this chimpanzee a human cortex and that this primate would exhibit some capacities relevant to human dignity within the limits imposed by the rest of its body.

Therefore, to ensure that this unlikely scenario will not occur, it is important to transfer only separated or dissociated human neural stem cells to nonhuman embryos. The available evidence suggests that these human cells would organize in response to the environment into which they enter and would be controlled by the nonhuman hosts. Such human neural stem cells, it appears, can be transferred in limited numbers to nonhuman embryos without raising ethical concerns about the development of human-nonhuman chimeras with human brains and the sorts of distinctive human functions and capacities that are pertinent to human dignity.

Karpowicz, Van der Kooy, and I recommend that when carrying out studies involving the transfer of differentiated human neural stem cells into prenatal animals investigators, keeping in mind that the nonhuman host's neurological networks are just developing, should (1) limit the number of stem cells transferred to the animal to the smallest number necessary to reach reliable scientific conclusions; (2) choose a host animal that is not closely related, either structurally or functionally, to humans; and (3) transfer only dissociated human neural stem cells, rather than whole masses of organized tissue, to prenatal nonhuman hosts.[89] These limitations are directed toward avoiding the possibility that the resulting chimera would develop capacities and characteristics that are associated with human dignity.

To these recommendations, I would now add that as studies involving human neural stem cells proceed, the guidelines of the Stanford ethics advisory committee should be adopted. That is, researchers engaged in studies involving the insertion of specialized human neural stem cells into nonhumans should follow a step-by-step approach, gradually increasing the number of human neural cells transferred to the nonhuman hosts and gradually expanding the areas of the nonhuman brain into which they are inserted, until these studies reach a preset end point that is commensurate with the needs of such studies and ethical requirements.

For instance, in a hypothetical experiment, stem cell investigators could inject human neural stem cells into a nonprimate prenatal mammalian model (e.g., the mouse) of Parkinson's disease to see whether these neural cells would infiltrate the developing substantia nigra and, if so, whether this is accompanied by a change in the symptoms of Parkinson's disease in the hosts. They would begin with small numbers of these human cells and insert them into only one small area of the prenatal nonhuman brain. They would then closely observe the developing brain structures and functions of these prenatal animals at each step. If no signs of human structures and functions appeared in them at the preset first stopping point, they would go on to the next step in this sequential process—for instance, increasing the number of inserted cells and assessing the outcomes at the next preset stopping point, and so on. This procedure would provide a carefully planned approach to research involving the insertion of human neural stem cells into animals that would avoid the development of human-nonhuman hosts with human-like brains.

Limits to Transferring Unspecialized Human Embryonic Stem Cells into Prenatal Nonhuman Hosts

Human embryonic stem cells have the ability to transform into almost any specialized cell of the human body. Therefore, ethical concerns arise when the transfer of these sorts of human stem cells to nonhuman hosts is under consideration, since these cells are more flexible than differentiated stem cells and might transform into human neural cells and invade the animal brain or else specialize into human germ cells and produce human gametes in the nonhuman host. These possible outcomes are of particular concern when the use of human embryonic stem cells in early prenatal nonhumans is under consideration, for the human embryonic stem cells might be incorporated into the brain and/ or germline of nonhuman embryos from their very beginning and completely take over the brain and/or gonads.

Possibility of Overwhelming Brain of Nonhuman Hosts

First, let us consider the possibility that such unspecialized human stem cells would overwhelm the brain of the nonhuman host. Thus far, the available evidence slowly being developed suggests that this does not occur. For instance, Goldstein and colleagues, in a study mentioned above, inserted human embryonic stem cells into early chick embryos to test the ability of these human cells to differentiate into a variety of types of cells within a living nonhuman system.[90] They found that the human embryonic stem cells differentiated and integrated with the tissue of the host chicks in ways that were controlled by the hosts. No humanized chicks resulted. The more recent study from the Salk Institute, also noted above, in which human embryonic stem cells were inserted into the brain ventricles of embryonic mice,[91] revealed that these cells integrated with the cells of the adult mouse forebrain but did not alter the ways in which that brain functioned. These studies suggest that the insertion of human embryonic stem cells into prenatal nonhuman subjects will not result in human-nonhumans with human-like brains.

The guidelines of the National Academies of Science (NAS) address the question of whether researchers should conduct research involving the transfer of unspecialized human embryonic stem cells into nonhumans at any stage of their development. They recommend that human embryonic stem cell research oversight committees at these researchers' institutions focus on the following considerations:

> The number of hES [human embryonic stem] cells to be transferred, what areas of the animal body would be involved, and whether the cells might migrate through the animal's body. The hES cells may affect some animal organs rather than others, raising questions about the number of organs affected, how the animal's functioning would be affected, and whether some valued human characteristics might be exhibited in the animal, including physical appearance.[92]

These guidelines also address in particular the insertion of human embryonic stem cells into nonhuman blastocysts (early embryos at five or six days after fertilization in which the inner cell mass has formed). The discussion section of the guidelines of the National Academies notes that if human embryonic stem cells were incorporated into a mouse blastocyst,

> the human cells [could] contribute extensively to any mouse that arises from implantation of such a chimeric blastocyst.... Potentially the inner cell mass, the progenitor of the fetus, would consist of a mixture of human and mouse cells. It is not now possible to predict the extent of human contributions to such chimeras. If the recipient blastocyst were from an animal that is evolutionarily close to a human the potential for human contributions would appear to be greater. For these reasons, research that involves the production of such chimeras should be performed first using nonhuman primate ES [embryonic stem] cells in mouse blastocysts before proceeding to the use of hES cells. The need for the use of blastocysts from larger mammals would need to be very clearly justified and nonhuman primate blastocysts should not be used at this time.[93]

The final guidelines set out by the NAS working group explicitly prohibit "research in which hES cells are introduced into nonhuman primate blastocysts or in which any ES cells are introduced into human blastocysts."[94]

In short, the discussion text of the guidelines, together with the guidelines themselves, indicate that stem cell investigators should start with the transfer of nonhuman primate embryonic stem cells, rather than human embryonic stem cells, into nonhuman blastocysts. At a point that researchers believe is warranted by their research with nonhuman primate blastocysts, they can switch to inserting human embryonic stem cells into nonhuman embryonic hosts—except not into nonhuman primate blastocysts.

However, it is not clear that it is enough to prohibit the transfer of human embryonic stem cells into primate embryonic blastocysts. If the entire inner cell mass of a nonhuman blastocyst host were completely replaced with human embryonic stem cells, this would result in an inner cell mass composed entirely of human cells that would be surrounded by a nonhuman trophectoderm. This, in theory, could lead to the production of a human individual or of a human-nonhuman chimeric individual with distinctive capacities associated with human dignity. Although the risk of producing such untoward results appears to be greater if the inner cell mass of a primate blastocyst is used, since primates are developmentally similar to humans, it is also theoretically possible—albeit highly unlikely due to developmental, space, and other considerations— that if the inner cell mass of large mammalian embryo were replaced with human embryonic stem cells, a human individual or a human human-nonhuman chimeric being with distinctive capacities associated with human dignity might be produced. As the NAS guidelines cited above point out, "It is not now possible to predict the extent of human contributions to such chimeras. If the recipient blastocyst were from an animal that is evolutionarily closer to a human [than the mouse], the potential for human contributions would appear to be greater."[95]

Because of this uncertainty, it would be wise to apply the same precautionary principle behind the prohibition of the NAS guidelines of the transfer of human embryonic stem cells to nonhuman primate embryos and to restrict the insertion of human embryonic stem cells into *any* nonhuman embryos in one of the following two ways. Either (1) prohibit the total suffusion of the entire inner cell mass of nonhuman blastocysts with human embryonic stem cells, or (2) permit the insertion of a small number of human embryonic stem cells into nonhuman blastocysts with the proviso that this number could gradually be increased in subsequent studies until before the point of total suffusion if no evidence of the emergence of human-like structures appeared as neural development took place in these hosts.

It is important to place limitations on research involving the insertion of human embryonic stem cells into *all* nonhuman blastocysts, not just those of primates, because we do not now know what the extent of human contributions to such blastocysts might be. These proposed restrictions do not provide specific stopping points that can be measured in detailed ways; instead, establishing them involves matters of judgment. They take the precautionary principle and extend it to the transfer of human embryonic stem cells to any sort of nonhuman blastocyst.

More generally, those proposing any study involving the insertion of unspecialized human embryonic stem cells into prenatal nonhumans should first provide a compelling rationale to show that the study is necessary to achieve important scientific knowledge. Next, the recommendations of the Stanford ethics advisory committee should come into play, as they did in the case of proposed studies involving specialized neural stem cells. That is, researchers engaged in studies involving the insertion of human embryonic stem cells into prenatal nonhumans would follow a step-by-step approach. They would gradually increase the number of human embryonic stem cells transferred to the prenatal nonhuman hosts and gradually expand the areas of the nonhuman into which they were inserted, until these studies reached a predefined end point commensurate with the needs of such studies and with ethical requirements. They would closely observe the developing brain structures and functions of these prenatal animals at each step. If no signs of human structures and functions appeared in the nonhuman hosts at the preset first stopping point, they would gradually increase the number of human embryonic stem cells transferred to the nonhuman prenatal hosts in subsequent studies. Indeed, it would be wise to start at later stages of prenatal development rather than the blastocyst stage and, if no untoward results occured, to move back to increasingly earlier stages of development of the nonhuman hosts, carrying out the same procedures and taking the same precautions outlined above.

For instance, stem cell investigators could inject a small number of human embryonic stem cells into a fetal mammal and gradually increase their number and the areas into which they were inserted in subsequent studies if no human structures and behaviors appeared in the fetal hosts. If the nonhuman fetal hosts were to show any signs that human structures or behaviors might develop or were beginning to develop at one of the stopping points, the study would be stopped. If no untoward results appeared, researchers would move to earlier stages of development of such prenatal mammalian nonhumans, repeating this approach. When they reached the nonhuman mammalian blastocyst stage, they would, as recommended above, either refrain from totally suffusing such hosts with human embryonic stem cells or transfer a small number of such cells to them, gradually increasing their number in subsequent studies if no human structures and behaviors appeared in the blastocyst hosts.

This general working procedure for studies involving unspecialized human embryonic stem cells in prenatal mammalian nonhumans would, as it did in the case of stem cell research involving the use of specialized human neural stem cells, provide a cautious approach to such research that would avoid the possibility that human-nonhuman chimeras with human-like brains would develop.

Possibility of Developing Human Gametes in Nonhumans

Another major ethical concern raised by research involving the transfer of human embryonic stem cells to nonhuman embryos is that these human stem cells might spread to the gonads of the developing nonhumans and differentiate into cells that generate human sperm or eggs. There is a theoretical possibility that some of these human gamete-producing chimeric primates might mate and produce a human child.[96]

Many would reject such a scenario as contrary to our basic convictions about how children should be brought into the world. As discussed above, not all social taboos are unjustified. One of our warranted social taboos is grounded in the belief that the act of bringing children into the world should take place within the human context. We retain this taboo in order to protect the personal and social significance of bringing children into the world and the children themselves.[97] We see procreation as a meaningful human experience that defines, in part, who we are as individuals and as a community. Moreover, we recognize that being born of human-nonhuman chimeras might have untoward physical, emotional, and social effects on any children who might result. Consequently, we set limits to the extent to which we are willing to alter modes of human procreation. Producing human children as an accidental byproduct of scientific studies that have an altogether different goal from reproduction as a result of the mating of human-nonhuman chimeras is well beyond those limits. Therefore, we would reject any such scenario as unethical.

In most instances, any human-nonhuman chimeras that result from the insertion of human embryonic stem cells into prenatal animals would be sacrificed at birth or shortly afterward. If the goals of research can be reached only by keeping these chimeras alive, however, then appropriate steps to avoid reproduction, such as isolation, should be taken. The NAS guidelines, which are in accord with this line of thought, assert that "no animal into which hES cells have been introduced at any stage of development should be allowed to breed."[98]

A Human Dignity Approach to the Creation of Human-Nonhuman Chimeras

The mingling of bodily materials from different sorts of living beings has become more acceptable since the ancients first developed the notion of the monstrous chimera. However, what is at issue today is not the mixing of materials from members of different species, which is accepted as ethical in several different research contexts. It is whether the transfer of certain sorts of human materials, such as specialized neural stem cells or unspecialized human embryonic stem cells, to nonhuman prenatal hosts would result in the creation of human-nonhuman chimeras.

Arguments against the transfer of such human stem cells to nonhumans, including the contrary to nature, species integrity, and social taboo arguments, do not succeed in exhibiting that it would be wrong in principle to develop human-nonhuman chimeras. Indeed, if these arguments were to succeed, we would have to cease all interspecies procedures and research, including xenotransplantation, transgenic modifications, and the manufacture of insulin and erythropoietin. The human dignity argument, however, explains what is at issue ethically in carrying out stem cell studies that might result in the creation of human-nonhuman chimeras. It maintains that it would be wrong to create human-nonhuman chimeras with human brains because these chimeric individuals would not be able to exercise their distinctive human dignity-related capacities since they would be set within a non-human physical system that lacks the structures to support the workings of the human brain. To create such chimeras would diminish or eliminate the distinctively human capacities associated with human dignity. Further, to develop nonhumans that might harbor human sperm or eggs and, in theory, could mate to create human children, would violate our sense that our children should not be produced as unanticipated side-effects of scientific studies.

The goal of stem cell chimeric studies is to support, rather than to denigrate, both human dignity and human well-being. The transfer of human stem cells to prenatal nonhumans, if carried out according to ethical guidelines such as those outlined above, would allow those pursuing such studies to reach toward these goals. Such studies need not threaten the belief at the core of our social ethic that human beings have a certain distinctive dignity, but instead could, if conducted according to carefully developed ethical guidelines, uphold that central conviction.

6

International Stem Cell Research and Research Cloning: Three Contrasting Approaches

Recent advances in stem cell research have led a surprising number of countries around the globe to grapple with the question of whether to engage in research on these novel cells.[1] These countries have responded in different ways to the ethical and policy challenges posed by stem cell research, depending on their history, cultural traditions, prevalent ethical and religious values, degree of technological optimism, and attitudes toward economic development through innovative scientific research.

Some, galvanized by the strong scientific, therapeutic, ethical, and economic pull of this research, have resolved to pursue stem cell research vigorously. The United Kingdom, Japan, China, Israel, Singapore, and South Korea are among them. They have not only embraced both embryonic stem cell research and research cloning but also set out to become the premier centers of stem cell research in the world. However, they have not allowed such research to proceed willy-nilly. Instead, they have established guidelines and regulations to govern it. I term their approach to stem cell research a "permissive" one.

Meanwhile, certain other countries, such as Canada and Spain, have been more reluctant to initiate stem cell investigations, since they consider them ethically and scientifically questionable in certain respects—and yet ethically and scientifically sound in others. Consequently, they have authorized only certain forms of embryonic stem cell research and have rejected research cloning altogether. Moreover, they have tended to place greater substantive and procedural conditions on the sorts of stem cell research that they allow than have countries adopting a permissive approach. I term their approach to this research a "moderate" one.

Still other nations, such as Italy, Austria, Ireland, and Germany, either place extremely strict constraints on embryonic stem cell research and ban research cloning entirely or else prohibit both as unethical and unnecessary. I term their approach a "restrictive" one.

Stem cell research policies adopted by countries around the globe have not been static, however. Since the turn of the twenty-first century there has been a trend to loosen them in some countries and to restrict them in others. As a result, conflicting sets of shifting regulations currently govern this research internationally. This renders any overall judgments about the global shape of stem cell research policy tentative.[2] Even so, it is instructive to consider how a few countries that have developed different approaches to stem cell research have grappled with the issues at stake before we consider the reasons for the development of stem cell research policy in the United States. We must grasp those matters about which countries that take a stance regarding stem cell research agree and those about which they differ and why they develop certain policies regarding this research rather than others before we can begin to realize the hope of developing scientifically sound and ethically responsible stem cell research policies that will be respected not only in the United States, but also globally.

In this chapter, I focus on the stem cell research policies adopted in the United Kingdom, Germany, and Japan. Each has taken a somewhat different position about whether, why, and how to proceed with this research. I chose these three countries to illustrate that such factors as history, cultural traditions, ethical and religious values, attitudes toward the use of technology, and economic policies do not inevitably carry the same weight in each country. Careful consideration of the reasons for the development of the stem cell policies of these countries can provide a sense of which among these factors play leading roles in the decisions of various countries regarding the development of a stem cell research policy framework. This sort of analysis will aid in assessing the long-run possibility of developing coordinated international stem cell research policies that will advance and safeguard human health while seeking to uphold ethical and social values that are important to the United States and countries around the world.

Stem Cell Research in the United Kingdom

Both embryonic stem cell research and research cloning have been approved in the United Kingdom (U.K.). Investigators can use embryos remaining at in vitro fertilization (IVF) centers in stem cell research, and they are allowed to develop embryos for research through IVF, cloning, and parthenogenesis. Cloning for reproductive purposes, however, remains off limits. In short, the U.K. has developed a permissive stem cell research policy. Yet it also requires all stem cell investigators to obtain licenses to pursue research projects and monitors their adherence to detailed stem cell research guidelines. This approach to stem cell research is largely the result of the country's relatively long engagement with the ethical and policy questions surrounding research with human embryos and of its parliamentary form of government, which invests considerable policy control in the hands of the government.

The Warnock Report and the Moral Significance of Human Embryos

The backdrop to the stem cell research policy in effect in the U.K. today can be found in the 1984 recommendations of the Committee of Inquiry into Human Fertilisation and Embryology.[3] The birth of the first child resulting from the use of IVF in the U.K. in 1978 had generated a wave of concern about whether this new reproductive technology was being carried out in ways that safeguarded the health of women and children and were consistent with ethical standards for research and treatment. In response, a committee of inquiry chaired by Mary Warnock, a prominent philosopher, was charged by the Conservative Party government with "consideration of social, ethical, and legal implications" of the application of methods of assisted reproduction and embryo research in the U.K. and to recommend policies for their use.[4]

No doubt, the most contentious issue with which the Warnock Committee had to grapple was whether research on human embryos should be allowed in order to study the causes of infertility and, if so, under what conditions. Warnock stated in the introduction to the committee's report published in book form in 1985 that "all the other issues we had to consider seemed relatively trivial compared with this one, concerned as it is with a matter which nobody could deny is of central moral significance, the value of human life."[5]

The committee, falling back on a Humean theory of moral sentiments, aimed to capture the feelings of the public about the moral consideration owed to the human embryo through extensive hearings. After these hearings concluded, some committee members stated that they believed that an embryo is a human being or potential human being from the time of fertilization forward and should therefore be treated as if it were no different from a child or an adult.[6] However, the majority of the committee held, to the contrary, that the stage of development of the embryo makes an important difference to the degree of protection that it should be afforded. These members indicated that "a collection of four or sixteen cells was so different from a full human being, from a new human baby or a fully formed human foetus, that it might quite legitimately be treated differently."[7] They asserted in the Warnock Report that although the human embryo is entitled to some measure of respect beyond that of nonhuman subjects, that respect is not absolute and may be weighed against the benefits arising from research. They immediately added that human embryos should not be used frivolously or unnecessarily in research, but only for research that promises advances in treatment and medical knowledge. Moreover, such research should be subject to stringent controls and monitoring.[8]

Given this majority view, the commission considered whether a specific cutoff point in the development of an embryo should be set after which research on it should be prohibited. The committee decided that it was important to set such a mark. The point chosen, near the lowest limit of embryonic age recommended to it by those who had testified in favor of such research, was at fourteen days after fertilization, when the primitive streak forms and an individual being is considered to have begun the process of development.[9] (See chapter 3.) Before this time, research on human embryos should be allowed, the committee recommended; after that time, such research should be banned.[10]

The Warnock Committee went on to recommend the use of spare embryos remaining after IVF treatment for research on the condition that the couples for whom those embryos had been generated had consented to this research use of them.[11] There was greater dissension among committee members about whether to approve the creation of human embryos solely for research by means of IVF using donated gametes. At the end of the day, the argument that succeeded was that to bar research on embryos generated for research would mean that "it would not be possible to undertake any research on the process of fertilisation itself using human eggs and sperm since this process would necessarily result in some cases in the generation of an embryo."[12] A slim majority of the committee thereupon recommended that research should be allowed on any embryo created by IVF, no matter whether it was generated for reproductive purposes or for research into infertility, up to the end of the fourteenth day after fertilization.[13]

Human Fertilisation and Embryology Act

The Warnock Report received strong backing from the government but a more mixed general response. After its publication, the *Times* of London featured a dramatic headline that read "Warnock: Ethics Undermined."[14] Others, however, gave it wholehearted support. John

Habgood, the Archbishop of York, a leading theologian of the Church of England, testified in favor of its recommendations at a subsequent parliamentary hearing.[15] The report precipitated a parliamentary struggle that led the government to postpone consideration of legislation to implement it. However, by the late 1980s, a parliamentary majority for passage had fallen into place, backed by a coalition of scientific and patient advocacy groups, as well as leaders from within the Church of England.[16] The argument that treatments for infertility were extremely important to the future of the family in Great Britain gradually overcame opposition from antiabortion groups, and the government adopted the basic recommendations of the Warnock Committee.[17]

As a result, a sweeping law, the Human Fertilisation and Embryology Act, was enacted in 1990.[18] This law established the Human Fertilisation and Embryology Authority (HFEA), a centralized agency that licenses all IVF procedures in the country and governs human embryo research as well. The agency is composed of seventeen members, a majority of whom must not be scientific experts. Policies developed by the HFEA govern the creation, use, storage, and disposal of human embryos formed for reproductive purposes.[19]

Embryonic Stem Cell Research and Research and Reproductive Cloning

Although the Warnock Committee had envisioned several future scientific developments, it had not considered the possibility that human embryonic stem cells might be developed or that research cloning might prove a useful source of these cells.[20] However, after embryonic stem cells were successfully cultured in 1998, the U.K. was the first major nation to address whether to allow research on human embryonic stem cells and, if so, how it should proceed and be regulated.

The government set up an expert group under the chairmanship of the chief medical officer, Professor Sir Liam Donaldson, to assess the issues raised by stem cell research and research cloning. In its 2000 report, the Doanldson Committee recommended that the categories of licensed research covered by the Human Fertilisation and Embryology Act should be extended to include embryonic stem cell research and research cloning.[21] (See chapter 2.) It emphasized that such research should be subjected to rigorous scientific and ethical review. In addition, it declared that stem cell research should be conducted primarily with embryos remaining after the completion of IVF treatment but that the generation of embryos for research by means of somatic cell nuclear transfer (cloning) should also be allowed when necessary to develop treatments for patients who needed immunologically compatible stem cells. The Donaldson Committee contended that the "slippery slope" argument—that allowing research cloning would be a first step down a precipitous path toward reproductive cloning—was not realistic because of the stringent controls over the licensing of research on human embryos that would be imposed on researchers in the U.K.

The government accepted the Donaldson Report, and in 2001 Parliament amended the Human Fertilisation and Embryology Act to bring stem cell research and research cloning within the regulatory scope of the HFEA. It expanded the indications for human embryonic stem cell research and wrote a permissive approach to research cloning into law. Yet it also enacted strict regulations to govern research cloning. There was some opposition to this expansion of the act, but it was not sufficient to overcome the majority position that the government held in Parliament. No one can conduct stem cell research in the U.K. without a license from the HFEA. Investigators must obtain a license from this agency if they plan to generate embryos for stem cell research and to derive pluripotent stem cells from donated embryos. The HFEA will not grant a license for such research if it is not satisfied that the use of an embryo is necessary and that the embryo will be used for no other purpose.

In 2001, the Pro-Life Alliance, an antiabortion organization, challenged this amendment to the Human Fertilisation and Embryology Act in court, claiming that the act's definition of an "embryo" did not include an organism created by somatic cell nuclear transfer. It reasoned that because of this definitional lacuna, both research and reproductive cloning were not covered by the act and were completely unregulated in the United Kingdom. Some argued that the alliance had brought this claim in hopes of forcing a full parliamentary debate about research and reproductive cloning that would result in the prohibition of both.[22] The claim of the alliance was denied on appeal. To make the prohibition of human reproductive cloning in the U.K. crystal clear, Parliament passed the Human Reproductive Cloning Act in 2001, in which it expressly banned cloning human embryos for reproductive purposes.[23]

Current State of Stem Cell Research in the U.K.

The government in the U.K. is keenly aware of the research and therapeutic potential of stem cell research and, spurred on by competition from such other research hubs as the bond-financed center developing in California (See chapter 7), is marshalling its financial forces in order to excel in the field of stem cell research. At the end of 2005, it increased its funding of this research from the equivalent of $85 million to $170 million.[24] A government-appointed U.K. Stem Cell Initiative recommended that the country spend at least the equivalent of $1 billion on this research between 2006 and 2015. The U.K. Stem Cell Foundation, a nonprofit organization, has set out to raise a significant sum of money to augment government funding for stem cell research.[25] Since 2001, the HFEA has approved of research projects that have resulted in well over thirty-five human embryonic stem cell lines.[26]

As of this writing, licenses to carry out research cloning as a part of embryonic stem cell research have been granted to investigators at two British centers, Newcastle University and the Roslin Institute in Edinburgh. In May 2005, Alison Murdoch and her colleagues in Newcastle announced that they had developed the country's first cloned human embryos for research purposes.[27] (See chapter 2.) However, the cloned embryos did not last long enough to allow the investigators to derive stem cells from them.

In March 2003, the House of Lords allowed the licensing of parthenogenesis, a technique that involves stimulating unfertilized eggs to develop into an early embryo without the use of sperm, for research purposes.[28] (See chapter 2.) A few months later, the HFEA granted a license to the Roslin Institute to create human embryos for stem cell research by means of this technique. Clearly, the United Kingdom plans to be on the cutting edge of stem cell research and is open to the use of novel techniques that promise to produce new sources of stem cell lines.

U.K. Stem Cell Bank

In 2004, the United Kingdom established the world's first stem cell bank as the major source of stem cell lines for researchers around the world. The National Institute for Biological Standards and Control, which administers the bank, received the equivalent of $4 million over three years, three-quarters from the Medical Research Council and one-quarter from the Biotechnology and Biological Sciences Research Council.[29]

The Stem Cell Bank will provide scientists in the U.K. and abroad with shared access to "ethically sourced, quality controlled human stem cell lines from all sources (adult, fetal and embryonic) on a single site" for research on a noncommercial basis.[30] Not only is the bank a repository for stem cell lines, but it also disseminates research findings and best practices, undertakes research on the characterization of stem cells, carries out safety testing of these cells, and develops methods for their preservation.[31]

Those donating stem cell lines to be stored at the bank must demonstrate that they have obtained informed consent for the generation and
use of those lines. Researchers seeking access to stem cell lines must
document that their research project has been approved by a research
ethics board before any lines are released to them. Scientists at the bank
have been characterizing human embryonic stem cell lines made available to them from around the world and developing rigorous standards
to ensure that they are of good quality.

Future Outlook for Stem Cell Research in the U.K.

No doubt the U.K. is eager to maintain its position at the forefront of
stem cell research throughout the world. The country has a tradition
of openness to scientific innovation and biotechnological change; the
current cultural climate is one of technological optimism. The government of the U.K. is also mindful of the economic opportunities offered
by such innovative scientific areas as stem cell research and has
provided significant financial support for this research in hopes of
reaping its potential economic benefits.

In political terms, a broad coalition of government, scientific, patient
advocacy, Church of England, and biotechnology forces that had
supported the 1990 Human Fertilisation and Embryology Act also
favored the extension of that law to embryonic stem cell research and
research cloning. Antiabortion and religious groups within the country
that had opposed the earlier law were weakened in the interim between
these laws by infighting and lack of public support and were therefore
not able to mount much of a fight against the legalization of this
research. Polls taken in 2005 to ascertain the views of Britons regarding
human embryo research indicate that approximately 75 percent of
those surveyed support it.[32]

In effect, the Warnock Report set the subsequent terms of debate
about research on human embryos, stem cell research, and research
cloning in the U.K.—and, indeed around the world. It allowed the
government to adopt a permissive approach to embryonic stem cell
research and research cloning, as well as to sanction the use of parthenogenesis. The country has developed a strict but research-friendly
regulatory environment for stem research in the sense that it allows
wide scope to this research, but it requires that anyone in the country
who plans to pursue stem cell research must obtain a license from
the HFEA. This regulatory agency has developed detailed requirements for such licensing and carries out follow-up monitoring of
laboratories around the country to ensure that these requirements are
met. Centers for research in regenerative medicine have spring up at

several locations with government financial assistance. Moreover, some stem cell scientists have immigrated into the U.K. from countries with more restrictive stem cell research policies in order to pursue this form of scientific investigation. The country plans to continue to invest considerable resources and funds into its endeavor to retain its place as a leading global stem cell pioneer.

Stem Cell Research in Germany

Germany has a strong scientific tradition. German scientists, for instance, played a significant role in the inception and growth of modern embryology and developmental and cell biology.[33] The country's outstanding reputation in these and other scientific fields would lead observers to suppose that it would eagerly adopt new forms of scientific endeavor such as stem cell research. However, Germany's history in the first part of the twentieth century has made many within the country extremely wary of the possible misuse of its scientific capabilities. Because of the horrific Nazi experiments carried out in the name of science and the eugenic health of the German people, many citizens are leery of reproductive and genetic interventions that aim to alter the natural course of human development, even for therapeutic ends.[34] Kathrin Braun explains that the German social ethos, "which is derived from the historical experience of the Nazi crimes, incorporates a common will not to be the sort of people who distinguish between a life worth living and a life not worth living."[35] Although embryonic stem cell research does not pose an obvious eugenic threat within Germany, it raises concerns among the German public about the devaluation of early human life. To sanction the destruction of human life at any stage of growth in the course of a scientific investigation, for many within the country, is to repeat the sins of the past.

Germany therefore bans the creation of human embryonic stem cells solely for research within its borders. However, it allows stem cell investigators to import human embryonic stem cells from other countries for use within Germany within certain limits and oversees research conducted on such cells within its borders.

Nazism, Eugenics, and the German Constitution

To understand the current German approach to stem cell research, it is imperative to recall some of its recent history. Although many in Germany immediately after World War II were reluctant to acknowledge the crimes of the Nazi regime, this silence had lifted by the 1960s.

A collective memory of the Nazi eugenic program, which had encompassed the involuntary sterilization of the mentally ill and monstrous forms of human experimentation, led postwar Germans to feel a deep aversion to the use of medical science to control reproduction and to manipulate the bodies of human beings.[36] Eric Brown observes, "Shame for the German past was seen as the basis for a new German society. 'Never Again' became the rallying cry of a new generation of German social democrats."[37] Revulsion against the abuses of the Nazi regime was the key force behind the stem cell research policy developed in Germany.[38]

Postwar Germans felt that it was imperative to restore the shattered notion of human dignity to national thought. Therefore, the 1949 German constitution (*Grundgesetz* or Basic Law), which was designed to be a bulwark against the return of Nazism to that country, includes a specific call to recognize human dignity. Article 1 declares that "the dignity of man is inviolable. To respect and protect it shall be the duty of all public authority."[39] The constitution recognizes the sanctity of human life in affirming the right to life of every human being. That same right to life also inheres in implanted embryos and fetuses, it holds.[40]

Perception of the Moral Significance of Human Embryos

The issue of abortion had brought into the open a conflict between the constitutional right to life of embryos and fetuses and the right of every person to "free development of personality" enunciated in Article 2 of the Grundgesetz. Those who emphasized claims of human dignity were aligned against those who upheld the moral autonomy of individuals, particularly the right of pregnant women to personal and bodily self-determination. The German courts ultimately decided that the right to "free development of personality" of pregnant women should prevail and held that a woman who would face a serious threat to her life and health if she were to continue a pregnancy, had been raped, would have a child with severe anomalies, or was in a "general situation of need," could have an abortion during the first trimester.[41] Criminalizing all abortions in order to uphold the right to life of embryos and fetuses, the courts and legislature reasoned, would drive women to obtain illegal abortions rather than to seek counseling that could protect fetuses by convincing these women to continue their pregnancies.[42]

This mixed approach to abortion and to the moral significance of the embryo was reflected in the views that German citizens tended to adopt regarding research on human embryos. The practice of IVF, which involves the development and use of such embryos for reproduction, came to Germany in the 1980s and expanded fairly rapidly. However, when it came to public attention that embryos outside a woman's body in excess of reproductive needs were being used for research, this created a significant stir that focused on the dignity and right to life of extracorporeal embryos.[43] A coalition of feminists, members of the Green Party, and Christian groups called on the government to protect embryos from "abuse, instrumentalization, and destruction." They expressed a fear of a loss of significant societal values and argued that Germany had a duty to be cautious about the uses of embryos because of its history.[44] Although the German public was willing to tolerate a policy that allowed abortion when the right of a woman to "free development of personality" was at issue, when research on human embryos outside a woman's body, which does not involve such a right, was at stake, it tended to maintain that the right to life of the embryo should prevail.

This latter view was reinforced by what came to be known as the "Singer Affair." In the 1980s, interest in ethics in medicine and bioethics was increasing in Germany, and in June 1989, Peter Singer was invited there to give a lecture at a conference on "Bioengineering, Ethics, and Mental Retardation." Singer had published a book, *Practical Ethics*, in which he argued that we should maximize the preferences of rational, self-conscious beings, whom he labeled as "persons," regardless of their species. (See chapter 3.) In his view, to be a human being is not necessarily to be a "person," since some humans are not self-conscious and rational and therefore are not "persons."[45] Disabled newborns are among these nonpersons, Singer maintained. Therefore, such infants do not have a right to life, and parents concerned about their suffering should be legally able to request active euthanasia for them, he argued.

News of the invitation to Singer to speak in Germany led to fierce protests by disability rights advocates, members of the Green Party, and feminists. They argued that Singer would begin a push down a slippery slope within Germany toward the extermination of certain groups of human beings—a slope with terrible precedents in German history. They demanded that the invitation to him be withdrawn, and it was. Other lectures by Singer were canceled or disrupted by shouting so that he could not speak; violence broke out at some of them, and he was physically assaulted by angry demonstrators. In the aftermath of the Singer Affair, public debate in Germany increasingly centered on the issue of the moral protection owed to early human life, and dissident voices were subdued.[46]

Development of Stem Cell Research Policy

In 1990, with little opposition, the Bundestag passed the Embryo Protection Act, which gives human embryos the same legal rights as fully developed humans.[47] It prohibits nontherapeutic embryo research, egg donation, germline interventions, human cloning (both reproductive and research or therapeutic), and the creation of human-nonhuman chimeric embryos. Furthermore, it outlaws attempts to fertilize more eggs than can be transferred to a woman in one in vitro fertilization cycle. Consequently, there can be no "surplus" embryos in Germany. This embryo research policy is one of the most restrictive in the world.

Adoption of this law precipitated an even more ardent public debate about the moral consideration owed to human embryos, a debate that is still being pursued.[48] To some, the Embryo Protection Act unjustifiably limits scientific research that could serve significant therapeutic purposes and relieve the suffering of many. Some members of the Bundestag and some investigators at medical research institutes have pointed out the need to respect individual choice, as well as the constitutional guarantee of scientific freedom, in arguing that this legislation is misguided.[49] Others have responded that to manipulate human embryos in research threatens the very nature of human beings.

To Christian opponents, particularly those in the Roman Catholic and Lutheran churches, the pursuit of research that is not beneficial to human embryos wrongly challenges the sanctity of human life. To secular critics, embryo research denigrates the common ethos of honoring human dignity and solidarity that lies at the heart of German postwar society. Both opposition groups see the conflict as one between scientific and economic interests that are eager to exploit new biotechnologies and popular antieugenic forces that, they say, have learned the lessons of history about the good society.[50]

In the spring of 2001, Germany's research funding agency, the Deutsche Forschungsgemeinschaft (DFG), which has a high degree of autonomy, proposed allowing embryonic stem cell research to proceed within the country using stem cells imported from abroad.[51] This policy, it pointed out, would not violate the Embryo Protection Act, since that law prohibits research on human embryos, not embryonic stem cells. The DFG observed that this proposal required weighing the constitutional right to life of embryos against the constitutional guarantee of freedom of research found in Article 5. Such balancing, it found, could result in a decision to proceed with embryonic stem cell research using imported stem cells if that research were directed toward goals with high priority.[52] The DFG cited the legal concept of comity, which maintains that there is a presumption that decisions taken in other countries are acceptable; this presumption, however, can be overcome if the regulations or laws of other countries contradict those of one's own country. Since the derivation of human embryonic stem cells is lawful in certain other countries, the agency argued, there is a presumption that importing human embryonic stem cells from those countries should be allowed and that presumption, it maintained, should stand.[53] The DFG also recommended that if imported embryonic stem cells proved insufficient for achieving the intended research goals, the option of allowing German scientists to derive embryonic stem cells from human embryos within the country should remain open.

Two national commissions considered the guidelines proposed by the DFG and offered conflicting recommendations about whether to proceed with embryonic stem cell research using stem cells imported from abroad. The Bundestag decided that a consultation process was needed on this issue, and in March 2001, it established a Study Commission on Law and Ethics in Modern Medicine (Enquete-Kommission, "Ethik und Recht in der modernen Medizin"). This commission was composed of thirteen members of the Bundestag and thirteen experts from such fields as ethics, theology, and the sciences. In November 2001, it recommended against allowing human embryonic stem cells to be brought into the country for research. Meanwhile, a second advisory body established by Chancellor Gerhard Schröder in May 2001, the National Ethics Council (Nationaler Ethikrat), which was (and is) composed of scientists, theologians, legal experts, business executives, and philosophers, recommended in favor of importing these cells.[54]

The debate about the DFG proposal set Germany's president and chancellor, who were political allies, against one another. President Johannes Rau asserted in a speech that "certain possibilities and plans of biotechnology and genetic engineering run contrary to fundamental values of human life." He raised the specter of Nazism, warning that "no one should forget what happened in the academic and research fields" in Germany during World War II. "An uncontrolled scientific community did research for the sake of its scientific aims, without any moral scruples." In response, Chancellor Schröder defended stem cell research, declaring that "the ethics of healing and of helping deserve just as much respect as the ethics of creation." He maintained that embryonic stem cell research should not be banned but should proceed on a limited basis.[55] However, Schröder's view had only modest support within the Bundestag. There was no established legacy of embryo research in the country and no broad coalition of scientists, patient advocacy groups, biotechnology associations, and state religious bodies to argue in favor of this research, as there was in the U.K. at this time.

After intense debate about the conclusions of these commissions, the Bundestag passed the Stem Cell Act in January 2002.[56] This law enacts a restrictive stem cell research policy that allows investigators to import embryonic stem cells from abroad only if their research cannot be carried out with alternative sources, such as human adult stem cells or animal cells. Taking a cue from the U.S. policy established by President Bush, the Stem Cell Act requires that investigators demonstrate that the imported embryonic stem cells were derived before January 1, 2002, from embryos that were created for reproductive purposes but ultimately were not needed for this end. Scientists who break this or the earlier 1990 Embryo Protection Act face a fine of more than the equivalent of $60,000 and up to three years of imprisonment. The law also criminalizes cooperation with scientists in other countries who use stem cell lines derived after the German cutoff date. It establishes a national commission to review all proposals to import embryonic stem cells for research and determine which would be approved. The DFG issued guidelines for research on these stem cells in January 2002.

This policy leaves Germany in the peculiar position of prohibiting any manipulations of human embryos that are detrimental to those embryos within the country while allowing research on human embryonic stem cells within the country that have been derived elsewhere through the destruction of those embryos. Two German commentators explain the reasoning behind this policy:

> Utilizing the cells is viewed as not being tantamount to a moral approval of the destruction of human life required for the sourcing of the cells and, therefore, not being in conflict with human dignity. Still, those ES cell lines are acknowledged to be the result of fundamental moral wrongdoing and, therefore, caution has to be employed with regard to the utilization of these cells.[57]

One of the coauthors of the motion for accepting the Stem Cell Act explained that "we cannot cancel" the fact that embryos were already killed for existing cell lines.[58] Since the damage had already been done, she implied, it was ethically acceptable to gain some benefit from it after the fact. "At least no new embryos will die," a member of the Green Party declared.[59] Another said, "Things have changed and that is reality. You can't be against reality."[60] A common reaction of those who had urged that this research should proceed under a less restrictive standard was that the Stem Cell Act wrongfully establishes a double ethical standard, allowing others to destroy embryos that it is considered unethical for German scientists to destroy. This, they maintain, is hypocritical.[61]

Future Outlook for Stem Cell Research in Germany

Germany's stem cell research policy is grounded in the same vision of the moral significance of the human embryo as the Bush policy in the United States: human embryos should not be destroyed in research, for they are owed all the protections accorded to living human beings. However, German policy prohibits federally funded research on stem cells that have been destroyed within its borders and criminalizes the pursuit of privately funded stem cell research by any German researcher within the country or outside the country under almost all circumstances. Germany comes as close to banning embryonic stem cell research as it can—without actually doing so. Although the stem cell research policy finally etched out in Germany leaves it with one of the most restrictive policies in the world, it does not ban this research entirely.

The Bundestag had heard arguments in favor of outlawing this research and yet did not act on them. Instead, it left a relatively narrow path along which stem cell research could proceed. Why did it do so? It is arguable that the passage of the Stem Cell Act in 2002 came at a time of softening of German attitudes toward biotechnological change and that it can be taken to signal the beginning of resistance to postwar taboos grounded in Germany's Nazi past.

Since the 1990s, the link between Nazism and the eugenic misuse of medical research, it is arguable has been weakening somewhat in Germany. In 1991, Bettina Schöne-Seifert and Klaus-Peter Rippe were among an increasingly vocal group within Germany that contended that "a deeply rooted fear of a loss of societal values—a very German argument—leads to hasty and premature legal prohibitions," among which they included the Embryo Protection Law.[62] Germans have been paying increasing attention to the promise of cutting-edge research to aid, rather than deny human freedom and to cure, rather than eliminate, those who are desperately ill.[63] Moreover, a growing interest can be detected within Germany in retaining the country's position of leadership in international scientific research and improving its economic base through the development of new biotechnologies such as stem cell research. In 2005, former Chancellor Schröder repeated his earlier call to Germany to liberalize laws restricting the use of embryonic stem cells, saying, "We must not uncouple ourselves from progress in international research in biological and genetic technology."[64] A survey conducted in that year found that over 40 percent of Germans now favored loosening restrictions on embryonic stem cell research, 30 percent opposed easing the legislation, and the remainder were undecided.[65] This suggests that there is an increasing interest in the pursuit of stem cell research within the country.

However, fewer than expected of Germany's highly regarded stem cell investigators have applied to import and use imported embryonic stem cell lines,[66] and Germany has not become a scientific powerhouse in the area of stem cell research even though it has several distinguished researchers in this and related areas. This outcome reflects the reality that despite—or perhaps because of—the weakening of the Nazi taboo, the public is confused about just what is at issue. David A. Scott, an American theologian now living in Germany, observes:

> At the deepest level, people are morally bewildered. Intelligent, well-meaning people find themselves in a pluralistic, scientific technological society, a society in which every area, from sports to arts, is increasingly run by the market mechanism. In this social context, commentators try to find a convincing politically effective, intellectually coherent way of dealing with the emerging ability and willingness to remake our biological constitution. In general, the churches and secular ethicists stand before that fact and are morally *fassungslos*—a great German word that describes bewilderment and the feeling that humans don't know how to begin to deal with this new capacity to remake ourselves.[67]

This public confusion suggests that even though the link between embryonic stem cell research and Nazism appears to be diminishing, it seems unlikely that German citizens will unite in calling for changes in the country's approach to this research in the foreseeable future. Indeed, Germany's Education and Research Minister in the administration of Chancellor Angela Merkel has reiterated her strong support for Germany's current embryonic stem cell law,[68] making it clear that the government will not recommend modifying it soon.

The question whether to relax Germany's current stem cell research policy will not be answered until those within the country respond to even more basic questions. Germany is being pushed by the potential of stem cell research to ask old ethical and metaphysical questions anew about what it is to be human and on what foundations the idea of human dignity rests. It will take more time to work out answers to these questions in ways that take account of Germany's past before any changes in its current stem cell research policy appear on the horizon.

Stem Cell Research in Japan

Japan, in contrast with Germany, but in accord with the United Kingdom, has adopted a permissive policy with regard to embryonic stem cell research and research cloning. The country provides significant public funding for the development of new stem cell lines derived from spare embryos created for reproductive purposes and from embryos created for research. In 2004, a national bioethics committee specifically approved of allowing investigators to engage in research cloning. Guidelines for stem cell research and research cloning have been developed slowly, however. All in all, Japanese stem cell investigators carry out their research in a permissive but increasingly regulated context.

Why has Japan been able to set out a policy that promotes stem cell research with relatively little discord, whereas Germany, and to a lesser extent, the United Kingdom, have reached their distinctive stem cell research policies only after heated debates? An eagerness to move forward with technological innovation, along with recognition of the economic benefits of stem cell research, has affected legislative and policy decisions regarding stem cell research in Japan, as they have in the United Kingdom. However, the basic factor explaining the lack of dissension in Japan is that its cultural framework is more homogeneous than those of the United Kingdom and Germany. The underpinnings of the Japanese worldview lie in a mixture of Buddhist and Shintoist beliefs and practices, as well as ancient social customs that, in combination, provide a widely accepted way of thinking, particularly about the human embryo. These traditional Japanese religious, social, and cultural mores have shaped the policy framework that Japan has adopted for the pursuit of human embryonic stem cell research and enabled that country to move relatively smoothly to enact legislation allowing such research.

Traditional View of the Moral Significance of Human Embryos

That human embryos might be destroyed in stem cell research represents a moral difficulty for those in Japan, but it is not same kind of moral difficulty that many in Germany and several other Western countries grapple with regarding the fate of human embryos. This difference is due to the reality that the Japanese do not conceptualize human embryos in ways that are akin to those found in Western bioethics today. That is, they do not ask whether the human embryo is a biologically separate individual human being, a potential or developing human being, or a clump of cells. The Japanese do not ponder whether embryos can have "interests," are "sentient," or have achieved "moral status." They are not given to fixing on these sorts of hard distinctions and fixed demarcations but, instead, see the world as flowing in process. Therefore they are prone to think about embryos in fluid terms.[69]

Yet they do not dismiss human embryos and fetuses as nothing. Far from it. William LaFleur observes:

> Japanese are for the most part much less ready than persons in the West to refer to an unborn fetus in terms that suggest it is something less than human or even less than sentient. The Japanese tend to avoid terms like "unwanted pregnancy" or "fetal tissue." That which develops in the uterus is often referred to as a "child"—even when there are plans to abort it.[70]

The embryo/fetus is a child that is developing within the body of a woman. The child/embryo/fetus that has died, been miscarried, or been aborted is considered still to exist by many Japanese. It is termed a *mizuko*, which means "water child" or "child of the waters," for it is regarded as suspended in water, where it is in the stages of becoming, rather than existent as a discrete embodied being.[71] It is not surprising that a people who live on islands encircled by water, as do the Japanese, envision the origin of human life as from some sort of watery substance.

The concept of the *mizuko* came into use during the Tokugawa era in Japan (1603–1867) and initially referred to a child who had died after birth.[72] However, it was gradually broadened to include an embryo/fetus that had been miscarried or aborted.[73] Once the *mizuko* died, it did not vanish. It remained a sort of spirit and dwelt in another world with the Buddhas and gods (*kami*). There it hovered over this world and related to those within it while awaiting rebirth.[74] In Japanese thought, there is a sense that the *mizuko* has been "returned" to the gods, will be formed once again, and will then return to this world.[75]

In seventeenth-century Japan, embryos/fetuses did not warrant any sort of special attention from the community. Harrison observes:

> In pre-modern Japan, it was thought that a child did not become a real "person" until some time after birth; the evidence for this lies in the many customs which distinguished a newborn baby from other "people," such as not giving it a name and not putting its arms through sleeves for a certain number of days after birth.[76]

Further, the child who died before the age of seven was usually not given a funeral, whereas those who died at an older age did receive that communal recognition.[77] Thus, at that time, infants and young children were not full members of the community and there was no sense of the loss of an individual human being that attached to aborted or miscarried embryos/fetuses.

The Japanese belief during the Tokugawa era that abortion was an acceptable practice also reveals their traditional beliefs about the moral consideration owed to the embryo/fetus. During this period, both induced abortion or *datai* ("disturbing the womb") and infanticide or *mabiki* ("clearing out space") were accepted as ways of regulating fertility. Although there is debate about whether these practices were routine or used only in times of famine, recent scholarship suggests that *mabiki* was practiced in order to preserve blood and family lines among the upper classes and to retain a desired standard of living among other classes.[78] The significant points are that abortion was not condemned on grounds that it involved the killing of a human being and that it was accepted as necessary at times.

In the nineteenth century, however, abortion began to be represented as a danger to the continuing prosperity of the family and the nation. Aborted embryos/fetuses represented a threat to familial and social well-being, for dead children continued to exist in the spirit world but often in a malevolent relationship to the living. According to one nineteenth-century block-print text, "If you 'return' [i.e. abort] your child, there will be many calamities in the family and the parents' physical condition will deteriorate from the ill will of the child."[79] Such children had to be appeased through private religious acts and the social prohibition of abortion and infanticide.

By the late nineteenth century, under the Meiji government, which had succeeded the Tokugawa shogunate, unborn fetuses, as well as living children, were viewed as extremely important to the nation. The country was entering into years of war that did not end until 1945. Soldiers were needed to fight in this war, and the government therefore actively encouraged the Japanese people to have large families to produce needed warriors.[80] For the same reason, the government adopted a policy in 1880 of increasing the population by officially banning induced abortion and infanticide.[81] After World War II, however, when military forces were decreased, there was a return to the older view that abortion is acceptable, and the practice was made legal in Japan under certain prescribed circumstances.[82] Since then, it has been used as the primary method of birth control in the country.[83]

The Japanese acceptance of abortion in much of traditional and contemporary religious and cultural thought, seems to contradict the First Precept of Buddhism, the leading religion of Japan, which declares, "I will not willingly take the life of a living thing." It is not that the Japanese believe that the embryo/fetus is "nonlife" and that the First Precept therefore does not apply to abortion.[84] It is that they do not see themselves as morally compromised by allowing abortion when it seems necessary. As LaFleur observes, "There are a lot of adjustments between the strict ethical axioms that are laid down at the base of a tradition and the moral realities of everyday life in the present. There have to be. And these adjustments that take place 'in between' *are*, in

fact the tradition."[85] Abortion is considered acceptable and even necessary to preserve a woman's health, to space children, and to avoid
falling into poverty, among other circumstances. Yet it is not carried
out with total disregard of the embryo/fetus. Japanese culture has long
evinced a concern about the effect of spirits of the dead.[86] This concern,
as noted above, came to extend to children and embryos/fetuses, who,
although dead, were viewed as in a continuing relationship with the
living.[87]

In the 1970s, a practice began of caring specifically for aborted and
miscarried embryos/fetuses through Buddhist religious ceremonies ded-
icated to them. A ritual known as the *mizuko kuyō* developed as a
memorial service for the embryo/fetus or child that had been aborted,
had miscarried, or was stillborn. The ceremony persists today. Its
object is to appeal to the deities for the well-being of the dead *mizuko*
through spiritual practices that hasten its way to a felicitous rebirth and
that communicate regret to it and to the deities for its loss.[88] Part of the
ritual refers back to the premodern belief that the embryo/fetus is
wandering through the spiritual world intent on *tatari*, or retribution
for having been evicted from its body. To appease it and render it a
benevolent influence, women and their relatives give offerings.[89] However, this ceremony does not necessarily indicate that women who have
had an abortion believe that they made a moral mistake in doing so.
Abortion continues to be considered regrettable, but at times necessary,
and *mizuko kuyō* provides a way of coping with this spiritually and
psychologically.

Thus, a belief that it is always wrong to destroy the embryo/fetus is
not inherent in Japanese traditional beliefs. Moreover, Japanese law
gives no special protection to the embryo/fetus.[90] Consequently, there
are no cultural or legal barriers to the pursuit of embryonic stem cell
research in Japan. Yet the destruction of the *mizuko* is not accepted
without regret, and attempts are made to ameliorate the situation into
which the embryo/fetus has been thrust by its destruction. As a result,
there is still an undercurrent of hesitation about the pursuit of embryonic stem cell research in Japan.

Attitudes toward Eugenics

Just before it entered World War II, Japan passed the National Eugenics Law of 1940, which aimed to repopulate the country with genetically
healthy Japanese stock to ensure that Japan would remain strong.[91]
The government's slogan was "Give Birth and Increase the Population" (*Umeyō, fuyaseyō*)—a population that had to be of good quality.

The law allowed abortion for two reasons: to eliminate embryos/fetuses with deleterious genes and to save the life of the pregnant woman.

After World War II, the government aimed to stabilize the population, rather than to increase it, and passed a revised version of the 1940 law entitled the Eugenics Protection Law of 1948. This statute broadened the conditions under which women could undergo abortion to include pregnancies caused by rape and, curiously, those initiated in families with leprosy. In 1949, an additional condition was added under which abortion was allowed in cases in which the continuation of a pregnancy would significantly harm a woman's health for either physical or economic reasons.[92] The result was a liberal abortion law. In 1996, this law was amended to eliminate the eugenic articles, and its title was changed to "Mother's Body Protection Law."[93]

This law was originally enacted to increase the population and keep it racially homogenous rather than to assure the fate of human embryos. As Shinryo Shinagawa observes, "almost nothing is written on the embryo and the fetus" in the act.[94] The Japanese had only opened a window to the West in the late nineteenth century and were still somewhat leery of including those who did not fit their racial profile within the community. Consequently, this and other laws did not stand in the way of the development of stem cell research, as did the Embryo Protection Act of 1990 in Germany, and Japan moved forward with this research without legal repercussions.

Laws and Guidelines for Embryonic Stem Cell Research and Research Cloning

No major country in modern history has been free of the misuse of human subjects in research, and Japan is no exception. It conducted egregious research programs before and during World War II in which human subjects were severely abused and subjected to unethical experiments.[95] A decision was made by the American Army command in postwar Japan to grant the Japanese scientists involved in these experiments immunity from prosecution in order to cover up certain similar experimental practices in which the United States had been involved.[96] The Japanese government also kept its experimental abuses hidden; these experiments have not been publicized within Japan or abroad. Consequently, the Japanese people have been unaware of them and have not been as motivated as the German people, who did learn about experimental abuses of human subjects that took place in their country during World War II, to face their past and ensure that no such heinous manipulations of human beings in horrific experiments would ever occur again.

Despite its secrecy about past unethical experimentation, Japan has taken pains to carry out stem cell research according to established canons of medical ethics. It did not allow human embryonic stem cell research to proceed until it had established careful oversight measures for this research. These were put into effect in 2001 when the government's key science policy organization, the Council for Science and Technology, released a set of guidelines for this research that had been developed by a Subcommittee of Human Embryo Research of the Bioethics Committee.[97] These guidelines endorse a permissive policy toward research on human embryonic stem cells, allowing it to proceed using stem cells derived from surplus embryos remaining after IVF treatments have ended.[98] They require donor consent, as well as prior review and approval by an institutional review board. Moreover, they prohibit human reproductive cloning. These guidelines apply to both publicly and privately funded research.

Later in 2001, the legislature enacted these recommendations into the Law Concerning Regulation Relating to Human Cloning Techniques and Other Similar Techniques, which permits stem cell research on surplus embryos and requires guidelines for the creation of embryos for research.[99] Article 1 of the law states that reproductive cloning "could have a severe influence on preservation of human dignity, safety for human life and body, and maintenance of social order," and the law therefore prohibits it. It also bans the generation of hybrid embryos (produced by inserting a human cell into an enucleated animal egg or an animal cell into an enucleated human egg) and the generation of chimeric embryos (produced by fusing early human and animal embryonic cells). A breach of this law is criminally punishable by up to ten years' imprisonment and a fine of about the equivalent of $93,000.[100]

The legal framework in Japan incorporates ongoing review of the regulations governing stem cell research. Accordingly, in 2003, a Japanese bioethics panel recommended that, in addition to acquiring institutional review board approval for embryonic stem cell research, such research proposals should also pass muster with an oversight body that resembles the HFEA in the U.K.[101] However, the bioethics panel had greater difficulty in reaching agreement about accepting and regulating the pursuit of research cloning. It released an interim report in 2003 that revealed that half of its members supported research cloning, while the other half supported either a full ban or temporary suspension of such research. Among members of the public who responded to the committee's request for comments, in contrast, 64 percent favored research cloning.[102] In June 2004 the bioethics panel, apparently moved by public opinion, set aside its internal divisions and recommended approval of research cloning by a vote of ten to five, and the

Japanese Council for Science and Technology Policy, chaired by Prime Minister Junichiro Koizumi, subsequently approved of this report in July 2004.[103]

Attitudes toward Biotechnology and Economic Growth

Japan has been more receptive to scientific, medical, and biotechnological endeavors—stem cell research in particular—than Germany since World War II. A significant majority of Japanese respondents indicated in polls over the last decade that they overwhelmingly (in the range of 95–98 percent) favor the pursuit of science and technology.[104] This openness to technological advancement included the development of human embryonic stem cell research. However, 41 percent of respondents indicated that they were very worried about the possible use of reproductive cloning. There is a sense in Japan, as there is in Germany and in many other nations, that the use of this form of cloning would in some sense diminish human beings.

The perception of biotechnology as a powerful stimulus of economic growth is pervasive in Japan.[105] The government has invested handsomely in two centers, the RIKEN Center for Developmental Biology in Kobe and the Frontier Institute of Biomedical Research at Kyoto University, which are designed to be the premier research institutes in regenerative medicine in the country. Investigators at these centers are pursuing fundamental research into the differentiation and application of a wide variety of cells from embryonic stem cells. In 2003, researchers at Kyoto University produced the first Japanese human embryonic stem cell line from one of ten frozen human embryos.[106] Since then, the same researchers have developed at least three more lines.[107] Moreover, biotech companies in Japan that are focused on stem cell research are attracting support from those seeking to invest in this promising area of scientific research.[108]

Future Outlook for Stem Cell Research in Japan

Japanese culture has not been shaped by historical factors that would lead to skepticism about engaging in stem cell research and research cloning. No organized pro-life lobby, feminist movement, or Green Party exists in Japan, as was the case in Germany, to press legislators to ban embryonic stem cell research. The forces that support and oppose these forms of research did not become involved in a public brouhaha, and the Diet did not have to negotiate between rival interests and concerns in the debate about stem cell research. Consequently, Japanese stem cell research policy, by and large, was not forged through extensive negotiations, as it was in Germany and to a lesser extent in the United Kingdom.

Furthermore, Japan, unlike Germany, did not emerge from its wartime experiences with grave misgivings about possible misuses of biotechnology and medical science. As a result, the country is more open to the benefits of biotechnology than is Germany. The Japanese people see the pursuit of scientific research as important to the maintenance of a robust economy. In short, Japan brought an historical and cultural perspective to the question of whether to engage in stem cell research that exhibited a legislative and popular openness to the pursuit of this research.

Japan has therefore adopted a permissive approach to stem cell research. Its laws and regulations regarding stem cell research are considerably less restrictive than those developed in Germany and draw from the British guidelines in many respects. Its use of guidelines, as in the U.K., allows for flexible regulation of this research while setting out specific monitoring, regulation, and ethical requirements that investigators within the country must meet that are reminiscent of those in the U.K. However, a recent report suggests that the Japanese oversight establishment is still somewhat hesitant to allow human embryonic stem cell research to proceed. In this report, leading Japanese stem cell investigators claim that overzealous institutional review boards have been much slower to make decisions about their research protocols than the equivalent boards in other countries. Curiously, one researcher said that these Japanese boards, "want to know exactly how important you think the cells are; it's as if they have a soul."[109] This observation provides a hint that the traditional view that the *mizuko* that has been destroyed is alive in another world where it will need to be tended to, and even assuaged, still lingers in Japan. The Japanese science ministry indicates that it is attempting to improve the institutional review board system so that it will carry out its reviews more rapidly.

Major Issues in Stem Cell Research Policy Faced in Common by the U.K., Germany, and Japan

The historical, cultural, religious, and political differences among the U.K., Germany, and Japan are striking. Therefore, it is not surprising that even though they have faced some of the same ethical and policy issues, they have responded to them in different ways with somewhat different rationales. But it is somewhat surprising that, despite their differing answers to the same questions, two of these countries, the U.K. and Japan, have adopted stem cell research policies that are remarkably alike and that Germany, a world leader in science, would abdicate that role and allow other countries to move ahead of it in the case of stem cell research. These observations call for a concluding look at the ways in which these countries have broached several significant questions related to the development of human embryonic stem cell research policy.

The question of the moral consideration owed to the human embryo has been an issue of concern in all three countries. Yet it is framed in different ways in each and this has affected the ways in which government policies with regard to stem cell research have been reached and justified in them. Both the U.K. and Germany devoted considerable time to legislative and public debates about this question; Japan did so to a lesser extent, for it is more inclined to have such decisions made at the upper levels of government with limited public input.

In the U.K., the view that emerged was that, while early embryos are owed respect, this must be balanced against the benefits of stem cell research. These benefits, according to the prevailing view in Parliament and among the public, overcome the moral weight of such embryos. The government therefore concluded that embryonic stem cell research should proceed.

In Germany, in contrast, a coalition of forces sought to protect human embryos. Some among them regarded human embryos as human beings on the basis of religious beliefs, while others maintained that destruction of human embryos would fly in the face of environmental and feminist concerns. Their mutual understanding of the human embryo as besieged and in need of protection from overzealous researchers was linked to a historical sense that if biotechnology were not reined in, it would run rampant in the country, leaving some—be they embryos or born human beings—dead and others injured for life. The view of this coalition prevailed, and a highly restrictive stem cell research policy was enacted in Germany primarily on the basis of the prevalent view of the moral and social significance of early human embryos.

This was not the case in Japan. Although the traditional view considers the human embryo to be a spirit child in some sense, it is a child that at times may regretfully be destroyed for the good of others. However, such destruction is not forever. This child will be reborn in the future and will have the opportunity to live a full life. Therefore, the stem cell research policy adopted in Japan, which seems to be affected by this traditional view, allows the destruction of human embryos in research that might provide scientific and therapeutic innovations. Even so, there are hints that there is some resistance to this policy among some in Japan who are mindful of the import of the *mizuko* in traditional Japanese thought and that stem cell research is being slowed down in practice, although not in policy, as a result.

Another major difference between these countries lies in their attitudes toward the employment of scientific endeavors to foster their country's economic health. The U.K. and Japan are quite open to the use of biotechnological innovation as an engine of economic progress and are actively pursuing stem cell research in order to move ahead in economic development. However, they consider it important to establish regulations and guidelines for stem cell research and are keen to ensure that those carrying it out are licensed and monitored. Their embrace of biotechnological and economic growth is not unlimited.

Germany, in contrast, is much more skeptical about using this research as a tool to bolster its economy. Economic power, it has maintained, should not be purchased at the cost of runaway science. It is also skeptical about the use of biotechnology to improve humankind, concerned that this might lead it into a new form of eugenics. Here, too, its history during the Nazi era when science was misused to bolster wrongful social goals hovers in the background. As a result, it allows some embryonic stem cell research to proceed—but under heavily regulated and monitored conditions.

International Stem Cell Research Policies and the Possibility of Rapprochement

Given that Germany has developed a highly restrictive stem cell research policy, while the U.K. and Japan have carved out more permissive policies, and that countries around the world that engage in stem cell research have adopted widely varying stem cell research policies, is there any hope that they will eventually overcome their differences and develop one international policy governing this research? The outlook is not promising. International attempts to harmonize policies in the area of biomedical ethics and human research, such as those of the Council of Europe and the United Nations, have not triggered global agreement about issues relating to stem cell research and research cloning. Yet there is some movement toward international accord with regard to stem cell research and science policy more broadly.

The Ethics Working Group of the International Stem Cell Forum, composed of nineteen members from seventeen countries, aims to clarify ethical issues and, where possible, harmonize ethical standards internationally.[110] It also seeks to share stem cell lines and develop an agreement on standards for the characterization and registration of stem cell lines. The working group, which carries out ongoing studies of the stem cell research policies of fifty countries, has concluded that, despite their differences, there are some common principles and professional norms that these countries share that may eventually provide a framework for an international approach to stem cell research.

The Hinxton Group, composed of sixty participants from fourteen countries, met in 2006 and produced a set of principles to guide stem cell research across nations.[111] One of the principles it enunciated is that restrictions on stem cell research should be rare, justified, and flexible so that changes in this area of research can be accommodated rapidly. In addition, the group maintained that scientists should be free to pursue research that is banned in their own country elsewhere, apparently in an effort to change current policy in countries such as Germany. In effect, the report reflects a permissive approach that leaves out of the remit of its principles those countries that take a restrictive or a moderate approach. It is unlikely that such countries would sign on to this report. It also seems unlikely that the Hinxton group's report would lead to international agreement on a regulatory framework for this research because of significant differences among nations regarding how rapidly and vigorously human embryonic stem cell research should proceed that are grounded in their different histories, cultural traditions, religious and ethical values, degrees of technological optimism, and attitudes toward economic development.

Yet, as the Ethics Working Party of the International Stem Cell Forum, the Hinxton Group, and others rightly point out, it is essential eventually to adopt common scientific and ethical standards for stem cell research and research cloning in order to protect the health, safety, and rights of research subjects and patients around the globe.[112] As stem cell research develops in various parts of the world, there will be increasing cooperation among scientists in those nations that embrace it. They will exchange information about research design, results, materials, and personnel. It is important that they also share information and reach agreement about such patient-centered issues as the need for ethical standards for informed consent for embryo and gamete donation and for the transfer of stem cells to patients in therapy. Issues with ethical implications, such as those of quality control of embryonic stem cells, privacy, and financial conflicts of interest, among others, will need to be addressed in the policies of many nations that pursue stem cell research in mutually compatible ways. To protect research subjects and, ultimately, patients who receive stem cell therapies, it is imperative that countries engaging in this research aim to develop common scientific and ethical standards for its pursuit, even in the face of significant historical, cultural, religious, economic, and other differences.

7

The Development of National Policy on Stem Cell Research in the United States

Stem cell research was being carried out in a fairly low-key way by scientists in various parts of the world until 1998, when news of the isolation and cultivation of human embryonic stem cells burst onto the national scene. Public, scientific, and legislative interest in this novel and promising research surged immediately around the world. The question whether it should proceed with federal support in the United States became the subject of explosive debate in the halls of Congress and among members of antiabortion groups and patient advocacy organizations, as well as the general public.

President William J. Clinton responded affirmatively to this question and was poised to allow federal funding of research with human embryonic stem cells when the George W. Bush administration came into office in 2000. The new president initiated a more restrictive policy regarding such research than the Clinton administration had planned, allowing it to proceed with federal funding on a limited number of human embryonic stem cell lines. Bush continued to provide federal support for research on adult stem cells and stem cells found in umbilical cords, placental blood, and bone marrow.

As a consequence, the United States today finds itself in a peculiar position with regard to stem cell research. It places strict limits on funding provided by the federal government for human embryonic stem cell research but allows such research to proceed unimpeded in the states and the private sector. Only twenty-two stem cell lines that were created before August 2001 can be studied with federal funding. However, any and all human embryonic stem cell lines can be explored with state or private monies. In effect, it falls to the states, academic research institutions, and private corporations to decide whether to pursue a broad range of stem cell research and, if so, according to what ethical standards.

The National Research Council and the Institute of Medicine of the National Academy of Sciences (NAS) stepped in to provide guidelines that address some of the difficult ethical questions posed by human embryonic stem cell research. These guidelines have opened the door to more consistent ethical oversight of stem cell research within the states and those institutions that adopt them. Yet, with their emphasis on newly established embryonic stem cell oversight committees that may devise differing institutional standards for carrying out embryonic stem cell research, they may indirectly help to perpetuate the current national patchwork of clashing ethical guidelines for this research—and the uncertainty that comes with them.

Stem cell investigators are not clear about whether and where they can carry out this research and according to what ethical guidelines. This leaves some perplexed about whether they can set up stem cell research programs in their state without incurring civil or even criminal penalties. Moreover, charitable and commercial groups are uncertain about how the current pastiche of ethical guidelines for embryonic stem cell research developing state by state, research institution by research institution, and company by company will affect this area of medical research. Consequently, they are being cautious about investing in this research. Although some investigators and potential funders have set aside these uncertainties and have forged ahead with this research, many others have held back, waiting for the ethical and legal dust to settle.

In this chapter, I examine how and why the current collection of uncoordinated and sometimes conflicting policies regarding human stem cell research—particularly embryonic stem cell research—have emerged on the national and state levels in the United States. I give special attention to the ethical and political reasoning used by the Clinton and Bush administrations to decide whether to support this research. I then trace the varying paths that state stem cell research policies are taking as they lurch into place. I go on to consider the reaction of the business community to these national and state policies and the ways in which patent policy regarding this research is evolving. Finally, I ask whether the patchwork of policies regarding embryonic stem cell research emerging in the United States will lead to sound and ethically warranted oversight of this research or whether a national stem cell review panel is needed to provide such oversight of this research for the country.

The Clinton Stem Cell Research Policy

In 1998, when scientists first announced that they had isolated and cultured human embryonic stem cells, President Clinton directed the National Bioethics Advisory Commission (NBAC), which he had established in 1995,[1] to conduct a "review of the issues associated with...human stem cell research, balancing all ethical and medical considerations."[2] He also charged NBAC with presenting recommendations about whether to pursue human embryonic stem cell research on the national level. The commission was designed to be broadly representative of the range of views about this issue found around the country, although it is arguable that it was weighted toward what are often termed progressive and moderate views, rather than conservative ones.[3] Its members were not exclusively scientists but hailed from a variety of disciplines; the commission also included individuals garnered from among the general public.[4]

In July 1999, word leaked out that NBAC planned to recommend in its final report that federal funding should be provided not only for research on already existing human embryonic stem cells but also for the derivation of such cells from embryos in excess of clinical need remaining at IVF clinics.[5] Whether to allow the destruction of human embryos in stem cell research with federal funds, which is a necessary consequence of deriving embryonic stem cells from them, had been the subject of heated debate in Congress and among various lobbying groups ever since the 1998 announcement of the isolation of these stem cells.[6] Since it appeared that allowing embryo destruction in federally funded research would violate the Dickey-Wicker Amendment, which prohibits the use of federal funds for research in which human embryos are destroyed,[7] the Clinton administration responded cautiously. The White House issued a statement saying that no federal funding would be allocated for research to derive embryonic stem cells from human embryos for research. It added that the administration's full-fledged human embryonic stem cell research policy would be presented in future guidelines being developed at that time by the National Institutes of Health (NIH), the leading federally funded research body in the country. The administration appeared to be backing away from the reported probable recommendation from NBAC to provide federal funding of research to derive human embryonic stem cells from embryos remaining at IVF clinics because it viewed that recommendation as legally and politically perilous.

The volatile debate among members of Congress about federal funding of research on human embryonic stem cells prompted the NIH to seek a legal opinion from its General Counsel about whether the Dickey-Wicker Amendment banned the use of federal funds to conduct research on human embryonic stem cells derived through a process that involved the destruction of early human embryos. The NIH General Counsel issued an opinion in January 1999 declaring that human stem embryonic cells are not human embryos within the statutory definition.[8] An embryo is defined in the Dickey-Wicker Amendment as an organism that is capable of becoming a human being when it is implanted in the uterus, and the General Counsel reasoned that human embryonic stem cells are not organisms according to this definition, since they are not capable of becoming human beings. Therefore, she concluded, the Dickey-Wicker Amendment does not prohibit federal funding for research on human embryonic stem cells already derived from human embryos. This meant that research on human embryonic stem cells could proceed with federal funding as long as the cells themselves were derived from human embryos with private or state, rather than federal, funding.

NBAC's Report on Stem Cell Research

Meanwhile, NBAC continued its work and released its final report on stem cell research in the fall of 1999. This report specifically addressed the burning issue of the day: What sort of moral significance should be attributed to the early human embryo? The commission, perhaps influenced by the reasoning of the British Warnock report (see chapter 6), declared that it had adopted "an intermediate position, one with which many likely would agree: that the embryo deserves respect as a form of life, but not the same level of respect accorded persons."[9] In reaching this conclusion, the commission drew from an argument developed by a legal philosopher prominent in the United Kingdom and the United states, Ronald Dworkin, who maintained that the exceptions often condoned by those who hold that abortion is wrong, such as their willingness to allow abortion when the life of the pregnant woman is at stake, reveal that abortion opponents do not, in fact, maintain that the fetus is a person with a right to life.[10] His explanation for this startling conclusion was that if they did believe that the fetus has a right to life, they would find it morally imperative not to kill the fetus by means of abortion, even to save the life of the woman. Since they do not take this stance, he argued, they do not view the fetus as equivalent to a living human being.

NBAC reasoned along the same lines, maintaining that "conservatives [who] allow such exceptions implicitly hold with liberals that very early forms of human life may sometimes be sacrificed to promote the interests of other humans." Conservatives, to be logically consistent,

NBAC declared, would have to make a more general exception to their belief that the fetus and embryo have a right to life and agree that "it also is permissible to destroy embryos when it is necessary to save lives or prevent extreme suffering." NBAC concluded that "research that involves the destruction of embryos remaining after infertility treatments is permissible when there is good reason to believe that this destruction is necessary to develop cures for life-threatening or severely debilitating diseases and when appropriate protections and oversight are in place in order to prevent abuse."[11]

On the basis of this argument, the commission recommended—as had been predicted by the press—the use of federal funds for both the derivation and the use in stem cell research of embryos remaining after IVF treatment. However, NBAC set certain conditions on research using spare embryos. These included that the specific decision to discard spare embryos should be made separately from the specific decision to donate those embryos for research on grounds that "this separation will reduce the chance that potential donors could be pressured or coerced into donating their embryos for stem cell research." NBAC also maintained that buying and selling embryos should be prohibited. It further recommended against providing federal funds to create human embryos for research by means of in vitro fertilization or by somatic cell nuclear transfer (research cloning).[12]

Despite NBAC's attempt to bridge the gap between those who favored federal funding of human embryonic stem cell research and those who were opposed to such funding, its final report was greeted with mixed reviews. Not surprisingly, in many instances these broke down according to the positions already taken by respondents. Even so, NBAC's deliberations did broaden the national debate. The commission emphasized the importance in a democratic polity of grounding recommendations of a nationally constituted body in commonly accepted views and publicly shared beliefs that can be supported by reasoned argument, rather than in a single point of view or ideology held by only some within that polity.[13]

NIH Guidelines for Stem Cell Research

It took almost two years for the NIH to devise guidelines for human embryonic stem cell research; these were issued in August 2000.[14] (See appendix A.) They declared that research involving stem cells derived from human embryos could be conducted using NIH funds only if these cells had been derived from embryos that had been created for fertility treatment without the use of federal funds and were in excess of the clinical needs of those seeking this treatment. Thus, the guidelines made it clear that human embryos would not be destroyed using federal monies in the course of this research. They stated further that certain research was ineligible for NIH funding. This included research in which human embryonic stem cells were combined with animal or human embryos; were used for human reproductive cloning; were derived using somatic cell nuclear transfer (cloning); or were derived from human embryos created for research, rather than reproductive, purposes.

The NIH began to accept grant applications for research projects using human embryonic stem cells soon after publication of the guidelines. These applications were to be reviewed by the NIH Human Pluripotent Stem Cell Review Group, a new group established at the NIH to ensure compliance with its guidelines. Although the names of the members of this review group were not announced officially, newspaper stories stated that they represented a wide range of scientific, ethical, and theological expertise and opinion.[15] Once research proposals had been approved by this group, they were to go through the usual NIH review process.

The first meeting of the Human Pluripotent Stem Cell Review Group was scheduled for April 25, 2001, at which time it was to review already existing human pluripotent stem cell lines in the United States to assess whether their use in stem cell research was eligible for federal funding. However, George W. Bush had taken office as president of the United States in January 2001, and that meeting was postponed until the new administration could complete a review of the stem cell research situation.[16] The review group never met.

The Bush Stem Cell Policy

Once in office, President Bush did not make an immediate decision about whether and how to proceed with embryonic stem cell research but, instead, spent time during his first year quizzing scientists, ethicists, and religious leaders about human embryonic stem cell research and reading related materials prepared for him by his staff.[17] This year provided time for considerable speculation and intensive lobbying campaigns by various groups that either favored or opposed human embryonic stem cell research. They included secular and religious antiabortion groups opposed to what they saw as the immoral destruction of human embryos in this research and patient advocacy groups, scientific associations, still other antiabortion groups, and religious bodies that viewed embryonic stem cell research as ethically sound—indeed, ethically mandatory, according to some. Those who objected to this research reminded the president that he had run as the candidate of the pro-life community and had pledged during his campaign to oppose federal funding for research that involved the destruction of human embryos. In their appeals to the president, supporters of this research focused on the needs of those who were suffering from serious diseases, such as Alzheimer's disease and childhood diabetes, for whom this research offered immense promise.

In early July 2001, the president requested that NIH administrators provide him with an estimate of the number of stem cell lines already in existence. They initially reported back that there were thirty such lines, but then apparently found thirty more.

On August 9, 2001, in a nationally televised speech, President Bush announced that he had decided to restrict federal funding of research with human embryonic stem cells to the use of approximately sixty cell lines that were already in existence as of the date of his speech. (See appendix B.) This meant, he stated, that the federal government would not be a party to funding the destruction of human embryos, for "the life and death decision has already been made." He declared that this decision "allows us to explore the promise and potential of stem cell research without crossing a fundamental moral line, by providing taxpayer funding that would sanction or encourage further destruction of human embryos that have at least the potential for life."[18] The president also indicated that the federal government would continue to support research on stem cells derived from other sources, such as umbilical cord blood, placentas, and adult and animal tissues.[19] He did not issue an executive order in which he set out this new policy but simply announced it in a speech. No notice of this new policy was issued by the National Institutes of Health and published for public comment in the *Federal Register*, as would have been the case for new regulations set out by federal agencies. Although this left the legal status of the Bush policy in limbo, it was enforceable through the implicit threat that federal employees who did not comply with it could lose their jobs.

The guidelines for stem cell research that had been developed and published by the NIH in August 2000 were withdrawn in November 2001. (See appendix C.) Under the Bush guidelines, federal funds can only be used for research on stem cell lines that (1) have been derived with the informed consent of their donors, (2) have been obtained from embryos created for reproductive purposes prior to August 2001 that were no longer needed for such purposes, (3) have not been donated as a result of financial inducements, and (4) have not been derived from embryos created solely for research purposes.[20] (See appendix D.) Those who develop these stem cell lines are required to provide a written statement to the NIH asserting that their lines meet these conditions.

The NIH established an internal panel to implement this new policy composed of scientists affiliated with its various institutes; it includes no ethicists or community members. Apparently, it is believed that members from the latter categories are not needed, since the ethical decisions have been made by the president, and only scientific questions remain.

Ethical Justification for the Bush Policy

In his speech, President Bush took pains to avoid the charge of complicity (meaning cooperation with evil) in the destruction of early human embryos. He believed that it was wrong to engage in such destruction and therefore offered federal funding only for research on human embryonic stem cell lines existing as of August 9, 2001, for which the "life and death decision" had already been made. This policy, he claimed, drew "a fundamental moral line" in that it did not encourage the further destruction of human embryos, for it made it clear that research on human embryonic stem cell lines derived from spare embryos after the August date would not be supported with federal funds. He argued that he had adopted a policy that would not induce the destruction of additional human embryos in the future and that his administration therefore was not complicit in the destruction of early human embryos.[21]

President Bush's approach indicates that he was attempting to meet tests set by the traditional Roman Catholic theory of complicity.[22] According to this theory, cooperation with evil can be either formal or material. "Formal" cooperation involves both intending to participate in the wrongdoing of another and actively doing so. President Bush and the federal government were not complicit in the destruction of human embryos in this sense (on the assumption that it is wrong to destroy early embryos in stem cell research), for they did not intend or actively participate in such destruction. They came upon the scene after the fact of embryo destruction and allowed stem cells to be derived with federal funds only on embryos that had already been destroyed.

"Material" cooperation, in contrast, occurs when a person contributes to the wrongdoing, even though he or she does not intend to do so. Such contribution may be carried out through an action that is morally neutral or even good. The basic question raised for the president with regard to material cooperation, then, was whether the federal policy that he established would contribute to the destruction of human embryos.

To answer this question a further distinction is required between material cooperation that is immediate and that which is mediate. When material cooperation is "immediate," the person acting is directly involved in the wrongdoing. Clearly, the president and the federal government were not involved in immediate material cooperation, for they did not participate in the destruction of embryos that had occurred before August 9, 2001.

When material cooperation is "mediate," the person acting contributes to the wrongdoing of another. This contribution need not take place at the time of the other's wrongdoing, but can occur afterward. Mediate material cooperation is not always wrong; it can sometimes be justified. Whether it is justified depends on two factors: (1) whether the good sought morally outweighs the evil involved and (2) how closely linked the good to be achieved is to the evil that is committed. If the good sought morally outweighs the evil involved and the evil act is not required to achieve the good end, then it is morally acceptable to use the benefits of an evil act. In such circumstances, one is not complicit in that act.

Was the administration involved in mediate material cooperation with those who had destroyed human embryos by funding embryonic stem cell research that depended on the destruction of human embryos? That is, was the president complicit in destroying human embryos by accepting the benefits of such destruction?

With regard to factor (1) above, the question is whether the good of saving human lives and alleviating human disease and suffering is so great that it outweighs the evil of killing an innocent human being (on the presumption that the early embryo is a human being). Here the Bush policy falters on this theory of complicity, for according to the Roman Catholic moral theology from which this theory of complicity is drawn, the good of saving lives cannot outweigh the evil of killing an innocent human being, no matter how great that good is.

With regard to factor (2) above, the issue is whether there is a close and necessary relation between the destruction of human embryos and the use of embryonic stem cells. Here, too, the Bush policy does not pass muster on this theory of complicity, since the death of the embryos was essential for obtaining embryonic stem cells. Thus, there was proximity of cooperation between the destruction of human embryos and the use of stem cells derived from these embryos. Consequently, on the theory of complicity adopted by the president, the stem cell lines for which he provided research funding were ethically tainted by their origins in the deliberate destruction of embryos (on the assumption that it is wrong to destroy early embryos in stem cell research), and the president's policy made him and the federal government complicit in the destruction of human embryos through their financial support of this research.

This conclusion is confirmed by the view expressed by the Pontifical Academy for Life of the Vatican, which had addressed complicity in the context of embryonic stem cell research before President Bush enunciated his stem cell research policy. In response to the question, "Is it morally licit to use ES [embryonic stem] cells, and the differentiated cells obtained from them, which are supplied by other researchers or are commercially obtainable?" the Pontifical Academy gave the following response: "The answer is negative, since: Prescinding from the participation 'formal or otherwise' in the morally illicit intention of the principal agent, the case in question entails a proximate material cooperation in the production and manipulation of human embryos on the part of those producing or supplying them."[23] That is, those who use human embryonic stem cells derived from embryos by others at the cost of destroying those embryos materially cooperate in that destruction. They benefit from the destruction of human embryos and are therefore complicit in that destruction, according to the Pontifical Academy.

It is sufficient to establish the complicity of stem cell investigators, on this theory, that the stem cells that they use could not have existed without the destruction of embryos, even though they did not bring about this destruction. Thus, whether a policy discourages the destruction of embryos in the future, the claimed justification for the Bush human embryonic stem cell research policy, is not the defining question that establishes complicity, according to the Pontifical Academy. The moral question at issue is whether those who use human embryonic stem cells benefit from their destruction. Clearly, stem cell investigators do benefit from such destruction. Therefore, according to the Pontifical Academy's view of complicity, they are complicit in the destruction of the embryos that they use in stem cell research.

Although the Pontifical Academy's moral condemnation did not explicitly cover those who finance embryonic stem cell research, it did encompass them, for these financiers provide the material support that allows stem cell researchers to engage in their putatively complicitous acts. Richard M. Doerflinger, of the National Council of Catholic Bishops, in an article written before the Bush policy had been put into effect, used the theory of complicity to argue against federal funding of stem cell research as follows:

> Therefore, it seems clear that a government agency that funds such research is directly promoting the destruction of embryonic human life. Even if it engages in a bookkeeping exercise to allow private funds to subsidize the act of destruction itself, that act is nonetheless an integral part of the research protocol—it is a *sine qua non* for the subsequent work on stem cells.[24]

Consequently, according to the very theory of complicity adopted by President Bush, his decision to provide federal funds for embryonic stem cell lines made him and the federal government complicit in the destruction of those embryos. The president and his advisers appear to have misunderstood and misapplied the theory of complicity that they adopted and therefore to have developed a flawed ethical justification for their stem cell research policy. The theory of complicity that they adopted does not distinguish between causing a putative wrong and benefiting from the putative wrong done by another and therefore condemns those who benefit from the use of human embryos.

Significant Factors Affecting the Bush Policy Decision

Why did the president base his entire stem cell policy on this Roman Catholic theory of complicity when other interpretations of complicity have been set out in recent times in the literature?[25]

This was not just an ethically difficult decision for the president, but a politically difficult one as well. No matter which way he turned, he risked alienating voters and members of Congress. If he backed unrestricted support for embryonic stem cell research, he might well win favor with millions of people who were sick and suffering, as well as medical researchers attempting to develop treatments for them, but would alienate much of his conservative base. If he cut off all federal funding of this research, he would keep the trust of conservatives but would appear to have cast off those with serious diseases and injuries, along with those attempting to find treatments for them.

The White House had been engaging in weekly telephone conferences with U.S. Roman Catholic Church leaders who were opposed to embryonic stem cell research during the time that he was pondering a decision about the pursuit of federally funded human embryonic stem cell research.[26] The president and his staff were also in frequent touch with significant figures within the conservative Protestant movement who also condemned this research.[27] Clearly, he hoped to retain their good will and that of others who opposed human embryonic stem cell research. Yet he also needed to respond to the majority of Roman Catholic voters who had indicated in polls that they favored embryonic stem cell research and to address the concerns of many Protestant, Jewish, and Muslim voters, moderate Republicans, many Democrats, patient advocacy groups, and scientific bodies and researchers who supported it. Moreover, he had to consider the congressional front. There is some evidence that if he had banned federal funding for all human embryonic stem cell research, the Senate would have passed legislation to overrule him, sending the debate to an uncertain fate in the House.[28]

President Bush needed a theory with moral overtones that would allow him to finance some human embryonic stem cell research—but not all such research. A newspaper report of July 8, 2001, states that three leading Roman Catholic thinkers had indicated to White House staff at that time that the stem cell research policy that President Bush later adopted would be a "morally acceptable compromise" that would comport with Catholic teachings.[29] However, these thinkers later denied that they had told him this. Therefore, it is not clear whether the president and his advisors thought that the policy that he finally proclaimed fell within the strictures of those teachings.[30] This theory of complicity had been accepted either directly or indirectly by various conservative Protestant leaders,[31] and they appeared amenable to the president's interpretation of it. Therefore, it appeared that they, too, would not object to the policy that he proposed to adopt. Thus, the final Bush policy that emerged was a compromise that not only seemed acceptable to many of his major conservative religious supporters but also gave something to those on the other side of the debate by allowing some embryonic stem cell research to proceed—even though it was grounded in a misinterpretation of the very theory that was said to give the president's policy its moral basis.

Responses to the Bush Policy

This new policy stirred intense controversy.[32] Some who favored proceeding with embryonic stem cell research applauded it, since it allowed at least some human embryonic stem cell research to proceed. They maintained that there were sufficient numbers of usable embryonic stem cell lines available around the world to allow this research to move ahead rapidly. Some who opposed this research also praised the Bush policy because it discouraged the future destruction of human embryos in stem cell research.[33] Since the policy was designed as a compromise, it is not surprising that it also evoked criticism from those on both sides of the debate. Some thought that the president had not gone far enough, while others thought he had gone too far.

Criticism from supporters of embryonic stem cell research centered on concerns that the number and quality of stem cell lines approved for use would be inadequate for research. There were not sixty or more usable stem cell lines to be found throughout the world, they argued.[34] To understand the full potential of these stem cells, Douglas Melton, a stem cell investigator at Harvard University, said, scientists needed to work with cells from between 100 and 1,000 embryos.[35] In addition, those who favored pursuing this research indicated that because the approved cell lines came from relatively few donors, they offered only a small sample size for determining how individual variation in genetic makeup affects the way in which stem cell progeny differentiate. A greater number of stem cell lines that were more diverse genetically would be needed to treat patients. Further, they argued, all of the stem cell lines eligible for funding under the Bush policy had been developed in a medium using animal tissues and serum[36] and therefore might be contaminated with animal viruses and proteins that could pose significant risks to patients. (See chapter 1.) Those who favored federal funding for embryonic stem cell research also declared more broadly that the Bush policy would diminish the standing of the United States within the international scientific and biotechnology communities and undermine both medical progress and national interests. They argued that it was imperative to make a broader range of stem cell lines eligible for federal funding to avert these outcomes.

Meanwhile, some who opposed the pursuit of human embryonic stem cell research also rejected the Bush policy because it violated the traditional theory of complicity. They declared that it made the government complicit in moral wrongdoing because it allowed research to proceed on embryos that had already been destroyed. The very persons who had destroyed embryos in order to derive embryonic stem cell lines from them, they argued, were now eligible to profit from their putative evildoing by receiving federal funds for research on those cell lines. Moreover, the Bush policy, these opponents held, also made the federal government complicit in these earlier immoral acts because it encouraged and rewarded the destruction of embryos after August 9, 2001, by allowing this research to proceed with state and private funding.[37]

Effect of the Bush Policy on Subsequent Stem Cell Research

Despite these various criticisms, the Bush policy remains in place as of this writing. The NIH, as instructed, has created a registry of stem cell lines that meet the criteria set out by the president.[38] Scientists have found that the twenty-two stem cell lines available for NIH-funded research are not well characterized and somewhat unstable.[39] They indicate that these lines tend to acquire significant numbers of genetic mutations that cause them to malfunction and grow tumors.[40] (See chapter 1.) Further, it has been difficult to obtain federal funding for research on these stem cell lines. As of the end of 2003, the NIH had awarded $60 million over a three-year period for human embryonic stem cell research, whereas it had provided $345 million in one year alone for human adult stem cell research.[41] When government funding

for an area of biomedical research is scarce, this discourages researchers from entering that area and consequently limits the research carried
out in that area.

Many scientists in stem cell research and related fields continue to
maintain that the Bush policy has slowed the pace of stem cell research
in the United States and put the country behind. They observe that
scores of new embryonic stem cell lines are being developed outside the
United States, as other countries seek to take the lead in this research.
A 2004 estimate maintained that over 100 of the 150 well-characterized
stem cell lines found worldwide cannot be used in federally funded
research in the United States because they were developed after August
9, 2001, or because they are not available for transfer to the United
States for a variety of technical or legal reasons unique to other
countries.[42] The political uncertainties in the United States, particularly the uncertainty about whether engaging in stem cell research
and research cloning will be made federal or state criminal offenses,
have made some scientists reluctant to enter the field, and this has
also slowed down the pace of this research.

On a practical level, this policy has increased the administrative
costs of pursuing stem cell research with federal funding. Several stem
cell investigators have had to build second laboratories wholly separate
from their original laboratories to meet the requirements of the Bush
policy. For instance, the Harvard Stem Cell Institute, which banks a
significant number of stem cell lines developed after August 9, 2001, has
built an entirely new laboratory so that its privately funded work can be
kept separate from its research on federally funded stem cell lines.[43]
Investigators have had to make major adjustments to their laboratories
in terms of equipment, personnel, and accounting measures in order to
adhere to the Bush policy. To meet the requirements of that policy, they
have had to segregate and allocate costs for supplies, materials, space,
equipment, and staff associated with stem cell research that is not
federally funded from work on stem cell lines that is federally funded.[44]
These additional requirements are time-consuming and burdensome,
stem cell investigators find, and slow down the pace of their research.

The President's Council on Bioethics Monitors Stem Cell Research

The President's Council on Bioethics entered the national stem picture
in 2001 after President Bush had already announced his stem cell
policy. Its mission, President Bush declared, was "to undertake fundamental inquiry into the human and moral significance of developments
in biomedical and behavioral science and technology." The president

asked the council to develop "a deep and comprehensive understanding [of the issues it investigated]...without an overriding concern to find consensus."[45] Thus, the council was not to attempt to seek out publicly shared beliefs, as NBAC had sought to do, but was to develop a deep comprehension of the ethical questions raised by stem cell research on the basis of which it was to reach justifiable conclusions.

This meant that the President's Council had to be composed of profound thinkers capable of going beyond the lowest common denominator to engage in "fundamental inquiry." Of the eighteen members initially selected for the council, seventeen were academics, including fourteen who held or had held named university chairs; another was a Nobel Prize winning political commentator. They were drawn from science and medicine, law and government, philosophy and theology, and several other areas of the humanities and social sciences. The President's Council did not include any community representatives. All of this suggests that it was designed as an elite panel. Although the political persuasions of the council's members are not known publicly, they have often been perceived as being predominantly conservative.

The president instructed the council to "monitor" stem cell research.[46] The council apparently took this to mean that it was not to recommend whether and how far human embryonic stem cell research should be pursued, whether the presidentially imposed deadline on stem cell lines eligible for research complied with the theory of complicity, or whether this research was receiving adequate ethical review once stem cells had been drawn from the approved stem cell lines, for it came to no conclusions about these matters. Instead, it focused on explaining the president's policy and updating readers about developments in the ethical and policy debates after the president's policy had come into force. The council had discussed the primary ethical question raised by human embryonic stem cell research, that of the moral standing of human embryos, in its 2002 report on reproductive and research cloning.[47] In that report, it had already given special attention to the question of the moral significance of early human embryos in the context of discussing research cloning.

The majority of the council had reached a surprising conclusion about the moral significance of human embryos in that earlier cloning report, in view of the group's reputed conservative bias; some among this majority maintained that early human embryos have "intermediate" moral standing (the position taken by NBAC), while others held that they have no special moral standing whatsoever.[48] A minority of the council had adopted the stance taken by President Bush, maintaining that early human embryos have the same moral standing as living persons. This group held that "it is morally wrong to exploit and destroy developing human life even for good reason."[49] In view of their severe differences about the moral significance of early human embryos, the council as a whole could not reach agreement about whether to recommend the pursuit of research cloning in stem cell research, although the majority appeared ready to endorse it.

A vote on this question was averted when the question at issue was changed during the last council meeting before the final section of the council's cloning report was written. Instead of asking the council to vote on the issue of the moral legitimacy of engaging in cloning for research purposes, the question posed to the group was whether it should recommend a four-year moratorium on such cloning or propose a ban on it altogether. No reason was given by anyone affiliated with the council for this change from the question that had been the focus of the council's discussions until this time. A formal vote was taken on this question, and the majority of the council   a different majority from that which had indicated that the embryo has either intermediate moral standing or no special moral standing—recommended imposing such a moratorium on research cloning.[50] Those favoring this conclusion argued that more time was needed to discuss the scientific and ethical merits of proceeding with such research. Thus, despite its extensive discussion of the moral significance of the early human embryo, the council came to no final conclusions or recommendations about this major issue in its earlier cloning report.

There is only a brief discussion of the question of the moral significance of early human embryos in the council's stem cell research report, which was published two years after its cloning report. Perhaps the council decided that there was no reason to repeat its earlier exploration of this question. Or it may be that the impasse that the council had come to in the earlier discussion of the moral significance of human embryos in its cloning report had discouraged it from returning to that issue in any depth in its stem cell research report. In any case, the council did not attempt to reach any final conclusions about this central question for stem cell research or to develop any new stem cell research policy recommendations for the president or the Congress in its later stem cell research report.

The writings and discussions of the President's Council on Bioethics concerning the ethical issues raised by research cloning and human embryonic stem cell research in these two reports stimulated considerable discussion among media commentators and those in disciplines concerned about this research. However, they appear to have had little effect on decisions by the president and Congress. The council's exploration of the moral significance of the human embryo received little notice from these officials, and they appear to have ignored its recommendation to establish a four-year moratorium on research cloning. The council experienced a similar lack of legislative success in its call for a complete ban on human reproductive cloning. Thus, although the President's Council on Bioethics played an important educational role regarding some of the underlying ethical issues related to stem cell research and research cloning, it was less successful in bringing about changes in public policy regarding stem cell research and research cloning through these two reports that it argued were important and necessary.

Congressional Attempts to Modify the Bush Policy

In the years since President Bush issued his order limiting federal funding to stem cell lines that predated his August 2001 speech, well over three dozen stem-cell related bills have been introduced into the House and the Senate. Members of Congress who introduced bills to expand the number of embryonic stem cell lines available for federally funded stem cell research were unsuccessful in gaining political traction on these bills until 2005. In that year, the Stem Cell Research Enhancement Act (H.R. 810) passed the House. This bill would have overruled President Bush's policy by authorizing federal funding for research using stem cell lines that were obtained from spare embryos remaining at IVF clinics, regardless of the date on which the stem cells had been derived from those embryos. The Senate passed an identical bill (S. 471) in 2006.[51] However, the president kept a promise he had made to veto such a bill.[52] (See appendix E.) It is unclear as of this writing whether another attempt to pass such legislation will succeed in the next Congress.

There is no federal legislation in effect that allows or prohibits either reproductive or research cloning because of a split between those who maintain that both of these forms of cloning should be banned and those who would prohibit only reproductive cloning. Although the House passed a bill in 2005 that would have permanently banned both forms of cloning, the Senate did not do the same. The House bill, the Human Cloning Prohibition Act (H.R. 1357) would have imposed a criminal penalty of imprisonment for not more than ten years and a civil penalty of not less than $1 million for carrying out either form of cloning. It would also have banned the import of any product into the United States derived from an embryo created by means of cloning. Concerns were raised about whether this would mean that any citizen of the United States who had received treatment with progeny of human embryonic stem cells derived from cloned embryos abroad would face legal difficulties when returning to the country on grounds that he or she was importing a product created by means of cloning. A companion anticloning bill (S. 658) was introduced into the Senate in 2005 that was similar to the House bill, except that it did not include the ban on importing products derived from research cloning. An opposing bill, the Human Cloning Ban and Stem Cell Research Protection Act (H.R. 1822 and S. 876) was introduced into the House and Senate in 2005. It would have banned reproductive cloning but allowed research cloning, provided that the latter was conducted in accordance with federal regulations regarding the protection of human subjects, received institutional review board approval, and provided patient privacy protections. These bills, however, expired at the end of that Congress.

The Human Chimera Prohibition Act (S. 1373) which was introduced into the Senate in 2005 but was not enacted, would have prohibited the creation of a human chimera. (See chapter 5.) This bill defined a chimera in multiple ways, including: a human embryo into which non-human cells had been introduced, a human-animal embryo produced by fertilizing a human egg with nonhuman sperm, an embryo produced by introducing a human nucleus into a nonhuman egg, a nonhuman life form engineered such that human gametes develop within the body of a nonhuman life form, and a nonhuman life form engineered such that it contains a human brain or a brain derived wholly or predominantly from human neural tissues. This bill was endorsed by President Bush in his 2006 State of the Union speech and was referred to the Senate Committee on the Judiciary, where it expired.

Emergence of State Laws and Policies Regarding Stem Cell Research

Ever since the decision of the Bush administration to provide federal funding for research on a limited number of embryonic stem cell lines, there has been a paradigm shift in the funding sources of biomedical research. Before the Bush decision, the primary sources of money for basic life sciences research were federal agencies, particularly the National Institutes of Health. Now some of the states are moving into a perceived funding gap for biomedical research and are endorsing and supporting embryonic stem cell research in particular. Bills to this effect have been passed in several state legislatures and are pending in others, even as bills to prohibit this research have been introduced into a few state houses.[53] The primary reasons for this upsurge of interest in the pursuit of stem cell research among the states are both scientific and economic.[54] However, the question of whether to support, quash, or ignore human embryonic stem cell research because of the moral significance that some attribute to early human embryos hangs over all such legislation.

After voters had approved a ballot initiative in California that provided funding for stem cell research and research cloning and established a constitutional right to conduct stem cell research (see below), lawmakers in other states known to promote the life sciences became alarmed about the possibility that scientists, as well as non-profit supporters and venture capitalists interested in promoting stem cell research, might move to California in considerable numbers. Providing state funding for embryonic stem cell research seemed to them a way to retain stem cell investigators as well as private industry. The head of a California start-up company spoke for many private entrepreneurs about the economic significance of state support for this research, saying, "For us, it's far nicer to look at an additional source of potential funding than just one, which is the National Institutes of Health. But it's not just us. Many others who have been looking to the NIH or private equity investments now have another place to look. This could drive a lot of companies into this space."[55]

Therefore, various bills regarding stem cell research and research cloning have been introduced into more than thirty state legislatures across the country, initiating intense debate and persistent lobbying by groups on both sides of the question. In 2005, approximately 180 bills on stem cell research came before state lawmaking bodies. In some states, there has been a standoff among opposing legislators, and no policy has been adopted regarding these forms of research; in others, laws that move toward either permission or prohibition have been passed. As a result, a varied patchwork of state laws regarding stem cell research is developing across the United States.

State Decisions Regarding Stem Cell Research

South Dakota is the only state that has explicitly chosen to prohibit all embryonic stem cell research and has criminalized it. It is a misdemeanor to conduct research that destroys a human embryo or that subjects a human embryo to substantial risk of injury or death in that state.[56] Furthermore, researchers in South Dakota may not use cells that have been generated elsewhere for stem cell research.

Certain other states, such as Arkansas, Iowa, Louisiana, Michigan, Nebraska, North Dakota, and Virginia, limit stem cell research by law in various ways. Michigan, for instance, prohibits research on live embryos.[57] This would seem to prohibit the derivation of new human embryonic stem cell lines in that state. Missouri legislators have introduced bills calling for restrictions on embryonic stem cell research for several years in a row without success. Their efforts have indirectly affected the conduct of embryonic stem cell research in that state, for a major in-state research institute donated $6 million to the Harvard Stem Cell Institute rather than attempt to expand its stem cell research efforts in Missouri.[58]

Several other states, including California, Connecticut, Illinois, Maryland, Massachusetts, New Jersey, and Washington, endorse stem cell research and are providing state funding to develop stem cell research centers within their borders.[59] For instance, in May 2006, Connecticut began to award grants to scientists from a ten-year $100 million fund approved by the state legislature in 2005.[60] Still other states plan to follow suit.

Research cloning has been an even more contentious issue for the states. At least seven states, Arkansas, Indiana, Iowa, Michigan, Rhode Island, North Dakota, and South Dakota, ban both reproductive and research cloning; an effort to do the same is under way in Mississippi.[61] Virginia law does not expressly prohibit research on cloned embryos, but it does forbid the possession of the product of human cloning. Several other states, including California, Connecticut, Maryland, Massachusetts, New Jersey, and Wisconsin, allow research cloning.[62] Some among them provide state funding for scientific investigators pursuing such research.

The California Stem Cell Research Initiative

California was one of the first states to designate funds for stem cell research and research cloning. Its policy framework for such research provides one model of how individual states might do this. In November 2004, California voters approved Proposition 71, the California Stem Cell Research and Cures Bond Act of 2004, which amends the state constitution and health and safety code to endorse the right to conduct stem cell research on both pluripotent and progenitor cells. In addition, the act created a $3 billion bond initiative for stem cell research, research cloning, the development of therapies using stem cells, and clinical trials of proposed stem cell therapies that offers funding for research projects and facilities.[63] The California Institute for Regenerative Medicine (CIRM) was created to oversee the initiative and grant awards using funds derived from bond sales. This institute is authorized to distribute an average of $295 million a year over a ten-year period to scientists or facilities affiliated with California universities and other advanced research facilities in the state.[64] This amounts to more funding for stem cell research in a year than the NIH has provided in this decade.

However, a program to award grants to stem cell investigators was delayed by legal challenges to various components of the new act initiated in 2005 by several groups opposed to embryo research.[65] These challengers argued that there is a lack of state oversight of the distribution of the funds for stem cell research, since the state decided to exempt parts of the CIRM from many of the rules that government entities must follow, including how they spend money. They also maintained that some CIRM board members who represent several of the institutions and companies applying for state funds have conflicts of interest.[66] These lawsuits were resolved in the state's favor at the trial level in early 2006, but appeals were not expected to to be resolved until late 2007.[67] Meanwhile, in the spring of 2006, CIRM authorized up to $200 million in loans to state stem cell research programs through the sale of "bond anticipation notes" and funded sixteen university and nonprofit stem cell research centers with $12 million.[68] Additional funds for such loans were allocated in November 2006 from the state's general fund by Governor Arnold Schwarzenegger and from nine philanthropic groups and individuals. After reviewing applications from stem cell investigators, the CIRM plans to disburse these funds to additional applicants in 2007.

Several institutions within the state are developing collaborative efforts among themselves and with stem cell research institutes abroad. The University of California, San Diego, for instance, will work with scientists from Monash University and the Australian Stem Cell Centre to bring together more than 300 leading scientists in regenerative medicine and stem cell science.[69] They will focus on embryonic stem cell biology, neurological disorders, and the treatment of blood disease, cardiac regenerative medicine, and diabetes. Under the agreement among them, the institutions will organize scientific exchanges, host joint workshops, develop joint grant applications, share equipment and materials, and establish joint clinical trials and commercial developments. These multi-institutional and international endeavors, Californians hope, will bring the state enormous scientific and economic benefits.

Current Status of State Stem Cell Research Policies

Legislatures in many of the states in which stem cell bills are pending are at a standoff about whether to pursue embryonic stem cell research; they have not enacted either permissive or restrictive policies regarding this research. Legislators in such states are being are lobbied persistently by scientific organizations, patient advocacy associations, venture capitalists, feminist groups, antiabortion groups, and religious bodies of varying persuasions, who are urging them to enact legislation in support of their preferred policy option regarding stem cell research. The debate taking place in many state houses regarding bills focused on stem cell research is heated and volatile. However, a trend appears to be developing to endorse and fund stem cell research in such states.

States that have proceeded with plans to develop and support stem cell research have been attempting to develop ethical guidelines to govern its pursuit. Some have adopted the stem cell guidelines set out by the National Research Council and the Institute of Medicine of the National Academies.[70] These will be filled in by Embryonic Stem Cell Research Oversight Committees (ESCROs) and institutional review boards at research institutions within those states. (See chapter 8.) There is concern, however, that even though specific research centers may develop ethical standards for embryonic stem cell research and research cloning based on these guidelines, institutional ethics guidelines will conflict with one another. In addition, some maintain that ethical oversight of such research within states will not be as thorough as federal oversight would be because of conflicts of interest that those serving on ESCROs might have. These conflicts could result from such factors as their professional relationships with stem cell research colleagues at their institution and the hope of increasing the prestige and prominence of their institution through this research.[71]

Private-Sector Approaches to Stem Cell Research

Stem cell investigators, in response to the perceived limitations of the Bush policy, have turned to philanthropic groups and entrepreneurs in hopes of obtaining financial support for their research. Several university research groups have succeeded in such efforts and have developed additional human embryonic stem cell lines with the aid of private funding. For instance, in early spring of 2004, Douglas Melton at Harvard University announced that he had developed seventeen new embryonic stem cell lines with support from the Juvenile Diabetes Association and the Howard Hughes Medical Institute.[72] This nearly doubled the worldwide supply of embryonic stem cell lines available for research at that time. The Harvard Stem Cell Institute, one of nine privately funded research institutes in the United States, is planning to raise $100 million in private donations in order to continue to carry out its stem cell research.[73] Rutgers University, the Rockefeller University, and the University of Wisconsin have announced similar fund-raising efforts.[74] This sort of backing by nonprofit and business groups could bring about more rapid development and expansion of this research, some commentators maintain.[75]

However, other observers report that the Bush stem cell policy has had a chilling effect on potential funders.[76] The head of the investment arm of a major bank pointed out in 2005 that venture capitalists had invested $300 million up to that time in stem cell companies, whereas they had put $20 billion into other technology platforms.[77] Venture capitalists have been leery of investing in stem cell research for several reasons. They believe that the Bush stem cell research policy is undercutting the progress of this research from the laboratory to the marketplace, and this is making it less attractive to them. Private corporations must now bear the costs of funding basic stem cell research should they go forward with it, costs that have been covered by federal funds in other sorts of basic research in the past. Therefore, potential investors are worried about whether they would receive an adequate return on the initially large payout needed to develop the scientific end of this research. Add to that issue concerns about market fragmentation. They are worried that stem cell research projects will have to be approved state by state rather than by a single regulatory authority—and that states that ban embryonic stem cell research would also ban the importation or use of products resulting from this research, thereby limiting the market for potential commercial applications.[78] Venture capitalists are also unsure about how intellectual property questions that arise with regard to this research will be resolved; they are concerned that they might inadvertently cross patents in the course of stimulating stem cells to differentiate.(See below.) All of these concerns and uncertainties make many private investors hesitant to invest in human embryonic stem cell research.

The investment picture shifted somewhat in 2005, when the $3 billion stem cell research ballot initiative was approved in California. Before that, major business players had been hesitant to invest in this research for the reasons discussed above and for fear of shareholder protests and product boycotts. However, the Wisconsin Alumni Research Foundation (WARF), which holds patents on several widely used human embryonic stem cell lines, reported that as of mid-2005, it had issued eight commercial licenses to large companies, indicating that interest in this research was growing among them.[79] Apparently, as state support for embryonic stem cell research has continued to increase, some large companies have felt reassured that their pursuit of this research would be viewed as beneficial and moral by the public.

In short, this research is primarily being funded within private industry by small biotechnology firms and a few large publicly traded companies, some of which turn to small companies and universities to obtain supplies of embryonic stem cells. However, signs are that the race to develop stem cell research products and to get them into clinical testing ahead of the competition is heating up among both small and large companies.[80] It is unclear at this time whether companies in private industry will develop guidelines that provide ethical safeguards for carrying out this research. (See chapter 8.)

Patenting Stem Cells and Technologies Related to Stem Cell Research

The U.S. patent system has played a role that has been crucial to stem cell research efforts, regardless of whether these have been funded by the federal government, states, or private industry. Securing patent protection has become a critical aspect of participating in the biotechnological industries, where patent protection can provide an incentive to researchers to make new discoveries and to corporations to invest in such discoveries in hopes that they will receive sufficient return to cover the costs of research and development.

Intellectual property law functions by giving inventors a limited monopoly over their knowledge of how to make new and useful products, and over the products themselves, in order to stimulate innovation.[81] The right to exclude others from using materials and methods covered by patents in order to promote the progress of science is found in Article 1, section 8 of the U.S. Constitution. Yet inventors can choose to disclose new and useful information and products to others within the protections of their intellectual property rights.[82] All in all, the patent system that has developed in the United States is said by its supporters to provide a stable climate that facilitates economic growth and long-term investment in research.

Human embryonic stem cells (when isolated from their natural state and purified), as well as the methods for deriving and using them, are eligible for federal patent protection. Patents related to stem cells have been filed with the U.S. Patent and Trademark Office covering, for instance, methods of differentiating various types of stem cells, repairing damaged connective tissue using stem cells derived from human bone marrow, and transplanting neural stem cells into a host.[83]

Property rights secured to holders of patents having to do with stem cell research, such as the right to use certain types of cells or certain methods to derive and maintain stem cell lines, may be transferred to others through agreements involving exclusive or nonexclusive licenses. Those who want access to these patented cell lines or methodologies must negotiate licenses and related fees or royalties from patent holders for any commercial applications that result from research carried out by these licensees with the cell lines.[84] In *Madey v. Duke*,[85] decided in 2002, a federal court held that academic researchers who use technology patented by others are not protected against infringement of those patents by the fact that they are doing experimental work, even when that work may not have direct commercial applications. As a consequence, stem cell researchers must now seek licenses from patent holders not only for commercial applications of patented stem cell lines and techniques but also for almost all noncommercial research uses of patented stem cell inventions.

How Stem Cell Patenting Works: An Example

U.S. Patents Nos. 5,843,780 (December 1, 1998) and 6,200,806 (March 13, 2001) were filed by James Thomson of the University of Wisconsin to cover the composition of primate (including human) embryonic stem cells, as well as the methods used to derive them.[86] They provide intellectual property protection, not only for the process of isolating these stem cells from the inner cell mass of a blastocyst, but also for the resulting embryonic stem cells. These patents are very broad and appear to cover all human embryonic stem cell lines, regardless of who generates them or the methods that they use. The 2001 patent gives the Wisconsin Alumni Research Foundation (WARF), to which Thomson assigned these patents, the legal right to exclude everyone else in the country from making, using, selling, buying, or importing any human embryonic stem cells covered by these patents until 2016 and 2018.[87]

WARF established the WiCell Research Institute in October 1999 as a not-for-profit corporation to advance stem cell research.[88] This new institute also served as a vehicle for licensing others to practice the patented invention in exchange for royalties. Since the NIH had given Thomson federal grants to support the work that led to the 1998 patent, it had a license from WARF to use the claimed human embryonic stem cells for research. Thus, once the Bush stem cell research policy was put into place, the NIH was given a license to use human embryonic stem cell lines that had been developed by groups in the United States that were eligible for federally funded research. Those groups, in exchange, received grants from the NIH to facilitate the distribution of their human embryonic stem cell lines under a license from WARF. As part of this arrangement, WARF agreed that it would not require other not-for-profit institutions to meet more restrictive terms than the NIH. As a result, academic researchers who receive federal funds for embryonic stem cell research can gain access to materials and licenses to carry out research under the patent through WiCell for a fee of $500, a figure reduced from the original $5,000.[89] This fee has since been canceled.

WARF licensed cells to Geron Corporation, a California biopharmaceutical company that develops and commercializes cell-based therapies, for the commercial applications of the use of embryonic stem cell lines to develop neural, cardiac, and insulin-producing cells.[90] Geron was given this license because it had partially funded the research carried out by Thomson that was covered by the WARF patents. Other commercial groups that request access to these stem cell lines must negotiate a materials transfer agreement with WARF and Geron. If they want to pursue commercial uses of the stem cells or the methods for deriving them, they ordinarily must seek an additional license that involves sharing profits with WiCell or Geron, which hold what are known as "reach-through rights."[91] Even if a company wants to use human embryonic stem cells for basic research, it must still obtain a commercial license at a typical royalty rate of $125,000 and $140,000 in annual maintenance fees.[92] These sorts of restrictions are not unique to WARF but are imposed by patent holders in general.[93]

The WARF/Geron agreement has been criticized by legal scholars Arti Rai and Rebecca Eisenberg because of the exclusivity of its licensing arrangement. They declare that "although embryonic stem cells are precisely the type of broadly applicable enabling technology that, as a general matter, should be licensed nonexclusively in the interest of promoting future research...WARF chose to license exclusively some of the most important commercial rights under the patent." Since the patents state that they claim "a method of culturing human embryonic stem cells and composition of matter which covers any cells with the characteristics of stem cells," these patents could be interpreted as giving WARF control over any and all stem cells, they observe.[94] This presents a significant problem because WARF's stem cell patents set the standards for all patents on stem cell research and could therefore preclude many other related patent applications. Some other commentators have also expressed concern that the sorts of restrictions in WARF's patents are overly broad and will slow down the use of human pluripotent stem cells in therapy.[95]

Patrick Taylor observes that "despite these limitations, it should be acknowledged that these terms are less restrictive and overbearing than the most short-sighted and confiscatory forms of material transfer agreement that some companies would impose if they could."[96] For instance, WARF does not require its licensees to name it as owner of any invention that results from the use of its stem cell lines or to give it an exclusive commercial license to any such invention. Further, it does not set terms that impede the publication of results of research conducted with its lines.

Even so, the exclusivity and breadth of the WARF patents were challenged in a 2006 filing with the U. S. Patent and Trademark Office by the California-based Foundation for Taxpayer and Consumer Rights. CIRM, the California agency overseeing stem cell research, had decided to give the state of California 25% royalties on any inventions created through embryonic stem cell research that it funds. This would be viewed as the commercialization of such stem cell research and would mean that California would have to pay WARF at the much higher commercial rate for licenses to use its stem cell lines than it would have paid under a license granted to California researchers as academics affiliated with nonprofit organizations. A successful suit would relieve the citizens of California of having to pay WARF at this higher rate. More broadly, it would allow more companies to explore the technology for basic research and treatments that are marketed, according to those filing this suit.[97] If the Patent Office takes this case, it could take two years or more to rule on it. Therefore, the state of this suit is currently in limbo.

Ethical Issues Raised by Patenting Human Pluripotent Stem Cells

The long-term effect of the current system of patenting and licensing, several legal commentators argue, limits the availability of stem cell research findings and discourages the development of new therapies.[98] Some among them contend that the patent system encourages the "proliferation of fragmented and overlapping intellectual property rights," thereby discouraging innovation.[99] This problem, they maintain, is too complex to be resolved simply through market forces. The NIH has also observed that in some contexts "intellectual property rights can stifle the broad dissemination of new discoveries and limit future avenues of research and product development."[100] Therefore, the NIH has urged the nonexclusive licensing of unique research materials and has recommended that the NIH-approved Uniform Biological Materials Transfer Agreements be used in order to minimize obstacles to the transfer and use of research materials.

With regard to the patenting of human embryonic stem cells in particular, Peter Mikhail argues that "development of technology based upon stem cells is of such fundamental interest that exclusive licenses should not be permitted without any evaluation of the consequences.... The combination of patenting and exclusive or unchecked free market licensing can foreclose research and development in crucial fields."[101] Rai and Eisenberg have suggested expanding the NIH's discretion to determine licensing requirements and intellectual property protection to commercially funded biomedical research. They argue that a partnership between government sources of funds and private investors is needed if stem cell research is to proceed at a rapid pace.[102] In their report on the intellectual property rights of genomic and proteomic research,the National Academies of Science recommended related measures that seek to achieve an appropriate balance between protecting research discoveries and granting access to them.[103]

The patent system currently allows questions of access and ethics relevant to embryonic stem cell research to be decided by the market-place. Yet there is no guarantee that the marketplace will go beyond the implementation of the revenue incentive to address such questions,[104] even though there is concern that research is being delayed or aban-doned because of patents and proprietary technologies.[105] Consider-ation of modifying the current system governing intellectual property rights in order to broaden access to data and materials should be a high priority for the federal government and for those who are commercia-lizing stem cell research in order to assure the public that this research is being conducted responsibly and is not being impeded by quasi monopolistic practices.

Summing up the Current Status of Stem Cell Research Policy across the Nation

The national policy that has been set in place with regard to embryonic stem cell research for the past several years is ethically incoherent. Moreover, it has minimal scope. The federal government has provided limited funding for this research and required little federal ethical oversight of it. The President's Council on Bioethics has been "moni-toring" stem cell research, observing its development in several states and in the private sector. There are no signs that it plans to reopen discussion of the current federal policy governing this research or to initiate consideration of its long-range ethical implications.

As of this writing, the current federal policy leaves it to the states, universities, and the biotechnology industry to pursue this research beyond the minimal federal approach and to develop ethical guidelines for conducting it. Several state legislatures that have not yet enacted policies supporting this research or guidelines for its development are poised to do so over the next several years. The volatility of the debate among various factions about embryonic stem cell research and re-search cloning, however, renders it difficult to make firm predictions about the future policy framework of this research on the state level. As some states follow the lead of California and build up stem cell research programs of their own, this research will develop in a fragmented way, resulting in a state-by-state patchwork of regulations and guidelines. States will duplicate efforts, multistate stem cell collaborations will be hampered by conflicts of laws and regulations, and access to findings and materials will be restricted.[106] Without some federal infrastructure that is specifically directed toward guiding this research, stem cell investigators spread across the states will remain unsure about whether and where they can carry out their work and according to what standards. In addition, private entrepreneurs will continue to be hesitant to invest in this research because state-by-state policy variations will offer no consistent regulation and ethical oversight of this research.

The National Research Council and the Institute of Medicine of the National Academies, as noted above, have provided guidelines for stem cell research[107] that may well be adopted by states that support human embryonic stem cell research, local research boards at academic institutions, and some private companies pursuing this research. These guidelines leave it to local institutional committees to render the guidelines specific to their research efforts and to respond to those ethical issues that the guidelines do not address. (See chapter 8.) Although these guidelines add to the ethical armamentarium available to those carrying out this research, they do not provide full-scale national guidelines and policy for stem cell research.

President Bush's policy has been increasingly challenged by some members of Congress, scientists, and patient advocacy groups who complain that this research is moving at a snail's pace without significant oversight. They argue that it needs the sort of federal financial support that the government gave to the Human Genome Project so that it can proceed more rapidly according to accepted ethical standards. The United States, they maintain, is threatened with the loss of its scientific and ethical edge in this field as a result of the continued presidential reluctance to fund embryonic stem cell research and to support a national ethics panel to review stem cell research as it moves beyond its initial stages. Polls reveal a growing sense among the public that this research should be expanded in both the public and the private sectors in order to learn whether its therapeutic promise can be fulfilled and to keep the United States at the forefront of this cutting edge area of science. A mid-2006 poll taken by the Coalition for the Advancement of Medical Research, for instance, indicates that 73 percent of Americans favor embryonic stem cell research.[108] A Harris poll taken in October 2005 found that 70 percent of all adults surveyed favored embryonic stem cell research.[109] Such polls provide an incentive for those in Congress who have been weighing its political pros and cons to authorize the pursuit of stem cell research more broadly with federal funds.

There is some evidence, as of this writing, that the number of those in the halls of Congress who have an interest in providing federal funding for research on a wider range of pluripotent stem cell lines continues to grow, despite President Bush's veto of a bill that would have accomplished this during the term of the last Congress. Should federal legislation expanding the scope of federally funded human embryonic stem cell research eventually pass and be upheld after another presidential veto, this would leave wide open the question of whether and how a coherent set of guidelines should be developed under a broadened national stem cell research policy.

8

In Pursuit of National Review and Oversight of Stem Cell Research in the United States

S tem cell research brings to the fore unique and fundamental ethical questions not only about whether to engage in research using early human embryos but also about a host of other issues that revolve around how we ought to use the regenerative powers that this research offers. These additional issues include such current questions as whether to employ some of the innovative techniques proposed for developing additional sources of human pluripotent stem cells, not only to treat those laid low by diseases, but also to bring babies into the world who would not have such diseases, and where to draw ethical boundaries around the transfer of human stem cells into nonhumans in the course of stem cell research designed to regenerate damaged human cells.

They also embrace more futuristic questions, such as whether we should seed human stem cells onto appropriately configured scaffolds[1] in order to grow new human tissue and organs to treat human beings, and to enhance their bodies, and whether to use genetically altered stem cells as vehicles for both therapy and enhancement.[2] Moreover, stem cell research will inevitably lead us to wrestle with questions of justice and access that haunt our current efforts to provide health care. Will those who are economically less well off be provided with stem cell therapies that have been developed in the public and private sectors at great financial cost? Will the development of banks of stem cell lines exacerbate demographic differences if the stem cell lines accepted for banking appear to favor certain groups of individuals over others? Clearly, stem cell research will increasingly force us to grapple with novel ethical issues whose resolution will have immense effects on the lives of many.

When an innovative area of scientific activity emerges that promises to provide significant discoveries about early human development, as well as new forms of medical therapy and enhancement, and yet is laced with unique ethical challenges, it becomes a societal activity.[3] That is, such scientific research is not only a private endeavor of a variety of teams intent on developing scientific understandings and medical treatments. It is also a public endeavor in that it offers biotechnological powers that, conjoined with similar powers, such as those provided by neuroscience, human genomics, and proteomics, promise to revolutionize the lives and health of many within society. Because it proffers these powers, such research appropriately becomes subject to public review. In a democratic republic, the degree of review of such technological power that is necessary needs to be assessed by a federal body that engages in open deliberations that are informed by significant public input. Such deliberation and public consultation is essential in that republic in order to avoid an undue conflation of state power and the blanket imposition of one viewpoint at the expense of all others.

In many countries where stem cell research is pursued, such as the United Kingdom, Canada, Japan, Singapore, and Germany, standing national stem cell review and oversight commissions authorized by the government play an important role in addressing the range of sensitive ethical issues that stem cell research poses for their societies. No similar national body currently carries out this function in the United States. Although federal agencies govern certain aspects of the conduct of stem cell research in this country, no one agency is responsible for ensuring that the full range of stem cell research is reviewed according to ethical guidelines grounded in shared values important to our republic. The President's Council on Bioethics, the successor to the National Bioethics Commission that developed guidelines for stem cell research, has developed no such guidelines for the ethical conduct of the whole range of stem cell research.

Given the lack of a national panel to guide and review ongoing stem cell research, investigators in that field, along with the infertility specialists working with them, have fallen back on guidelines for stem cell research developed by two private professional organizations. One is the National Academy of Sciences, which includes members from a wide range of the sciences chosen by current members, and the other is the American Society of Reproductive Medicine, whose membership is constituted by those specializing in the treatment of infertility-related conditions. The guidelines of these organizations overlap with one another in certain respects and yet conflict in others. This leaves scientific and medical professionals and the nation as a whole with a collection of varying and sometimes conflicting rules for the ethical conduct of stem cell research. Yet for many, the ethical questions raised by stem cell research overshadow the scientific, business, and other issues that surround it and require a consistent and coherent response that can come from formulating them and responding to them at the national level.[4]

In this chapter, I argue that there is a need for a national stem cell review panel in the United States, especially in view of a possible expansion of federal policy regarding human embryonic stem cell research by the new Congress. I discuss the possible functions, membership, and methods for engaging in public deliberation that such a national panel could pursue, reviewing these factors in light of the recommendations for the ethical conduct of stem cell research of the National Bioethics Advisory Commission and of four other groups that have considered or have developed ethics review panels for this specific purpose. I argue that such a panel would offer a way of assuring the public and the Congress that the novel issues that stem cell research raises are being addressed in ways that are ethically responsible and that build on broad public consultation and democratic deliberation.

Current State of Federal Regulation of Stem Cell Research

Stem cell research is currently regulated on the federal level by three bodies: the National Institutes of Health, the Office for Human Research Protections, and the Food and Drug Administration. These agencies are authorized to address only certain kinds of ethical questions that arise during preclinical (before use in humans) and clinical (involving humans) stem cell research. However, none of the three is responsible for grappling with the full range of unique ethical questions raised by this research. As a consequence, they do not jointly provide one coherent national stem cell research policy to guide those in the field and to assure the public that this research is being carried out according to shared ethical standards that take account of the range of views found in an open, pluralistic democratic society.

Role of the National Institutes of Health

As of this writing, a committee at the National Institutes of Health (NIH) appointed to "focus solely on the science" of stem cell research[5] decides which human embryonic stem cell lines are eligible for use by federally funded researchers on the basis of criteria set out by President Bush in 2001.[6] (See appendix B.) These standards require that (1) the embryonic stem cell lines to be used in stem cell research were derived with the informed consent of the donors, (2) they were obtained from embryos created for reproductive purposes before August 2001 that were no longer needed for such purposes, (3) no financial inducements were given to those who donated these embryos for this research, and (4) these stem cell lines were not derived from embryos created solely for research purposes. (See appendix D.)

These criteria have the advantage of being concise and definitive. However, they also have certain disadvantages. The most significant of these is that they do not apply to the numerous stem cell lines that have been developed in the United States without federal funding. A related problem is that they do not provide ethical guidance about the broad range of issues that are created by research and therapeutic uses of stem cells and their progeny once these cells have been drawn from the approved stem cell lines. Instead, they focus exclusively on the prelude to human embryonic stem cell research—that is, the derivation of these stem cell lines from human embryos (with federal funds)—and leave it to federal agencies that are not authorized to address basic ethical issues raised by this form of research to regulate their development. Moreover, these criteria do not cover research with other sorts of stem cells, such as adult and fetal stem cells, or take account of new scientific findings in stem cell research that raise novel ethical issues. Even more basically, these criteria do not enable anyone—on the federal level, within the field of stem cell research, or among the public—to develop a comprehensive picture of the current status of stem cell research and of the direction that ethical guidelines for its pursuit around the country could and should take. The narrowness of these criteria raises special concerns for the overwhelming majority of people in the United States who have indicated that they believe the presidential policy regarding stem cell research should be expanded to cover federally funded research on human embryonic stem cell lines derived after August 2001.[7]

In effect, the Bush criteria leave decisions about whether to go forward with a variety of different kinds of stem cell research in the hands of local institutional review boards. Yet these boards do not necessarily have members with specialized knowledge about the science of stem cell research or experience in grappling with the ethical issues that such research raises. In short, there is a wide range of stem cell research that is being undertaken in this country for which the presidential criteria that have been set out by the NIH are irrelevant.

Role of the Office for Human Research Protections

The Office for Human Research Protections, an agency of the Department of Health and Human Services, has a hand in the review of all stem cell research involving human volunteers. It administers the Common Rule, which provides the core federal regulations governing research on human beings at institutions receiving federal funds.[8] This rule applies to those who donate early embryos, gametes (sperm and eggs), or somatic (body) cells for stem cell research whose identities are readily ascertainable to those working with the resulting stem cell lines,[9] even though they are not "human subjects" in the usual sense.[10] Local institutional review boards (IRBs) must confirm that these donors have given informed and voluntary consent to the provision of such biological materials for stem cell research to the satisfaction of the Office for Human Research Protections, and they must review whether the donation was carried out in a way that posed no unreasonable risk (physical or privacy-related) to the donors, again to the satisfaction of the Office for Human Protections. The Office for Human Research Protections, therefore, has an important role in ensuring that those who donate biological materials to be used in stem cell research do so freely on the basis of accurate and complete knowledge of what this involves. The other area where the Common Rule applies to stem cell research involves ensuring that researchers maintain the confidentiality of any personal information about such donors collected from analyses of the reproductive materials they provide.[11] Here, too, local IRBs must confirm to the satisfaction of the Office for Human Research Protections that institutional investigators have taken steps to protect such confidential information.

Thus, the Office for Human Research Protections is responsible for ensuring that informed consent requirements for donating embryos, gametes, and other biological materials for federally funded stem cell research are met and that the confidentiality of information about such donors is protected as far as possible within the law. However, this agency is not authorized to address any other aspects of embryonic stem cell research that raise broader ethical issues.

Role of the Food and Drug Administration

Another agency, the Food and Drug Administration (FDA), is charged with responding to issues of safety and efficacy raised by stem cell research once it reaches the clinical stages and is applied to living humans. The scope of the FDA's regulatory responsibilities also extends to preclinical research that will ultimately have clinical applications in human beings. Those carrying out these forms of stem cell research have to meet its laboratory and donor screening requirements. The FDA has indicated that it will regulate the clinical use of stem cells and their derivatives in humans as cellular products. These are defined as "articles containing or consisting of human cells or tissues that are intended for implantation, transplantation, infusion, or transfer into a human recipient."[12] This means that it focuses on preventing the use of contaminated cells and tissues in humans and the improper handling of these materials, as well as demonstrating the clinical safety and effectiveness of using such cells and tissues in patients.

In 2006, the agency set out final comprehensive regulations covering the use of a wide range of cells and tissues and cellular and tissue-based products, including highly engineered cells and tissues such as stem cell-related materials.[13] This regulatory framework is based on a tiered structure in which the degree of communicable disease risk determines the degree of regulation. The higher the risk of communicable disease posed by cell and tissue-based products, the greater the regulation. Stem cells removed and then reimplanted in their donor or a close relative of the donor are considered to pose less of a risk than those that are implanted into unrelated patients.

This means, for example, that the Food and Drug Administration would be involved in review of any proposals to use stem cells or their progeny that have been cultivated from the human embryonic stem cell lines developed from embryos provided by donors and grown on beds of mouse "feeder" cells, since these "feeders" are suspected of carrying viruses that might be harmful to humans. (See chapter 1.) Donors who are not providing stem cells or their progeny for themselves or for a close relative have to be screened for risk factors and clinical evidence of communicable disease. Any use of such stem cells or their offshoots in humans also falls under Food and Drug Administration regulations governing the transfer of human materials that have had contact with nonhuman animal materials to living humans (xenotransplantation) because of their exposure to mouse "feeder" cells.

The Food and Drug Administration, however, is not authorized to wrestle with policy questions related to the ethical import of stem cell research during its preclinical or clinical stages.[14] Consequently, it would not be entitled or necessarily prepared to provide ethical review of stem cell research programs or to engage in interdisciplinary deliberation about ethical and social issues raised by this research.

Influence of These Three Agencies on Federal Review of Stem Cell Research

All in all, while there is some federal review of donor consent and confidentiality in human embryonic stem cell research during its pre-clinical stages provided by the Office for Human Research Protections and review of the safety and efficacy of stem cell research at the clinical stages that is provided by the Food and Drug Administration, and there is some degree of ethical review of stem cell research proposals by the NIH, the jurisdiction of federal agencies over ethical standards for stem cell research is limited. This leaves local institutional review boards to set such standards for stem cell research receiving federal funds, as well as for some privately funded research. However, these boards, which, as noted above, do not necessarily have any scientific or ethics background regarding stem cell research, must develop their own ethical formulas about how this research should proceed. As a result, stem cell research is currently being conducted across the country according to ethical standards that can differ from institution to institution. The fact that there are no federal ethical standards for stem cell research leaves stem cell investigators with a national patchwork of conflicting ethical requirements that is especially problematic for those attempting to engage in multi-institutional research programs with colleagues at other stem cell research centers.

Current State of Professional Review of Stem Cell Research

Stem cell investigators have therefore turned to professional bodies to assist them in sorting out the ethical issues raised by stem cell research. Yet the world of human embryonic stem cell research, in particular, cannot be viewed in isolation from the world of assisted reproduction, since they raise overlapping scientific and ethical questions. These questions will be heightened if the increasing interest expressed by many citizens in the United States in expanding federal stem cell research policy to include the use of stem cells derived from spare embryos remaining at assisted reproduction centers, regardless of the date on which they were derived, is written into national policy, as has been proposed.[15] Moreover, the developing movement to enlarge federal stem cell research policy to include the creation of human embryos for stem cell research by means of in vitro fertilization and even by human cloning for research, if successful, would also increase the scope and kinds of ethical questions raised at the intersection of stem cell research and assisted reproduction. Such changes would call for broader ethical guidelines for stem cell research.[16]

The landscape between the worlds of embryonic stem cell research and assisted reproduction constitutes ethical territory for which there are few guideposts in the United States. The major guidelines for it are the voluntary professional guidelines developed by the National Academies of Science (NAS)[17] and the American Society for Reproductive Medicine (ASRM).[18] But these guidelines come into conflict with one another in certain respects.

To gain a sense of how such conflict occurs and whether there is hope of reconciling these guidelines to form one unified national policy, I focus here on an issue of central ethical concern that arises in the territory between stem cell research and assisted reproduction: What are the requirements for obtaining informed consent from those who donate embryos for stem cell research? Focusing on this issue will help us gauge whether stem cell investigators and infertility specialists might find common ground between their professional guidelines more generally with regard to other issues that they jointly face.

Conflicts between Available Guidelines: Informed Consent for Embryo Donation

A fundamental ethical premise underlying any guidelines for the donation of spare human embryos for embryonic stem cell research is the principle of respect for prospective donors.[19] This respect is manifested by fully informing these persons about what donating their embryos would entail to them and to the recipients and then seeking their consent for this donation. Since this informed consent requirement is entirely dependent on what transpires at IVF clinics, stem cell investigators must seek out those IVF clinics that use informed consent standards for embryo donation that conform to the guidelines available to these stem cell investigators, which currently are those set out by the NAS. Yet infertility specialists at assisted reproductive centers are likely to obtain informed consent to embryo donation from patients in ways that conform to the guidelines set out by their professional organization, the ASRM. However, the guidelines of the ASRM and the NAS display significant differences.

Before I examine these differences and what they mean for the ethical conduct of stem cell research, it is important to set the context for informed consent from prospective donors by recalling why embryos that will not used for reproductive purposes remain at IVF clinics. (See also chapter 2.)

Why Spare Embryos Remain at IVF Clinics

The primary reason that spare embryos remain at IVF clinics is related to the fact that women understandably hope to avoid having to go through the onerous process of egg retrieval more than one time. The hormone injections required to stimulate the production of multiple eggs are uncomfortable, and the drugs used can sometimes create unpleasant side effects. In unusual instances, they can bring about ovarian hyperstimulation syndrome,[20] which involves the retention of fluids in a woman's abdominal cavity, causing it to swell and creating severe abdominal pain. This complication can usually be resolved by treatment after a few days.[21] However, in its most severe form, it is estimated that this syndrome affects 1 to 5 percent of women,[22] and in its moderate form between 1 and 20 percent of women.[23] The eggs that result from ovulation induction are then recovered for use in IVF procedures in a procedure that itself has certain minor risks, such as bleeding and infection.[24]

To avoid these risks and the discomfort associated with multiple cycles of egg production and retrieval, as well as to avoid the additional financial costs they would incur by repeating this procedure, those undergoing IVF treatment often elect to have as many eggs and embryos developed as is safe during an initial IVF attempt.[25] The fact that the transfer of more than three embryos to a woman's uterus increases her risks and those of any resulting children means that it may be inadvisable to use all of the embryos created in vitro in one IVF cycle. Therefore, some embryos may remain and be frozen for use in later attempts should the first IVF treatment be unsuccessful.[26] (Currently, human eggs cannot be reliably frozen for later use, although researchers appear to be close to developing a method for doing this.) As a result, when couples have finally completed or ended IVF treatments, they may have embryos remaining that they will no longer use for reproductive purposes. It was estimated in 2003 that there were over 400,000 such embryos stored in a frozen state in centers around the United States.[27]

Some couples who have learned about the possibility of using spare embryos in stem cell research are interested in donating their remaining embryos for this research.[28] Yet questions have arisen about just who should discuss the possibility of embryo donation with such patients, when this discussion should take place, and what sort of information they should be given.

Who Should Obtain Informed Consent for Embryo Donation?

There is disagreement among the available guidelines for informed consent to embryo donation for stem cell research about who should discuss this option with prospective donors—the fertility specialist treating them, or the stem cell investigator who will receive their embryos should they decide to donate them.

The guidelines of the ASRM state that "whenever possible, someone other than the treating infertility specialist should make requests for embryos for research purposes."[29] They explain that having the stem cell investigator or someone else not involved in the care of patients receiving treatment for infertility will ensure that the couples' reproductive needs are kept foremost by the treating professional. The guidelines of the NAS would seem to maintain the opposite. They declare that:

> Decisions related to the production of embryos for infertility treatment should be free of the influence of investigators who propose to derive or use hES cells in research. Whenever it is practicable, the attending physician responsible for the infertility treatment and the investigator deriving or proposing to use hES cells should not be the same person.[30]

Thus, they keep stem cell researchers and the investigator proposing to use embryonic stem cells derived from embryos contributed by patients at IVF clinics at arms length. They go on to maintain that "an IVF clinic or other third party [is] responsible for obtaining consent or collecting materials" from patients, thereby indicating that the treating physician or else his or her delegate, is responsible for obtaining consent for the donation of spare embryos by patients for research. Bernard Lo and colleagues agree with the NAS view, maintaining that the infertility specialist is focused on the patient's well-being, rather than on the potential scientific benefits of the research, making him or her the optimal person to inform possible embryo donors about what this involves.[31]

In effect, these two sets of guidelines, which are the only ones currently available to those in reproductive medicine and in stem cell research, differ about who should obtain informed consent from embryo donors. The infertility specialist following the guidelines recommended by the ASRM will be reluctant to obtain such consent, and yet the stem cell investigator following the NAS guidelines might well expect the infertility specialist to do just that.

When Should Informed Consent for Embryo Donation Be Sought?

These guidelines also disagree about when the option of embryo donation for research should be discussed with those undergoing IVF treatment.

The guidelines of the ASRM recommend that couples be asked to make a decision about donating embryos for stem cell research only after they have decided not to continue storing spare embryos: "Making separate decisions about no longer using embryos and donating them for research guards against pressure placed on couples to donate embryos."[32] This guideline draws on the proposed guidelines of the National Bioethics Advisory Commission. These maintained that the option to donate embryos for research should be presented to patients only at the time when it is clear that they have embryos remaining in order to address "concerns about coercion and exploitation of potential donors, as well as controversy regarding the moral status of embryos."[33]

Although the NAS guidelines recommend that informed consent should be obtained from embryo donors at the time of donation,[34] they neither prohibit nor require an earlier discussion of the disposition of any spare embryos that might remain. Therefore, the NAS guidelines are unclear about this point, apparently because they are more concerned about ensuring that final consent for such donation has been obtained than about obtaining consent during the complete treatment regimen of those undergoing IVF.

However, other guidelines regarding obtaining consent for embryo donation for stem cell research, such as those developed by Lo and colleagues, take a more wholisic view of those undergoing IVF treatment, maintaining that decisions about the disposition of embryos need to be made by patients at the beginning of treatment and throughout the assisted reproduction process.[35] Offering the option to donate embryos for research at the outset of treatment gives prospective embryo donors sufficient time to think about the decision, in their view. Reaffirmation of the decision to donate embryos for research at the time when treatments have ended and spare embryos remain, they argue, gives prospective donors the opportunity to change their minds.

Thus, currently available guidelines do not agree about just when embryo donors should be broached about the option of donating spare embryos for stem cell research. This, too, leaves infertility specialists and stem cell investigators to cope with conflicting recommendations from professional organizations and commentators about this issue.

What Kind of Information Should Be Provided to Prospective Embryo Donors?

Consent forms covering various aspects of IVF treatment vary from clinic to clinic in the kind and degree of specificity of the information they provide.[36] To attempt to remedy this problem, the guidelines of the ASRM recommend what sort of information should be given to prospective embryo donors. This includes standard requirements for informed consent to any sort of research involving human subjects, such as an explanation of the nature and purpose of the research and an exposition of its risks and benefits. Additional requirements are relatively sparse. They call for informing prospective embryo donors about the specific nature of the research project in which their embryos would be used when this is known, revealing that any resulting stem cell lines might exist indefinitely, and informing them of steps that will be taken to ensure their privacy, confidentiality, and anonymity.

The guidelines developed by the NAS cover a greater number and kind of elements of informed consent than those of the ASRM.[37] Several of these are similar to the requirements of the ASRM, but several differ, including the requirements to inform potential embryo donors about other options available for the donation of their embryos and to discuss the possible future uses of these embryos with them.[38]

Thus, it is clear that the guidelines of the ASRM and those of the NAS do not cover the same elements of informed consent and that the latter are more expansive than the former. Stem cell investigators and infertility specialists will be left to puzzle out which of these elements must be included in consent forms of those who donate embryos for stem cell research and how to reconcile two different sets of guidelines.

Import of Conflicting Guidelines for Researchers

These differences in informed consent requirements between the guidelines of these two professional organizations create a dilemma for stem cell investigators who are seeking donated embryos for their research. An IVF center with which they are in contact in hopes of obtaining embryos for research may follow ASRM guidelines (a strong possibility, given that these are the only guidelines available to infertility specialists at such centers). However, the local institutional review board that must review and approve their research may follow the NAS guidelines (very possible, given the scientifically specialized composition of such boards). The local institutional review board may therefore reject the informed consent processes that infertility specialists have followed to obtain embryos for their proposed stem cell research.

In such instances, stem cell investigators will be caught between a rock and a hard place. It is arguable that the guidelines of the NAS should prevail in such circumstances, for they are more wide ranging than those of the ASRM and take into account the most recent scientific and legal developments specific to stem cell research. Yet it could also be claimed that the guidelines of the ASRM should trump those of the NAS because they reflect more accurately the needs of patients who are caught up in the world of assisted reproduction. Stem cell investigators, therefore, are left with no clear answer about who should obtain consent from prospective embryo donors, when that party should do so, and what kind of information that party should provide. There is currently no body available to reconcile the differences between these guidelines on a national basis. The very fact that these guidelines differ from one another in significant respects highlights the need for a nationally constituted stem cell research review panel to develop common guidelines that would apply in the relevant ethical territory between stem cell research and assisted reproduction.

Shaping a National Stem Cell Research Review Panel

A national stem cell review panel could provide a coherent set of ethical standards for those conducting stem cell research. Moreover, it could provide a degree of expertise and experience in addressing novel ethical issues that arise in stem cell research that is not often found among local institutional review boards. Such a national stem cell research review panel, if constructed according to standards that reflect the need for both expert and ordinary citizen membership and with clear goals and functions, could provide public accountability for this far-reaching scientific endeavor.

It would be a mistake, however, to chisel stem cell research guidelines developed by such a national panel into law, for the law functions by prescribing standard responses to anticipated situations and is not prepared to address the rapid and novel sorts of changes that stem cell research promises. To make ethical requirements for stem cell research a matter of black letter law would result in a rigid set of requirements that would be difficult to modify in light of new discoveries and conditions. In contrast, guidelines set out by a nationally constituted ethics review panel that were written into regulations rather than law could be designed to offer standards that are more flexible and open to modification in light of new contexts and findings after appropriate notice and comment.

Two Possible Models for a National Research Review Panel

There are at least two models of national medical research review panels available that, although not focused exclusively on stem cell research, can provide us with insights into the functions and goals of such bodies: the United Kingdom's Human Fertilisation and Embryology Authority and the NIH's Recombinant DNA Advisory Committee.

The Human Fertilisation and Embryology Authority provides a research review and oversight model that has been adopted with some variations by several nations around the world. (See chapter 6.) This body is charged by the Parliament with licensing those engaged in stem cell research and with approving their research proposals before they initiate investigations. Its broad mandate includes identifying ethical problems related to stem cell research, developing guidelines for carrying on this research, monitoring this research as it proceeds, and drawing together data from this research in order to note developing scientific trends and any ethical problems that arise that would lead it to modify its guidelines.[39] The Parliament has not written laws and regulations that the Human Fertilisation and Embryology Authority must enforce but has left it to the Authority to develop guidelines for embryo research and practices related to assisted reproduction as needed. The Authority has held numerous public consultations about ethical issues that have arisen with regard to specific research programs and has developed guidelines to address them. This national review and oversight panel has provided a broad framework for review of all stem cell research in the United Kingdom, allowing ethical issues to be addressed as they arise and providing built-in adaptive mechanisms that prepare it to address new discoveries and conditions.

A similar national stem cell research review panel might initially seem useful in the United States as well. However, if a Human Fertilisation and Embryology Authority model were adopted in the United States, it would have to be modified in certain respects, given the different forms of government of the United Kingdom and the United States, our different histories, and our different approaches to the regulation of practices such as stem cell research and assisted reproduction. (See chapters 6 and 7.)

An alternative model for a national review body that incorporates some of the features of the Human Fertilisation and Embryology Authority is provided by the original Recombinant DNA Advisory Committee.[40] DNA research, which was nearly banned in the United States in the 1970s, was able to proceed mainly because it was monitored by this respected national body. The Recombinant DNA Advisory Committee served for many years as a national review board for proposals for gene transfer research. It was authorized by the NIH to provide mandatory review for publicly funded gene transfer research protocols and voluntary review for such research carried out in the private sector. Its guidelines regarding the wealth of possible applications of gene transfer research allowed that research to proceed according to sound ethical standards. This committee also served as a national ethics advisory board, encouraging discussion and debate of this ethically sensitive area of scientific research.[41]

The Recombinant DNA Advisory Committee served to assure the public that genetic research was being carried out with sufficient attention to relevant ethical considerations. However, there was concern among researchers that it did not move with sufficient rapidity to review research proposals and among outside commentators that its reviews of research proposals were too cursory. Consequently, it received a mixed evaluation for its work. Moreover, the fact that the NIH had responsibility for establishing this committee struck some as involving a conflict of interest, for the very body that was engaged in authorizing and funding this research was also responsible for overseeing and reviewing it.

With the positive and negative aspects of the models of the Human Fertilisation and Embryology Authority and the Recombinant DNA Advisory Committee in mind, we turn to other possible models for a national review panel specifically directed toward stem cell research.

Five Models for a Panel Specifically Directed toward Stem Cell Research

The idea of establishing a panel to review stem cell research on a national or local level has been developed by the following bodies:

1. The stem cell review panel recommended by the National Bioethics Advisory Commission in its 1999 stem cell research report.[42] (See appendix A.)
2. A federal stem cell research review board authorized by the director of the NIH on the recommendation of an ethics advisory group that had developed guidelines for stem cell research in

2000.[43] (See appendix A.) Authorization of this review board, however, was withdrawn in 2001 after a change in the federal administration.[44] (See appendix C.)
3. A stem cell review board established by the Geron Corporation in 1999.[45]
4. An ethics advisory board for stem cell research established by Advanced Cell Technology.[46]
5. A national review board for human embryonic stem cell research proposed by a working group of the NAS.[47]

These various proposed or established panels provide five somewhat different models for the review of the conduct of stem cell research. Some among them reflect aspects of the models provided by the Human Fertilisation and Embryology Authority in the United Kingdom and the Recombinant DNA Advisory Committee in the United States. I analyze them next in terms of their functions, membership, and methods of public deliberation.

Recommended Functions of a National Stem Cell Review Panel

The five panels envisioned by these groups were assigned a variety of different roles, ranging from the sole function of reviewing stem cell research proposals to a more extensive set of functions, such as collecting data regarding all stem cell research conducted in both the public and private sectors on a national basis and providing for their own evaluation after a period of service.

The functions of the national stem cell review body proposed by the National Bioethics Advisory Commission were wide ranging.[48] They included reviewing proposals for the derivation of human embryonic stem cell lines submitted by investigators seeking federal funding, maintaining a public registry of the lines that it had approved, developing a database that included all protocols that derive or use human embryonic stem cells (including those submitted by state and private sponsors on a voluntary basis in its initial phases), providing guidance to its sponsoring agencies regarding the social and ethical issues to be considered in reviewing human embryonic stem cell research protocols, and assessing the state of stem cell science in annual reports.

These recommendations by the commission were noteworthy in that they not only called for specific review of certain kinds of ethically controversial stem cell research proposals but also recognized the need to disseminate consolidated information about the pursuit of this research with both public and private funds around the country. Moreover, the commission was careful to ensure that the stem cell research review panel that it proposed would not usurp the functions of local institutional review boards. These local boards would have remained responsible for reviewing all protocols for stem cell research before sending those involving the derivation of stem cells from embryos to this national panel for further review. In addition, the National Bioethics Advisory Commission's recommendations encouraged private companies to submit proposals to derive embryonic stem cell lines to this panel, allowing proprietary information to be exempt from disclosure in order to make consultation with a national panel attractive to them. In a final stroke, the commission recommended that after a period not exceeding five years, this proposed national stem cell review panel should undergo an independent evaluation of its activities to determine whether it had adequately fulfilled its functions and should be continued. Thus, the commission envisioned a panel that went well beyond one whose sole purpose was to review some or all stem cell research proposals.

The stem cell research review body proposed by the NIH, in contrast, was designed exclusively to review stem cell research proposals submitted to it by federally funded investigators in order to ensure that their research conformed to NIH guidelines.[49] No distinction was made between proposals for the derivation and the use of stem cell research; this panel was to review all stem cell research proposals. Once such research was under way, the panel devised by the NIH would have had no monitoring or data-gathering functions.

Within the private sector, the ethics board initiated by Geron first developed general guidelines for stem cell research and then reviewed the company's developing research in light of them.[50] Its guidelines addressed the moral significance of early human embryos, analyzed informed consent requirements in the context of the donation of blastocysts for stem cell research, and prohibited reproductive cloning. The board went on to list four issues about which it hoped to stimulate public discourse, indicating that it, like the National Bioethics Advisory Commission and the Recombinant DNA Advisory Committee, saw one of its major functions as the encouragement of a national discussion of stem cell research policy. We have no similar indications of the functions of the privately authorized Advanced Cell Technology ethics board.[51]

The last of the five panels is that proposed in NAS guidelines. This body, which was appointed in 2006,[52] is to "serve as a forum for considering new developments in the scientific, clinical, and public policy issues surrounding hES research and for periodic review of the relevant guidelines."[53] Thus, it is charged with updating the NAS guidelines in light of new scientific and public policy findings. However, it appears that it will not review specific research proposals, establish ethical requirements that local review committees must follow, or collect the results of research in one national data bank, as the panel recommended by the National Bioethics Advisory Commission would have done. The relatively limited role that the NAS panel plays undoubtedly rests on the reality that it is a voluntary, rather than a legally mandated, body and does not have the legal authority to serve as a national stem cell review panel.

The combined model of the role and functions of a stem cell research review board that emerges from the recommendations of these groups is of a nationally constituted stem cell research review panel that would carry out some or all of the following functions:

- Develop ethical guidelines for engaging in stem cell research after internal discussion and debate and wide-ranging public consultations
- Expand and modify those guidelines as needed
- Review guidelines for the use of stem cells developed by local institutional boards and other local boards as needed
- Review proposals to generate new human embryonic stem cell lines in light of the conditions set out in the panel's guidelines after these proposals have been approved by local committees charged with reviewing stem cell proposals
- Review stem cell research proposals that raise especially challenging ethical questions
- Certify those stem cell lines that have been developed on the basis of protocols that the panel has approved
- Maintain a public registry of approved protocols and certified stem cell lines
- Establish a database of information linked to the public registry that includes all protocols that derive or use embryonic stem cells
- Use the database and other sources to track the history and uses of certified cell lines
- Develop an annual report that assesses the current state of stem cell science and recent developments in stem cell research and that summarizes emerging ethical or social concerns associated with this research
- Provide for a review and analysis of its own work

Each of these functions covers an important aspect of the oversight of stem cell research and is therefore included within the purview of the model that I propose for a national stem cell review panel.

The primary function of such a panel would to advise various stakeholders, including stem cell researchers and infertility specialists aiding them, other basic and medical researchers, legislators, the president, and the public, about the ethical issues raised by stem cell research proposals and to provide guidelines for carrying out this research that would be available to stem cell researchers and infertility specialists around the country. In providing such recommendations, this panel would also be developing policy for the pursuit of stem cell research throughout the country, either directly or indirectly, depending on the kind of authority that it was given and the reach of its guidelines. This national panel would also serve as a central point for coordinating available information about the current status of stem cell research that would be useful to researchers and those involved in policy formation.

At the outset, such a national panel would have to make clear just how it intended to function, explaining this in terms of its charge from the agency that authorizes it and in terms of how much it could realistically expect to accomplish. A serious concern is that it might be overextended if it were charged with carrying out the host of functions listed above. Therefore, a panel just starting out would do well to consider whether it could and should initially carry out all of these roles. If it determined that it could not do so at the start, it could prioritize its functions, selecting those that it considers most important to begin with and then moving into carrying out other functions once it believed that it had gained sufficient experience and could add others.

Recommended Membership of a National Stem Cell Research Review Panel

Who should serve on such a stem cell review panel? The composition of the group will reflect the features and needs of the area of research to which it is directed, as well as the special nature of the body as an ethics panel. It should also reflect the needs of a democratic polity that incorporates a wide range of viewpoints about this research in attempting to reflect shared values.

The panel proposed by the National Bioethics Advisory Commission was to be an interdisciplinary group that included members of the public.[54] Its membership would have had expertise in a variety of areas related to stem cell research (these were not spelled out) and would also have reflected the views and values of "ordinary" citizens.

The composition of the proposed NIH review group that never met was not described in the notice announcing its formation.[55] Since it was to be the successor to the working group that had developed these guidelines, word of mouth suggested that it, like that working group, would be an interdisciplinary panel with a mix of scientists, clinicians, ethicists, lawyers, patients, and representatives of patient interest groups. Its membership, therefore, would have combined expertise in areas especially relevant to stem cell research with the perspectives of members of the public.

The membership of two stem cell advisory boards established by private companies provides a useful contrast with that of the boards described above. The composition of the Ethics Advisory Board of Geron[56] was more narrowly drawn than that of the review bodies described above. It was composed of five members with expertise in the fields of religious studies and bioethics. This advisory board included no scientists, medical professionals or counselors with expertise in assisted reproduction, lawyers, or patient advocacy group representatives.

Advanced Cell Technology, a private company that developed an ethics board to review its program of research cloning, indicated in a 2002 publication that its members were "ethicists" and "clinicians."[57] Two were well-known bioethicists drawn from the field of religious studies; others, as far as can be determined, included scientists, physicians, and assisted reproduction counselors.

The NAS guidelines indicate that the advisory panel's "membership should include nationally and internationally recognized authorities in the scientific, medical, ethical, and legal issues associated with hES cell research, and representatives of the public."[58] At this time, it is the policy of the NAS that no stem cell investigators are eligible to serve on this panel. This decision was made to avoid the appearance of a conflict of interest that might result if stem cell investigators were to write the guidelines to which they would then be subject.[59] This group is currently composed of scientists in the biological sciences, genetics, and cell biology; medical professionals and medical school administrators; the former chair of the National Bioethics Advisory Commission; the head of a university bioethics program; academic lawyers familiar with stem cell research and patenting law who also have expertise in bioethics; and representatives of patient interest groups.[60] Thus, its membership is drawn from those in various disciplines with expertise relevant to stem cell research, as well as from among the public.

This analysis of the membership of five active or proposed stem cell review panels suggests that a national stem cell review panel should seek members who are well grounded in a variety of scientific fields related to stem cell research, as well as in ethics, public policy, and clinical counseling. It should also include those who bring the perspectives of "ordinary" citizens to its work, including those affected by diseases that stem cell therapies might treat. Members of the panel should be open to hearing from a variety of stakeholders, social groups, and experts so that its recommendations address all the relevant issues and alternatives.

It is arguable that membership on such a committee needs to be drawn more broadly than this. For instance, two public interest groups have criticized the membership of the NAS's review committee on grounds that its range of expertise is drawn too narrowly in the direction of the sciences.[61] These groups argue that the committee should include public health experts, bioethicists, and policy experts who have advocated caution and effective public review of stem cell research; professionals with expertise in the provision of women's health; and those with research experience and concern for access to health care for ethnic minorities and the economically vulnerable.

It is difficult to specify the sorts of expertise and interests that members of a national review panel should bring to its deliberations that will strike everyone as measuring up to their preferred ideal. The recommendations for expanding the membership of the NAS panel provided by these critics reflect the view that democratic deliberation needs to be carried out by a group that demonstrates a wider range of interests and expertise than the currently appointed panel. This was the approach taken by the National Bioethics Advisory Commission, which recommended that the membership of a nationally constituted stem cell review panel should be interdisciplinary and should include members of the public.

The Geron board is also open to possible criticism on grounds that its members were all from the same field and had insufficient expertise in areas related to stem cell science and in addressing the concerns of patients and the public. Yet this board issued a set of guidelines and presented an analysis of the issues that reflected an understanding of the science involved and of varying views about the ethics of conducting this research. It went on to reach conclusions for which it provided reasonable grounds. This suggests that while it is important to have a range of disciplines related to stem cell research represented on a review board, the lack of such representation can be balanced out in unusual instances by members who are themselves open to developing greater background in other disciplines and who represent a range of ethical views and interests.

Recommended Method(s) of Deliberation of a National Stem Cell Review Panel

The five groups that developed these panels did not specifically address the methods of deliberation that they expected them to employ. Even so, we have at hand two different models of how a national ethics panel should deliberate that are provided by the National Bioethics Advisory Committee and the President's Council on Bioethics. These at first seem to offer two wholly disparate models for public deliberation and decision by a national panel addressing pressing ethical issues. However, careful review of their modes of functioning reveals that one of these two models was eventually adopted by both of these national bioethics groups.

The National Bioethics Advisory Commission set out its method of deliberation in its 1999 report on stem cell research, in which it stated that public deliberation in a democratic republic involves seeking common ground among opposing views held by citizens—ground that rests on shared underlying values. It declared: "In our view, an appropriate approach to public policy in this arena is to develop policies that demonstrate respect for all reasonable alternative points of view and that focus, when possible, on the shared fundamental values that these divergent opinions, in their own ways, seek to affirm."[62]

Yet the commission did not blindly follow public opinion. In an area of moral controversy, it maintained, it is sometimes possible to identify common ground and to provide a reasonable statement of that ground on which to base the recommendations of a national bioethics panel. Thus, it did not seek to fix on the most popular beliefs but the most reasonable shared views among those held by the citizenry in reaching its recommendations. The commission used this deliberative method in its stem cell report to point the way to what it saw as an area of agreement among those with opposing views about the moral significance of human embryos. I will not repeat the commission's entire argument here but note that it focused on the belief held in common by both sides that human embryos should be accorded respect and should not be destroyed arbitrarily.[63] (See chapter 7.) The National Bioethics Advisory Commission went on to base its recommendations regarding the use of early human embryos in stem cell research on that area of common agreement between the two camps.

In its reliance on widely shared views supported by publicly available forms of reasoning, the commission drew from several thinkers who reflect, directly or indirectly, the thought of John Rawls. In brief, Rawls had observed that at the core of political arrangements in a well-ordered society of mutual respect and civility lies a set of values and principles that reasonable persons who embrace different, and sometimes conflicting, comprehensive views can publicly endorse.[64] He termed this "public reason" and maintained that it emerges from the shared fundamental interests of the citizens of a constitutional democracy, however divergent they might be in terms of philosophical and religious views. He held that those recommending public policy should provide grounds for their conclusions that cohere with public reason.[65]

Similarly, the National Bioethics Advisory Commission maintained that even though an area may be replete with moral controversy, national bioethics commissions should provide reasoned grounds for their conclusions about how to broach this area that cohere with the reasonable understandings shared by citizens with varying comprehensive views.[66] To do this, the commission must not only engage in deliberations in chambers but also invite public consultation and comment in various ways, including meeting in a variety of locations around the country.

The President's Council on Bioethics, in contrast, did not explicitly set out a method of public deliberation that it would pursue in its writings. Its deliberative approach must therefore be gleaned from its reports and from the writings and statements of its chair, Leon Kass, the primary author of its reports and spokesperson for the group.[67] Although the council's 2004 stem cell research report does not consider how a national bioethics group should broach public deliberation, its 2002 report on human cloning provides some indication of how its members envisioned the appropriate mode of deliberation of a national ethics panel. I draw from both Kass's writings and statements and the 2002 council report to detail the method of deliberation that this body eventually adopted.

Kass indicated, in the "Chairman's Vision" adapted from his opening remarks at the first meeting of the President's Council in 2002, that in carrying out public deliberation, the group would be freed from any method of reasoning that reflected "an overriding concern with consensus."[68] Instead, he maintained in the introduction to the council's report on human cloning that it would pursue arguments to their conclusion and not succumb to "a thin utilitarian calculus of costs and benefits or a narrow analysis based only on individual 'rights.'" Kass went on to explain in that introduction that "we have not suppressed disagreements in search of a single, watered down position. Instead, we have presented clear arguments for the relevant moral and policy positions on multiple sides of these difficult questions." The council's overarching aim, he declared, was "to convey the moral and social importance of the issue at hand and to demonstrate how people of different backgrounds, ethical beliefs, and policy preferences can reason together about it."[69]

Kass seemed to conceive of consensus building as a form of politically expedient negotiation directed toward producing the most efficient results; he saw it as a form of compromise or lowest common denominator formulation that subverts careful reasoning mindful of the moral and social implications of the issues addressed. Instead of seeking such consensus, he declared, the council would ground its reflections on "the broader plane of human procreation and human healing, with their deeper meanings."[70] Thus, the President's Council would proceed by principled reasoning about significant issues raised by human cloning based on insight into its long-range moral and social implications, rather than by weakening or abandoning guiding principles in order to reach agreement.

Kass's approach to public deliberation reflected to a certain degree the political philosophy of Leo Strauss, a professor of political philosophy with whom he had studied at the University of Chicago. Strauss's thought has recently come to prominence and been subjected to a variety of interpretations due to his oblique way of writing.[71] Strauss rejected post-Enlightenment thought and sought to return to a vision of nature and natural law that he maintained suffused classical Greek thought.[72] He likened contemporary society to Plato's republic and maintained that the guardians of today's republic have the ability to discern more clearly than others the nature of that which is truly human.[73] They have emerged from Plato's Cave into the light of the Sun to achieve a noetic vision of the Good and to establish rules for society grounded in traditional ideals, Strauss explained. Being completely devoted to the search for truth, these contemporary guardians grapple with fundamental questions about what it means to be human, veering away from relativism and subjectivism. They are entrusted with directing the republic toward proper human ends. Thus, the method of deliberation embraced by Strauss was that of philosophical reflection based on principle that would eventually emerge with objectively true moral judgments. Kass's call to address fundamental questions about what it means to be human, his concern to avoid relativism, and his belief in offering principled argument and substantive ideals unsullied by concern about consensus reflect, in great part, the views of Strauss.

Not all members of the President's Council adopted this approach to public deliberation. In the council's cloning report, for instance, members indicated that they did not all agree that a method of argument based on unbending principles provided the soundest basis on which to pursue public deliberation. Those in favor of the use of research cloning, who constituted a majority of the President's Council, joined in concluding that "on balance, the objections to cloning-for-biomedical-research are outweighed by the good that can be done for current and future individuals who suffer."[74] Public deliberation, in their view, should proceed by weighing and balancing opposing goods and seeking a moral balance among them, rather than by standing on unswerving principles. In contrast, those on the council who rejected research cloning, who constituted a minority of the group (and included Kass), maintained that no method of balancing could resolve the issue.[75] They held instead that the decision had to be made as a matter of principle. The principle involved was that it is morally wrong to exploit and destroy developing human life. This principle indicated that research cloning was clearly wrong, these members held. This left the President's Council with no common view of whether research cloning should be pursued and no method of public deliberation that all members could adopt.

Yet a curious transformation in the method of deliberation of the council appeared in the final section of the cloning report, where the question under consideration had been changed from whether to support research cloning to the question of whether to establish a limited moratorium on this form of cloning. There a different majority of members (including Kass) recommended a four-year moratorium on research cloning. This, they argued, would allow time "for further democratic deliberation and for seeking a consensus about whether this research should proceed."[76] This compromise, the new majority declared, "is perfectly warranted by the state of public opinion and justified by the supreme values in our democracy of informed and deliberate decision in matter of great moment."[77] Thus, somewhat surprisingly, the majority of the President's Council now embraced consensus seeking, consultation with the public, and the "supreme values" of informed and deliberate decision about significant issues. This was essentially the same method of public deliberation adopted by the National Bioethics Advisory Commission that had been rejected earlier as providing mere compromise in significant sections of the council's cloning report.

Method of Public Deliberation That Emerged from Both Bioethics Commissions

In the end, therefore, these two national bioethics groups emerged with a remarkably similar view of the way that public deliberation should proceed.[78] They both maintained that a national review body developing recommendations about new and unique sorts of research should seek to discern shared values and develop policies that are informed by reason that take these values into account.

This does not mean that both national bioethics groups insisted that there is only one legitimate way of engaging in public deliberation regarding substantive ethical issues such as those surrounding stem cell research. It means that they agreed that the goal of public reasoning and policy development in a pluralistic democratic polity should be to find areas of underlying agreement among those who express opposing philosophical and religious views.[79] The cost of resolving conflict about such issues as whether to carry out human embryonic stem cell research and human research cloning cannot be the elimination of disagreement by converting or forcing one side over to the other or else ignoring one side entirely. Instead, a national bioethics panel should seek mutual ground that opposing sides can acknowledge as reasonable and consistent with shared values. Ethical pluralism does not preclude reasonable agreement. Thus, the mode of public deliberation eventually adopted by these two presidential commissions on bioethics provides a model for how a national ethics panel should deliberate as it addresses pressing ethical issues in stem cell research.

Model for Stem Cell Review Panel That Emerges

The model of a national stem cell review panel that emerges from this analysis is that of a board that would have six major functions: it would (1) formulate guidelines for stem cell research, (2) review and approve of stem cell research proposals, (3) formulate policy regarding stem cell research, (4) provide public education about stem cells and research into them, (5) collect and make generally accessible data regarding stem cell research, and (6) arrange for an assessment of its own procedures and results. In carrying out these functions, it would conduct open discussions and engage in public consultations, and it would express its conclusions following lines of reasoning that are accessible to the public and that take into account shared public values. This panel would engage in consultation with local review boards regarding the continuing applicability of both national and local guidelines for this research in view of new scientific findings and changing conditions. It would also review stem cell research protocols that raise especially difficult ethical issues after they had been reviewed by local institutional review boards. In addition, this panel would develop a repository of information about available human embryonic stem cell lines in order to inform stem cell investigators and the public about the current status of this research and provide the basis for future policy formulation.

To carry out these functions, this panel would include members with expertise regarding the scientific, clinical, ethical, and policy issues related to stem cell research, as well as members of the public from a variety of backgrounds. It would also include "ordinary" citizens to its work, including those affected by diseases that stem cell therapies might treat. While this cannot be guaranteed, its membership would be drawn from among persons sensitive to the variety of views about the ethical and policy questions surrounding stem cell research held by people around the country and receptive to seeking common ground among them based on reasoned deliberation about shared values. To this end, members of the panel should be open to hearing from a variety of stakeholders, social groups, and experts so that its recommendations address all the relevant issues and alternatives.

Stem Cell Review Panels in Privately Held Biotechnology Companies

Private corporations may be reluctant to accept review of their stem cell research by a federally constituted ethics panel for a variety of reasons. For one, they may perceive government involvement in private industry as threatening to the vitality of scientific inquiry. In addition, such companies are founded on the desire to take the initiative in developing innovative technologies for the market and may well reject the possibility that a government body would intrude into their creative enterprise in ways that affect the bottom line. Furthermore, they may believe that competition-based pressures for secrecy would be undermined by consultation with a national stem cell review panel. Indeed, some among them may not wish to draw attention to proposed research that might undermine, rather than enhance, their interests because of its ethically controversial nature.

Some companies were able to overcome these concerns and to consult about their proposed research with the Recombinant DNA Advisory Committee, the body discussed above that provided oversight for federally funded research into gene transfer technology. They apparently found that approval of their research by this national panel not only was useful in resolving difficult ethical issues that they faced but also was desirable because it assured the public that their research met nationally recognized ethical guidelines.

Some companies, however, may prefer to develop their own stem cell review panels rather than consult with a nationally established one, believing that these offer certain advantages to those in the private sector. Such panels offer a way of suggesting to the public that companies are conducting their research in an ethically responsible manner. If a corporation plans to pursue research that some members of the public consider wrong, the very existence of an in-house ethics board could indicate that the ethics board has considered the issue and may suggest that the company is not pursuing such research solely for business reasons but is also attempting to meet shared ethical standards. Furthermore, establishing ethics panels at private stem cell research companies can lead to the identification of difficult ethical issues that might be raised by developments in stem cell science and medicine before they impinge on company research in negative ways.

Biotechnology companies would be well advised to select a multi-disciplinary review panel to oversee stem cell research that is composed of a range of experts from different disciplines who are not affiliated with the company, as well as some public members. This would provide for independent review of their research and would therefore make such review more credible. Such members should be appointed for a specific term and guaranteed tenure for the entire length of that term so that they are not in peril of being dismissed for taking stances that appear to work against the interests of the company. Their names should be publicly available, and minutes should be kept of their meetings so that there is a record of who took what stance and why. It would be useful for such panels, in developing stem cell research guidelines, to review available guidelines developed by academic institutions, professional associations, and other private and public agencies to gain a sense of their reasons for making recommendations. They could also review the guidelines of other companies and modify their own guidelines in light of the best of these.

There are certain steps that ethics panels in the private sector would have to take in order to perform in a way that would be viewed as ethically sound. They should require a clear guarantee from the company that their work will not be contravened by corporate officers concerned exclusively about business interests.[80] They should be informed about proposed stem cell research before it reaches the start-up phase in order to avoid becoming an approval, rather than a consultative, body. Further, members of a panel affiliated with a private biotech company would have to resolve any conflicts of interest of potential members, such as that generated when such persons own stock in the company, before they were appointed to the panel.

Compensation for the services of such panel members should not be excessive so as to avoid the perception of undue inducement. The remuneration provided could be equivalent to that provided to members of a national stem cell review panel or to those who serve as consultants to various NIH bodies.

A private company engaged in stem cell research could create a process that involves first carrying out a scientific and an ethics review of a research proposal by two separate panels and then sending that proposal for review by relevant administrative officers in order to check on legal compliance. Any proposed modifications in the proposal recommended by administrators would then be sent back to the initial scientific and ethics review panels for final consideration. Should they have reservations about administrative changes, some mutual accommodation would be sought that does not subvert the conclusions of either panel. This would promote institutional coordination between scientific, ethics, and administrative offices without compromising the decisions of the scientific and ethics panels.

Need for a National Stem Cell Research Review Panel

With each novel and more ingenious foray into stem cell research in the United States, the question of whether to set out a set of national guidelines to respond to the ethical issues that this research creates comes to the fore with increased force. An ancillary debate inevitably ensues about the proper forum for developing such guidelines. At times, it appears that in the absence of a federal review policy establishing such a body, the substantive ethical questions raised by stem cell research are lost in the debate about whether one group or another should be recognized as the premier stem cell research review body for the country. Yet the forum in which the available options for stem cell research are discussed and guidelines are recommended is as crucial to the development of sound ethical thought and public policy as are the conclusions themselves.

A national stem cell research review panel could serve to identify substantive ethical issues that this research raises and recommend guidelines that are responsive to them. Such a panel could reduce the current uncertainty caused by the existence of multiple sets of divergent guidelines across the scientific-cum-medical professions and the states. It could also develop guidelines in advance for emerging issues that we will have to confront as stem cell research moves into the clinical setting and develops ever more ingenious ways of restoring and enhancing the human body. Further, such a national panel could establish a repository of information about the current state of stem cell research that would provide the basis for future stem cell research and policy formulation. It would also provide review of stem cell research proposals to private companies pursuing this research, as requested. In an era of multiple contentious voices, a national stem cell review and oversight panel could develop considerable moral authority by proving to be both relevant and rigorous in its review of stem cell research and providing multiple opportunities for public participation in the development of national policies regarding this research.

Establishing such a national panel would be nothing new. Ample precedent for such bodies has been set, for instance, by the Belmont Report,[81] which shaped the Common Rule, and the Recombinant DNA Advisory Committee discussed above. The National Bioethics Advisory Committee recognized the need for a national board to review and oversee stem cell research in 1999, stating that "the need for national oversight and review of ES and EG cell research is crucial."[82] That need, if anything, has become more urgent as the scope of stem cell research continues to expand.

In the current political climate, which has been dominated by "the culture wars" and a failure of opposing groups to attempt mutual interchange and understanding, it may seem unlikely that agreement could be reached about establishing a national panel to address the substantive ethical issues that stem cell research raises. Many are leery of setting up such a body because of what they perceive to be the current politicization of science and the imposition of one ideological approach to the pursuit of this research on the rest of the country. However, this does not call for resignation to the status quo. We are increasingly recognizing the need to extricate ourselves from the current political wars and to develop a set of guidelines based on shared values and reasonable common ground that can keep pace with the ethical questions that this research raises.

As public opinion moves increasingly toward the expansion of national stem cell research policy and the depoliticization of science policy, and as federal legislation is in the offing that would expand the scope of this research, the door is opening to the establishment of a national stem cell review panel. If, instead of developing guidelines for stem cell research on the basis of substantive debate about the ethical issues that this research raises, we continue to play "liberals" or "progressives" against "conservatives" or "neoconservatives," we will fail to make ethical progress in guiding this research and will be left in the current state of uncertainty about whether and how to proceed.

To ensure ethical accountability for current efforts to expand the scope of stem cell research and plan for ways of addressing the ethical issues that this research will undoubtedly continue to raise in the future, we need to develop a federal panel to review this research in a climate that is open to broad forms of public consultation. Such a panel would, as the National Bioethics Advisory Commission maintained, assure the public and the Congress "that oversight can be accomplished efficiently, constructively, in a timely fashion, and with sufficient attention to the relevant ethical considerations."[83]

Appendix A

NIH Guidelines for Funding of Human Pluripotent Stem Cell Research, August 25, 2000

National Institutes of Health, "Guidelines for Research Using Human Pluripotent Stem Cells," 65 *Federal Register* 51975, August 25, 2000, available at http://stemcells.nih.gov/staticresources/news/newsArchives/fr25au00–136.asp

I. Scope of Guidelines

These Guidelines apply to the expenditure of National Institutes of Health (NIH) funds for research using human pluripotent stem cells derived from human embryos (technically known as human embryonic stem cells) or human fetal tissue (technically known as human embryonic germ cells). For purposes of these Guidelines, "human pluripotent stem cells" are cells that are self-replicating, are derived from human embryos or human fetal tissue, and are known to develop into cells and tissues of the three primary germ layers. Although human pluripotent stem cells may be derived from embryos or fetal tissue, such stem cells are not themselves embryos. NIH research funded under these Guidelines will involve human pluripotent stem cells derived: (1) From human fetal tissue; or (2) from human embryos that are the result of in vitro fertilization, are in excess of clinical need, and have not reached the stage at which the mesoderm is formed.

In accordance with 42 Code of Federal Regulations (CFR) 52.4, these Guidelines prescribe the documentation and assurances that must accompany requests for NIH funding for research using human pluripotent stem cells from: (1) Awardees who want to use existing funds; (2) awardees requesting an administrative or competing supplement; and (3) applicants or intramural researchers submitting applications or proposals. NIH funds may be used to derive human pluripotent stem cells from fetal tissue. NIH funds may not be used to derive human pluripotent stem cells from human embryos. These Guidelines also designate certain areas of human pluripotent stem cell research as ineligible for NIH funding.

II. Guidelines for Research Using Human Pluripotent Stem Cells That Is Eligible for NIH Funding

A. Utilization of Human Pluripotent Stem Cells Derived from Human Embryos

1. Submission to NIH

Intramural or extramural investigators who are intending to use existing funds, are requesting an administrative supplement, or are applying for new NIH funding for research using human pluripotent stem cells derived from human embryos must submit to NIH the following:

a. An assurance signed by the responsible institutional official that the pluripotent stem cells were derived from human embryos in accordance with the conditions set forth in section II.A.2 of these Guidelines and that the institution will maintain documentation in support of the assurance;

b. A sample informed consent document (with patient identifier information removed) and a description of the informed consent process that meet the criteria for informed consent set forth in section II.A.2.e of these Guidelines;

c. An abstract of the scientific protocol used to derive human pluripotent stem cells from an embryo;

d. Documentation of Institutional Review Board (IRB) approval of the derivation protocol;

e. An assurance that the stem cells to be used in the research were or will be obtained through a donation or through a payment that does not exceed the reasonable costs associated with the transportation, processing, preservation, quality control, and storage of the stem cells;

f. The title of the research proposal or specific subproject that proposes the use of human pluripotent stem cells;

g. An assurance that the proposed research using human pluripotent stem cells is not a class of research that is ineligible for NIH funding as set forth in section III of these Guidelines; and

h. The Principal Investigator's written consent to the disclosure of all material submitted under Paragraph A.1 of this

section, as necessary to carry out the public review and
other oversight procedures set forth in section IV of these
Guidelines.

2. Conditions for the Utilization of Human Pluripotent Stem Cells
Derived from Human Embryos

Studies utilizing pluripotent stem cells derived from human embryos may be conducted using NIH funds only if the cells were
derived (without Federal funds) from human embryos that were
created for the purposes of fertility treatment and were in excess
of the clinical need of the individuals seeking such treatment.

a. To ensure that the donation of human embryos in excess of
the clinical need is voluntary, no inducements, monetary or
otherwise, should have been offered for the donation of
human embryos for research purposes. Fertility clinics and/
or their affiliated laboratories should have implemented specific written policies and practices to ensure that no such
inducements are made available.

b. There should have been a clear separation between the decision to create embryos for fertility treatment and the decision
to donate human embryos in excess of clinical need for research purposes to derive pluripotent stem cells. Decisions
related to the creation of embryos for fertility treatment
should have been made free from the influence of researchers
or investigators proposing to derive or utilize human pluripotent stem cells in research. To this end, the attending physician
responsible for the fertility treatment and the researcher or
investigator deriving and/or proposing to utilize human pluripotent stem cells should not have been one and the same
person.

c. To ensure that human embryos donated for research were in
excess of the clinical need of the individuals seeking fertility
treatment and to allow potential donors time between the
creation of the embryos for fertility treatment and the decision
to donate for research purposes, only frozen human embryos
should have been used to derive human pluripotent stem cells.
In addition, individuals undergoing fertility treatment should
have been approached about consent for donation of human
embryos to derive pluripotent stem cells only at the time of
deciding the disposition of embryos in excess of the clinical
need.

d. Donation of human embryos should have been made without
any restriction or direction regarding the individual(s) who
may be the recipients of transplantation of the cells derived
from the human pluripotent stem cells.

e. Informed Consent

Informed consent should have been obtained from individuals who have sought fertility treatment and who elect to donate human embryos in excess of clinical need for human pluripotent stem cell research purposes. The informed consent process should have included discussion of the following information with potential donors, pertinent to making the decision whether or not to donate their embryos for research purposes. Informed consent should have included:

(i) A statement that the embryos will be used to derive human pluripotent stem cells for research that may include human transplantation research;

(ii) A statement that the donation is made without any restriction or direction regarding the individual(s) who may be the recipient(s) of transplantation of the cells derived from the embryo;

(iii) A statement as to whether or not information that could identify the donors of the embryos, directly or through identifiers linked to the donors, will be removed prior to the derivation or the use of human pluripotent stem cells;

(iv) A statement that derived cells and/or cell lines may be kept for many years;

(v) Disclosure of the possibility that the results of research on the human pluripotent stem cells may have commercial potential, and a statement that the donor will not receive financial or any other benefits from any such future commercial development;

(vi) A statement that the research is not intended to provide direct medical benefit to the donor; and

(vii) A statement that embryos donated will not be transferred to a woman's uterus and will not survive the human pluripotent stem cell derivation process.

f. Derivation protocols should have been approved by an IRB established in accord with 45 CFR 46.107 and 46.108 or FDA regulations at 21 CFR 56.107 and 56.108.

B. Utilization of Human Pluripotent Stem Cells Derived from Human Fetal Tissue

1. Submission to NIH
   Intramural or extramural investigators who are intending to use existing funds, are requesting an administrative supplement, or are applying for new NIH funding for research using human pluripotent stem cells derived from fetal tissue must submit to NIH the following:
   a. An assurance signed by the responsible institutional official that the pluripotent stem cells were derived from human

fetal tissue in accordance with the conditions set forth in section II.A.2 of these Guidelines and that the institution will maintain documentation in support of the assurance;

b. A sample informed consent document (with patient identifier information removed) and a description of the informed consent process that meet the criteria for informed consent set forth in section II.B.2.b of these Guidelines;

c. An abstract of the scientific protocol used to derive human pluripotent stem cells from fetal tissue;

d. Documentation of IRB approval of the derivation protocol;

e. An assurance that the stem cells to be used in the research were or will be obtained through a donation or through a payment that does not exceed the reasonable costs associated with the transportation, processing, preservation, quality control and storage of the stem cells;

f. The title of the research proposal or specific subproject that proposes the use of human pluripotent stem cells;

g. An assurance that the proposed research using human pluripotent stem cells is not a class of research that is ineligible for NIH funding as set forth in section III of these Guidelines; and

h. The Principal Investigator's written consent to the disclosure of all material submitted under Paragraph B.1 of this section, as necessary to carry out the public review and other oversight procedures set forth in section IV of these Guidelines.

2. Conditions for the Utilization of Human Pluripotent Stem Cells Derived from Fetal Tissue

a. Unlike pluripotent stem cells derived from human embryos, DHHS funds may be used to support research to derive pluripotent stem cells from fetal tissue, as well as for research utilizing such cells. Such research is governed by Federal statutory restrictions regarding fetal tissue research at 42 U.S.C. 289g-2(a) and the Federal regulations at 45 CFR 46.210. In addition, because cells derived from fetal tissue at the early stages of investigation may, at a later date, be used in human fetal tissue transplantation research, it is the policy of NIH to require that all NIH-funded research involving the derivation or utilization of pluripotent stem cells from human fetal tissue also comply with the fetal tissue transplantation research statute at 42 U.S.C. 289g-1.

b. Informed Consent As a policy matter, NIH-funded research deriving or utilizing human pluripotent stem cells from fetal tissue should comply with the informed consent law applicable to fetal tissue transplantation research (42 U.S.C. 289g-1) and the following conditions. The informed consent process should have included discussion of the following information with potential donors, pertinent to making the decision whether to donate fetal tissue for research purposes.

Informed consent should have included:

(i) A statement that fetal tissue will be used to derive human pluripotent stem cells for research that may include human transplantation research;

(ii) A statement that the donation is made without any restriction or direction regarding the individual(s) who may be the recipient(s) of transplantation of the cells derived from the fetal tissue;

(iii) A statement as to whether or not information that could identify the donors of the fetal tissue, directly or through identifiers linked to the donors, will be removed prior to the derivation or the use of human pluripotent stem cells;

(iv) A statement that derived cells and/or cell lines may be kept for many years;

(v) Disclosure of the possibility that the results of research on the human pluripotent stem cells may have commercial potential, and a statement that the donor will not receive financial or any other benefits from any such future commercial development; and

(vi) A statement that the research is not intended to provide direct medical benefit to the donor.

c. Derivation protocols should have been approved by an IRB established in accord with 45 CFR 46.107 and 46.108 or FDA regulations at 21 CFR 56.107 and 56.108.

III. Areas of Research Involving Human Pluripotent Stem Cells That Are Ineligible for NIH Funding

Areas of research ineligible for NIH funding include:

A. The derivation of pluripotent stem cells from human embryos;

B. Research in which human pluripotent stem cells are utilized to create or contribute to a human embryo;

C. Research utilizing pluripotent stem cells that were derived from human embryos created for research purposes, rather than for fertility treatment;

D. Research in which human pluripotent stem cells are derived using somatic cell nuclear transfer, i.e., the transfer of a human somatic cell nucleus into a human or animal egg;

E. Research utilizing human pluripotent stem cells that were derived using somatic cell nuclear transfer, i.e., the transfer of a human somatic cell nucleus into a human or animal egg;

F. Research in which human pluripotent stem cells are combined with an animal embryo; and

G. Research in which human pluripotent stem cells are used in combination with somatic cell nuclear transfer for the purposes of reproductive cloning of a human.

IV. Oversight

A. The NIH Human Pluripotent Stem Cell Review Group (HPSCRG) will review documentation of compliance with the Guidelines for funding requests that propose the use of human pluripotent stem cells. This working group will hold public meetings when a funding request proposes the use of a line of human pluripotent stem cells that has not been previously reviewed and approved by the HPSCRG.

B. In the case of new or competing continuation (renewal) or competing supplement applications, all applications shall be reviewed by HPSCRG and for scientific merit by a Scientific Review Group. In the case of requests to use existing funds or applications for an administrative supplement or in the case of intramural proposals, Institute or Center staff should forward material to the HPSCRG for review and determination of compliance with the Guidelines prior to allowing the research to proceed.

C. The NIH will compile a yearly report that will include the number of applications and proposals reviewed and the titles of all awarded applications, supplements or administrative approvals for the use of existing funds, and intramural projects.

D. Members of the HPSCRG will also serve as a resource for recommendations to the NIH with regard to any revisions to the NIH Guidelines for Research Using Human Pluripotent Stem Cells and any need for human pluripotent stem cell policy conferences.

Dated: August 17, 2000.
Ruth L. Kirschstein,
Principal Deputy Director, NIH.
[FR Doc. 00–21760 Filed 8-23-00; 8:45 am]

Appendix B

Speech by President George W. Bush regarding Human Stem Cell Research, August 9, 2001

George W. Bush, "Remarks by the President on Stem Cell Research," August 9, 2001, 8:01 P.M. CDT, available at http://www.whitehouse.gov/news/releases/2001/08/20010809-2.html

THE PRESIDENT: Good evening. I appreciate you giving me a few minutes of your time tonight so I can discuss with you a complex and difficult issue, an issue that is one of the most profound of our time.

The issue of research involving stem cells derived from human embryos is increasingly the subject of a national debate and dinner table discussions. The issue is confronted every day in laboratories as scientists ponder the ethical ramifications of their work. It is agonized over by parents and many couples as they try to have children, or to save children already born.

The issue is debated within the church, with people of different faiths, even many of the same faith coming to different conclusions. Many people are finding that the more they know about stem cell research, the less certain they are about the right ethical and moral conclusions.

My administration must decide whether to allow federal funds, your tax dollars, to be used for scientific research on stem cells derived from human embryos. A large number of these embryos already exist. They are the product of a process called in vitro fertilization, which helps so many couples conceive children. When doctors match sperm and egg to create life outside the womb, they usually produce more embryos than are planted in the mother. Once a couple successfully has children, or if they are unsuccessful, the additional embryos remain frozen in laboratories.

Some will not survive during long storage; others are destroyed. A number have been donated to science and used to create privately funded stem cell lines. And a few have been implanted in an adoptive mother and born, and are today healthy children.

Based on preliminary work that has been privately funded, scientists believe further research using stem cells offers great promise that could help improve the lives of those who suffer from many terrible diseases—from juvenile diabetes to Alzheimer's, from Parkinson's to spinal cord injuries. And while scientists admit they are not yet certain, they believe stem cells derived from embryos have unique potential.

You should also know that stem cells can be derived from sources other than embryos—from adult cells, from umbilical cords that are discarded after babies are born, from human placenta. And many scientists feel research on these type of stem cells is also promising. Many patients suffering from a range of diseases are already being helped with treatments developed from adult stem cells.

However, most scientists, at least today, believe that research on embryonic stem cells offer the most promise because these cells have the potential to develop in all of the tissues in the body.

Scientists further believe that rapid progress in this research will come only with federal funds. Federal dollars help attract the best and brightest scientists. They ensure new discoveries are widely shared at the largest number of research facilities and that the research is directed toward the greatest public good.

The United States has a long and proud record of leading the world toward advances in science and medicine that improve human life. And the United States has a long and proud record of upholding the highest standards of ethics as we expand the limits of science and knowledge. Research on embryonic stem cells raises profound ethical questions, because extracting the stem cell destroys the embryo, and thus destroys its potential for life. Like a snowflake, each of these embryos is unique, with the unique genetic potential of an individual human being.

As I thought through this issue, I kept returning to two fundamental questions: First, are these frozen embryos human life, and therefore, something precious to be protected? And second, if they're going to be destroyed anyway, shouldn't they be used for a greater good, for research that has the potential to save and improve other lives?

I've asked those questions and others of scientists, scholars, bio-ethicists, religious leaders, doctors, researchers, members of Congress, my Cabinet, and my friends. I have read heartfelt letters from many Americans. I have given this issue a great deal of thought, prayer, and considerable reflection. And I have found widespread disagreement.

On the first issue, are these embryos human life—well, one researcher told me he believes this five-day-old cluster of cells is not an embryo, not yet an individual, but a pre-embryo. He argued that it has the potential for life, but it is not a life because it cannot develop on its own.

An ethicist dismissed that as a callous attempt at rationalization. Make no mistake, he told me, that cluster of cells is the same way you and I, and all the rest of us, started our lives. One goes with a heavy heart if we use these, he said, because we are dealing with the seeds of the next generation.

And to the other crucial question, if these are going to be destroyed anyway, why not use them for good purpose—I also found different answers. Many argue these embryos are byproducts of a process that helps create life, and we should allow couples to donate them to science so they can be used for good purpose instead of wasting their potential. Others will argue there's no such thing as excess life, and the fact that a living being is going to die does not justify experimenting on it or exploiting it as a natural resource.

At its core, this issue forces us to confront fundamental questions about the beginnings of life and the ends of science. It lies at a difficult moral intersection, juxtaposing the need to protect life in all its phases with the prospect of saving and improving life in all its stages.

As the discoveries of modern science create tremendous hope, they also lay vast ethical mine fields. As the genius of science extends the horizons of what we can do, we increasingly confront complex questions about what we should do. We have arrived at that brave new world that seemed so distant in 1932, when Aldous Huxley wrote about human beings created in test tubes in what he called a "hatchery."

In recent weeks, we learned that scientists have created human embryos in test tubes solely to experiment on them. This is deeply troubling, and a warning sign that should prompt all of us to think through these issues very carefully.

Embryonic stem cell research is at the leading edge of a series of moral hazards. The initial stem cell researcher was at first reluctant to begin his research, fearing it might be used for human cloning. Scientists have already cloned a sheep. Researchers are telling us the next step could be to clone human beings to create individual designer stem cells, essentially to grow another you, to be available in case you need another heart or lung or liver.

I strongly oppose human cloning, as do most Americans. We recoil at the idea of growing human beings for spare body parts, or creating life for our convenience. And while we must devote enormous energy to conquering disease, it is equally important that we pay attention to the moral concerns raised by the new frontier of human embryo stem cell research. Even the most noble ends do not justify any means.

My position on these issues is shaped by deeply held beliefs. I'm a strong supporter of science and technology, and believe they have the potential for incredible good—to improve lives, to save life, to conquer disease. Research offers hope that millions of our loved ones may be cured of a disease and rid of their suffering. I have friends whose children suffer from juvenile diabetes. Nancy Reagan has written me about President Reagan's struggle with Alzheimer's. My own family has confronted the tragedy of childhood leukemia. And, like all Americans, I have great hope for cures.

I also believe human life is a sacred gift from our Creator. I worry about a culture that devalues life, and believe as your President I have an important obligation to foster and encourage respect for life in America and throughout the world. And while we're all hopeful about the potential of this research, no one can be certain that the science will live up to the hope it has generated.

Eight years ago, scientists believed fetal tissue research offered great hope for cures and treatments—yet, the progress to date has not lived up to its initial expectations. Embryonic stem cell research offers both great promise and great peril. So I have decided we must proceed with great care.

As a result of private research, more than 60 genetically diverse stem cell lines already exist. They were created from embryos that have already been destroyed, and they have the ability to regenerate themselves indefinitely, creating ongoing opportunities for research. I have concluded that we should allow federal funds to be used for research on these existing stem cell lines, where the life and death decision has already been made.

Leading scientists tell me research on these 60 lines has great promise that could lead to breakthrough therapies and cures. This allows us to explore the promise and potential of stem cell research without crossing a fundamental moral line, by providing taxpayer funding that would sanction or encourage further destruction of human embryos that have at least the potential for life.

I also believe that great scientific progress can be made through aggressive federal funding of research on umbilical cord placenta, adult and animal stem cells which do not involve the same moral dilemma. This year, your government will spend $250 million on this important research.

I will also name a President's council to monitor stem cell research, to recommend appropriate guidelines and regulations, and to consider all of the medical and ethical ramifications of biomedical innovation. This council will consist of leading scientists, doctors, ethicists, lawyers, theologians, and others and will be chaired by Dr. Leon Kass, a leading biomedical ethicist from the University of Chicago.

This council will keep us apprised of new developments and give our nation a forum to continue to discuss and evaluate these important issues. As we go forward, I hope we will always be guided by both intellect and heart, by both our capabilities and our conscience.

I have made this decision with great care, and I pray it is the right one.

Thank you for listening. Good night, and God bless America.

Appendix C

Withdrawal of NIH Guidelines for Research Using Human Pluripotent Stem Cells, November 2, 2001

Department of Health and Human Services, National Institutes of Health, "Withdrawal of NIH Guidelines for Research Using Human Pluripotent Stem Cells," 66 *Federal Register* 57107, November 2, 2001, available at http://stemcells.nih.gov/staticresources/news/newsArchives/fr14n001-95.asp

ACTION: Notice; withdrawal of NIH Guidelines for Research Using Pluripotent Stem Cells Derived from Human Embryos (published August 25, 2000, 65 FR 51976, corrected November 21, 2000, 65 FR 69951).

SUMMARY: The National Institutes of Health (NIH) announces the withdrawal of those sections of the NIH Guidelines for Research Using Human Pluripotent Stem Cells, http://www.nih.gov/news/stemcell/stemcellguidelines.htm (NIH Guidelines), that pertain to research involving human pluripotent stem cells derived from human embryos that are the result of in vitro fertilization, are in excess of clinical need, and have not reached the stage at which the mesoderm is formed. The President has determined the criteria that allow Federal funding for research using existing embryonic stem cell lines, http://www.whitehouse.gov/news/releases/2001/08/print/20010809-1.html. Thus, the NIH Guidelines as they relate to human pluripotent stem cells derived from human embryos are no longer needed.

FOR FURTHER INFORMATION CONTACT: NIH Office of Extramural Research, NIH, 1 Center Drive, MSC 0152, Building 1, Room 146, Bethesda, MD 20892, or e-mail DDER@nih.gov.

Dated: November 2, 2001.
Ruth L. Kirschstein,
Acting Director, National Institutes of Health.
[FR Doc. 01-28426 Filed 11-13-01; 8:45 am]
BILLING CODE 4140-01-P

Appendix D

NIH Criteria for Federal Funding of Human Pluripotent Stem Cells, November 7, 2001

NOTICE OF CRITERIA FOR FEDERAL FUNDING OF RESEARCH ON EXISTING HUMAN EMBRYONIC STEM CELLS AND ESTABLISHMENT OF NIH HUMAN EMBRYONIC STEM CELL REGISTRY

Release Date: November 7, 2001

NOTICE: NOT-OD-02-005, available at http://grants.nih.gov/grants/guide/notice-files/NOT-OD-02-005.html.

Office of the Director, NIH

On August 9, 2001, at 9:00 P.M. EDT, the President announced his decision to allow Federal funds to be used for research on existing human embryonic stem cell lines as long as prior to his announcement (1) the derivation process (which commences with the removal of the inner cell mass from the blastocyst) had already been initiated and (2) the embryo from which the stem cell line was derived no longer had the possibility of development as a human being.

In addition, the President established the following criteria that must be met:

- The stem cells must have been derived from an embryo that was created for reproductive purposes;
- The embryo was no longer needed for these purposes;
- Informed consent must have been obtained for the donation of the embryo;
- No financial inducements were provided for donation of the embryo.

In order to facilitate research using human embryonic stem cells, the NIH is creating a Human Embryonic Stem Cell Registry that will list the human embryonic stem cells that meet the eligibility criteria. Specifically, the laboratories or companies that provide the cells listed on the Registry will have submitted to the NIH a signed assurance. Each provider must retain for submission to the NIH, if necessary, written documentation to verify the statements in the signed assurance.

The Registry will be accessible to investigators on the NIH Home Page http://escr.nih.gov. Requests for Federal funding must cite a human embryonic stem cell line that is listed on the NIH Registry. Such requests will also need to meet existing scientific and technical merit criteria and be recommended for funding by the relevant National Advisory Council, as appropriate. Further guidance is accessible at http://grants.nih.gov/grants/guide/notice-files/NOT-OD-02-006.html.

Inquiries should be directed to the Deputy Director for Extramural Research DDER@nih.gov.

Appendix E

President George W. Bush's Veto of the Stem Cell Research Enhancement Act of 2005, July 2006

"Message to the House of Representatives," available at http://www.white house.gov/news/releases/2006/07/20060719-5.html#

TO THE HOUSE OF REPRESENTATIVES:
I am returning herewith without my approval H.R. 810, the "Stem Cell Research Enhancement Act of 2005."

Like all Americans, I believe our Nation must vigorously pursue the tremendous possibilities that science offers to cure disease and improve the lives of millions. Yet, as science brings us ever closer to unlocking the secrets of human biology, it also offers temptations to manipulate human life and violate human dignity. Our conscience and history as a Nation demand that we resist this temptation. With the right scientific techniques and the right policies, we can achieve scientific progress while living up to our ethical responsibilities.

In 2001, I set forth a new policy on stem cell research that struck a balance between the needs of science and the demands of conscience. When I took office, there was no Federal funding for human embryonic stem cell research. Under the policy I announced 5 years ago, my Administration became the first to make Federal funds available for this research, but only on embryonic stem cell lines derived from embryos that had already been destroyed. My Administration has made available more than $90 million for research of these lines. This policy has allowed important research to go forward and has allowed America to continue to lead the world in embryonic stem cell research without encouraging the further destruction of living human embryos.

H.R. 810 would overturn my Administration's balanced policy on embryonic stem cell research. If this bill were to become law, American taxpayers for the first time in our history would be compelled to fund the deliberate destruction of human embryos. Crossing this line would be a grave mistake and would needlessly encourage a conflict between science and ethics that can only do damage to both and harm our Nation as a whole.

Advances in research show that stem cell science can progress in an ethical way. Since I announced my policy in 2001, my Administration has expanded funding of research into stem cells that can be drawn from children, adults, and the blood in umbilical cords with no harm to the donor, and these stem cells are currently being used in medical treatments. Science also offers the hope that we may one day enjoy the potential benefits of embryonic stem cells without destroying human life. Researchers are investigating new techniques that might allow doctors and scientists to produce stem cells just as versatile as those derived from human embryos without harming life. We must continue to explore these hopeful alternatives, so we can advance the cause of scientific research while staying true to the ideals of a decent and humane society.

I hold to the principle that we can harness the promise of technology without becoming slaves to technology and ensure that science serves the cause of humanity. If we are to find the right ways to advance ethical medical research, we must also be willing when necessary to reject the wrong ways. For that reason, I must veto this bill.

GEORGE W. BUSH
THE WHITE HOUSE,
July 19, 2006.

Notes

Chapter 1

1. James A. Thomson, Joseph Itskovitz-Eldor, Sander S. Shapiro, Michelle A. Waknitz, Jennifer J. Swiergiel, Vivienne S. Marshall, Jeffrey M. Jones, "Embryonic Stem Cell Lines Derived from Human Blastocysts," *Science* 282 (1998): 1145–1147; Michael J. Shamblott, Joyce Axelman, Shunping Wang, Elizabeth M. Bugg, John W. Littlefield, Peter J. Donovan, Paul D. Blumenthal, George R. Huggins, John D. Gearhart, "Derivation of Pluripotent Stem Cells from Cultured Human Primordial Germ Cells," *Proceedings of the National Academy of Sciences USA* 95 (1998): 13726–13731.
2. Irving L. Weissman, "Stem Cells: Units of Development, Units of Regeneration, and Units in Evolution," *Cell* 100 (2000): 157–168.
3. National Institutes of Health, "Executive Summary," in *Stem Cells: Scientific and Future Research Directions*, June 2001, updated August 12, 2005, ES-8, available at http://stemcells.nih.gov/info/scireport; National Institutes of Health, "Stem Cells and Diseases," October 6, 2006, available at http://stemcells.nih.gov/info/health.asp. All web addresses were accessed in December 2006.
4. Raymond D. Lambert and Maria DeKoninck, *La conduite responsable de la recherche. Les cadres normatifs*, May 21, 2006, available at http://www.cours.fmed.ulaval.ca/a05/eth64841.
5. John Gearhart, "Medical Promise of Embryonic Stem Cell Research (Present and Projected)," Testimony before the President's Council on Bioethics, April 25, 2002, available at http://www.bioethics.gov/transcripts/apr02/apr25session1.html; National Research Council and the Institute of Medicine of the National Academies, *Stem Cells and the Future of Regenerative Medicine* (Washington, D.C.: National Academies, 2002); Irving Weissman, "Stem Cell Research: Paths to Cancer Therapies and Regenerative Medicine," *Journal of the American Medical Association* 294 (2005): 1359–1366.
6. National Institutes of Health, "3. The Human Embryonic Stem Cell and the Human Embryonic Germ Cell," in *Stem Cells: Scientific Progress and Future Research Directions*, June 2001, updated August 12, 2005, 18,

available at http://stemcells.nih.gov/info/scireport; National Institutes of Health, "11. Use of Genetically Modified Stem Cells in Experimental Gene Therapies," in *Stem Cells: Scientific Progress and Future Research Directions*, June 2001, updated August 12, 2005, 99, available at http://stemcells.nih.gov/info/scireport; Gearhart, "Medical Promise of Embryonic Stem Cell Research" (see note 5).

7. E. Kaji and J. M. Leiden, "Gene and Stem Cell Therapies," *Journal of the American Medical Association* 285 (2001): 545–550.

8. Clive Cookson, "Mother of All Cells," in "Special Report: The Future of Stem Cells," *Scientific American/Financial Times* 293 (2005): A6–10.

9. National Institutes of Health, "Stem Cells and Diseases" (see note 3).

10. Gunjan Sinha, "Human Embryonic Stem Cells May Be Toxicology's New Best Friends," *Science* 308 (2005): 1538.

11. National Institutes of Health, "Stem Cell Basics, VI: What Are the Potential Uses of Human Stem Cells and the Obstacles That Must Be Overcome before These Potential Uses Will Be Realized?" October 6, 2006, available at http://stemcells.nih.gov/info/basics/Stem Cell Basics.pdf; National Institutes of Health, "Executive Summary" (see note 3), ES-1.

12. National Institutes of Health, "Executive Summary" (see note 3), ES-5.

13. National Institutes of Health, "10. Assessing Human Stem Cell Safety," in *Stem Cells: Scientific Progress and Future Research Directions*, June 2001, updated August 12, 2005, 93, available at http://stemcells.nih.gov/info/scireport.

14. J. E. Till, E. A. McCulloch, L. Siminovitch, "Isolation of Variant Cell Lines during Serial Transplantation of Hematopoietic Cells Derived from Fetal Liver," *Journal of the National Cancer Institute* 33 (1964): 707–720; J. E. Till, E. A. McCulloch, L. Siminovitch, "A Stochastic Model of Stem Cell Proliferation Based on the Growth of Spleen Colony-Forming Cells," *Proceedings of the National Academy of Sciences USA* 51 (1964): 29–36; L. Siminovitch, E. A. McCulloch, J. E. Till, "The Distribution of Colony-Forming Cells among Spleen Colonies," *Journal of Cell Physiology* 62 (1963): 327–336.

15. National Institutes of Health, "4. Adult Stem Cells," in *Stem Cells: Scientific Progress and Future Research Directions*, June 2001, updated August 12, 2005, 25, 28–38, available at http://stemcells.nih.gov/info/scireport.

16. M. J. Evans and M. H. Kaufman, "Establishment in Culture of Pluripotential Cells from Mouse Embryos," *Nature* 292 (1981): 154–156; G. R. Martin, "Isolation of a Pluripotent Cell Line from Early Mouse Embryos Cultured in Medium Conditioned by Teratocarcinoma Stem Cells," *Proceedings of the National Academy of Sciences USA* 78 (1981): 7634–7638.

17. J. A. Thomson, J. Kalishman, T. G. Golos, M. Durning, C. P. Harris, R. A. Becker, J. P. Hearn, "Isolation of a Primate Embryonic Stem Cell Line," *Proceedings of the National Academy of Sciences USA* 92 (1995): 7844–7848.

18. A. Bongso, C. Y. Fong, S. C. Ng, S. Ratnam, "Isolation and Culture of Inner Cell Mass Cells from Human Blastocysts," *Human Reproduction* 9 (1994): 2110–2117.

19. Thomson et al., "Embryonic Stem Cell Lines Derived from Human Blastocysts" (see note 1).

20. Shamblott et al., "Derivation of Pluripotent Stem Cells" (see note 1).

21. Rebekah J. Jakel, Bernard L. Schneider, Clive Svendson, "Using Human Neural Stem Cells to Model Neurological Disease," *Nature* 5 (2004): 136–144; Yu-Tzu Tai and Clive N. Svendson, "Stem Cells as a Potential Treatment of Neurological Disorders," *Current Opinion in Pharmacology* 4 (2004): 98–104. In January 2007, a research group headed by Anthony Atala of Wake Forest University School of Medicine announced finding stem cells with characteristics similar to those of embryonic stem cells in the amniotic fluid of pregnant women. (See P. De Coppi, G. Barsch, Jr., M. M. Siddiqui, T. Xu, C. C. Santos, L. Perin, G. Mostoslavsky, A. C. Serre, E. Y. Snyder, J. J. Yoo, et al., "Isolation of Amniotic Stem Cell Lines with Potential for Therapy," *Nature Biotechnology* 25 [2007]: 100–106.) This report followed previous ones from the Atala group and another group in Taiwan. It was hailed by some who object to the use of early human embryos in stem cell research as providing a superior alternative to embryonic stem cells for such research. However, well-regarded stem cell investigators whom I consulted noted that the origin of these amniotic fluid stem cells is unclear and doubted that these cells can differentiate into as many types of cell types as human embryonic stem cells.

22. National Institutes of Health, "Stem Cell Basics" (see note 11); National Institutes of Health, "4. Adult Stem Cells" (see note 15), 23.

23. National Institutes of Health, "4. Adult Stem Cells" (see note 15), 25.

24. B. J. Cummings, N. Uchida, S. J. Tamaki, D. L. Salazar, M. Hooshmand, R. Summers, F. H. Gage, A. J. Anderson, "Human Neural Stem Cells Differentiate and Promote Locomotor Recovery in Spinal Cord-Injured Mice," *Proceedings of the National Academy of Sciences USA* 102 (2005): 14069–14074.

25. Rick Weiss, "Stem Cell Injections Repair Spinal Cord Injuries in Mice," *Washington Post*, September 20, 2005, A2.

26. National Institutes of Health, "Executive Summary" (see note 3), ES-1.

27. C. R. Bjornson, R. L. Rietze, B. A. Reynolds, M. C. Magli, A. L. Vescovi, "Turning Brain into Blood: A Hematopoietic Fate Adopted by Adult Neural Stem Cells In Vivo," *Science* 283 (1999): 534–537.

28. D. L. Clarke, C. B. Johansson, J. Wilbertz, B. Veress, E. Nilsson, H. Karlstrom, U. Lendahl, J. Frisen, "Generalized Potential of Adult Neural Stem Cells," *Science* 288 (2000): 1660–1663.

29. T. R. Brazelton, F. M. Rossi, G. I. Keshet, H. M. Blau, "From Marrow to Brain: Expression of Neuronal Phenotypes in Adult Mice," *Science* 290 (2000): 1775–1779; E. Mezey, K. J. Chandross, G. Harta, R. A. Maki, S. R. McKercher, "Turning Blood into Brains: Cells Bearing Neuronal Antigens Generated In Vivo from Bone Marrow," *Science* 290 (2000): 1779–1782; G. C. Kopen, D. J. Prockop, D. G. Phinney, "Marrow Stromal Cells Migrate throughout Forebrain and Cerebellum and They Differentiate into Astrocytes after Injection into Neonatal Mouse Brain," *Proceedings of the National Academy of Sciences USA* 96 (1999): 10711–10716.

30. D. Orlic, J. Kajstura, S. Chimenti, I. Jakoniuk, S. M. Anderson, B. Li, J. Pickel, et al., "Bone Marrow Cells Regenerate Infarcted Myocardium," *Nature* 410 (2001): 701–705; A. A. Kocher, M. D. Schuseter, M. J. Szabolcs, S. Takuma, D. Burkhoff, J. Wang, S. Homma, N. M. Edwards, S. Itescu, "Neovascularization of Ischemic Myocardium by Human Bone-Marrow-Derived Angioblasts Prevents Cardiomyocyte Apoptosis, Reduces

Remodeling, and Improves Cardiac Function," *Nature Medicine* 7 (2001): 412–413.

31. M. Dezawa, H. Ishikawa, Y. Itokazu, T. Yoshihara, M. Hoshino, S. Takeda, C. Ide, Y. Nabeshima, "Bone Marrow Stromal Cells Generate Muscle Cells and Repair Muscle Degeneration," *Science* 309 (2006): 314–317; E. Gussoni, Y. Soneka, C. D. Strickland, E. A. Buzney, M. K. Khan, A. F. Flint, L. M. Kunkel, R. C. Mulligan, "Dystrophin Expression in the mdx Mouse Restored by Stem Cell Transplantation," *Nature* 401 (1999): 390–394.

32. D. S. Krause, N. D. Theise, M. I. Collector, O. Henegariu, S. Hwang, R. Gardner, S. Neutzel, S. J. Sharkis, "Multi-Organ, Multi-Lineage Engraftment by a Single Bone Marrow-Derived Stem Cell, *Cell* 105 (2001): 369–377.

33. National Institutes of Health, "4. Adult Stem Cells" (see note 15), 33; Brazelton et al., "From Marrow to Brain" (see note 29); Krause et al., "Multi-Organ, Multi-Lineage Engraftment" (see note 32).

34. Y. Jiang, B. N. Jahagirdar, R. L. Reinhardt, R. E. Schwartz, C. D. Keene, X. R. Ortiz-Gonzalez, M. Reyes, et al., "Pluripotency of Mesenchymal Stem Cells Derived from Adult Bone Marrow," *Nature* 418 (2002): 41–49; M. Reyes, T. Lund, T. Lenvik, D. Aguiar, L. Koodie, C. M. Verfaillie, "Purification and Ex Vivo Expression of Postnatal Human Marrow Mesodermal Progenitor Cells," *Blood* 98 (2001): 2615–2625.

35. C. M. Morshead, P. Beneveniste, N. N. Iscove, D. van der Kooy, "Hematopoietic Competence Is a Rare Property of Neural Stem Cells That May Depend on Genetic and Epigenetic Alterations," *Nature Medicine* 8 (2002): 268–273.

36. L. B. Balsam, A. J. Wagers, J. L. Christensen, T. Kofidis, I. L. Weissman, R. C. Robbins, "Haematopoietic Stem Cells Adopt Mature Haematopoietic Fates in Ischemic Myocardium," *Nature* 428 (2004): 668–673; F. Norol, P. Meriet, R. Isnard, P. Sebillon, N. Bonnet, C. Caillot, C. Carrion, et al., "Influence of Mobilized Stem Cells on Myocardial Infarct Repair in a Nonhuman Primate Model," *Blood* 102 (2003): 4361–4368; A. J. Wagers, R. I. Sherwood, J. L. Christensen, I. L. Weissman, "Little Evidence for Developmental Plasticity of Adult Hematopoietic Stem Cells," *Science* 297 (2002): 2256–2259; R. F. Castro, K. A. Jackson, M. A. Goodell, C. S. Robertson, H. Liu, H. D. Shine, "Failure of Bone Marrow Cells to Transdifferentiate into Neural Cells In Vivo," *Science* 297 (2002): 1299.

37. D. D. Thiese, D. Kause, S. Sharkis, "Comment on 'Little Evidence for Developmental Plasticity of Adult Hematopoietic Stem Cells,'" *Science* 299 (2003): 1317; E. Mezey, A. Nagy, I. Szalayova, I., S. Key, A. Bratincsak, J. Baffi, T. Shahar, "Comment on 'Failure of Bone Marrow Cells to Transdifferentiate into Neural Cells In Vivo,'" *Science* 299 (2003): 1184; H. Blau, T. Brazelton, G. Keshet, E. Rossi, "Something in the Eye of the Beholder," *Science* 298 (2002): 363.

38. M. Alvarez-Dolado, R. Pardal, J. M. Garcia-Verdugo, J. R. Fike, H. O. Lee, K. Pfeffer, C. Lois, S. J. Motrrison, A. Alvarez-Buylla, "Fusion of Bone-Marrow-Derived Cells with Purkinje Neurons, Cardiomyocytes and Hepatocytes," *Nature* 425 (2003): 968–973; G. Vassilopoulos, P. R. Wang, D. W. Russell, "Transplanted Bone Marrow Regenerates Liver by Cell Fusion," *Nature* 422 (2003): 901–904; X. Wang, H. Willenbring, Y. Akkari,

Y. Torimaru, M. Foster, M. Al-Dhalimy, E. Lagasse, M. Finegold, S. Olson, M. Grompe, "Cell Fusion Is the Principal Source of Bone-Marrow-Derived Hepatocytes," *Nature* 422 (2003): 897–901; Q. L. Ying, J. Nichols, E. P. Evans, A. G. Smith, "Changing Potency by Spontaneous Fusion," *Nature* 416 (2002): 545–548; N. Terada, T. Hamazaki, M. Oka, M. Hoki, D. M. Mastalerz, Y. Nakano, E. M. Meyer, L. Morel, B. E. Petersen, E. W. Scott, "Bone Marrow Cells Adopt the Phenotype of Other Cells by Spontaneous Cell Fusion," *Nature* 416 (2002): 542–545.

39. D. Zipori, "The Stem Cell State: Plasticity Is Essential, Whereas Self-Renewal and Hierarchy Are Optional," *Stem Cells* 23 (2005): 719–726; M. Korbling and Z. Estrov, "Adult Stem Cells for Tissue Repair: A New Therapeutic Concept?" *New England Journal of Medicine* 349 (2003): 570–582; J. L. Abkowitz, "Can Human Hematopoietic Stem Cells Become Skin, Gut, or Liver Cells?" *New England Journal of Medicine* 346 (2002): 770–772; J. Frisen, "Stem Cell Plasticity?" *Neuron* 35 (2002): 415–418. See also Shane Smith, William Neaves, Steven Teitelbaum, Letter to editor, "Adult Stem Cell Treatments for Diseases?" *Science* 313 (2006): 439.

40. Jos Domen, Amy Wagers, Irving L. Weissman, "Chapter 2. Bone Marrow (Hematopoietic) Stem Cells," in *National Institutes of Health, Regenerative Medicine 2006*, August 2006, 24, available at http://stemcells.nih.gov/info/scireport/2006report.htm; Select Committee on Stem Cell Research, The United Kingdom Paliament, "Stem Cell Research, "Chapter 2: Stem Cells," February 13, 2002, 3–5, available at http://www.parliament.the-stationery-office.co.uk/pa/ld200102/ldselect/ldstem/83/8303.htm.

41. National Institutes of Health, "Executive Summary" (see note 3), ES-1.

42. Domen et al, "Chapter 2: Bone Marrow (Hematopoietic) Stem Cells" (see note 40), 24.

43. Ibid.

44. Robert S. Schwartz, "The Politics and Promise of Stem-Cell Research," *New England Journal of Medicine* 355 (2006): 1189–1191; Kenneth Chien, "Making a Play at Regrowing Hearts," *Scientist* 20 (2006): 35–39.

45. Orlic et al., "Bone Marrow Cells Regenerate Infarcted Myocardium" (see note 30).

46. A. Mathur and J. F. Martin, "Stem Cells and Repair of the Heart," *Lancet* 364 (2004): 183–192.

47. Volker Schächinger, Sandra Erbs, Albrecht Elsässer, Werner Haberbosch, Rainer Hambrecht, Hans Hölschermann, et al., "Intracoronary Bone-Marrow-Derived Progenitor Cells in Acute Myocardial infarction," *New England Journal of Medicine* 355 (2006): 1210–1221; Birgit Assmus, Jörg Honold, Volker Schächinger, Martina B. Britten, Ulrich Fischer-Rasokat, Ralf Lehmann, Claudius Teupe, et al., "Transcoronary Transplantation of Progenitor Cells after Myocardial Infarction," *New England Journal of Medicine* 355 (2006): 1222–1232; J. G. Cleland, N. Freemantle, A. P. Coletta, A. L. Clark, "Clinical Trials Update from the American Heart Association: REPAIR-AMI, ASTAMI, JELIS, MEGA, REVIVE-II, SURVIVE, and PROACTIVE," *European Journal of Heart Failure* 8 (2006): 105–110; R. A. Kloner, "Attempts to Recruit Stem Cells for Repair of Acute Myocardial Infaction," *Journal of the American Medical Association* 295 (2006): 1058–1060.

48. Ketile Lunde, Svein Solheim, Svend Aakhus, Harald Arneson, Michael Abdelnoor, Torstein Egeland, Knut Endresen, et al., "Intracoronary Injection of Mononuclear Bone Marrow Cells in Acute Myocardial Infarction," *New England Journal of Medicine* 355 (2006): 1199–1209; G. P. Meyer, K. C. Wollert, J. Lotz, J. Steffens, P. Lippolt, S. Fichtner, H. Hecker, et al., "Intracoronary Bone Marrow Cell Transfer after Myocardial Infarction: Eighteen Months Follow-Up Data from the Randomized Controlled BOOST (Bone Marrow Transfer to Enhance ST-Elevation Infarct Regeneration) Trial," *Circulation* 113 (2006): 1287–1294; D. Zohlnhöfer, I. Ott, J. Mehilli, K. Schomig, F. Michalk, T. Ibrahim, G. Meisetschlager, et al., REVIVAL-2 Investigators, "Stem Cell Mobilization by Granulocyte Colony-Stimulating Factor in Patients with Acute Myocardial Infarction: A Randomized Controlled Trial," *Journal of the American Medical Association* 295 (2006): 1003–1010; S. Janssens, C. Dubois, J. Boegarat, K. Theunissen, C. Deroose, W. Desmet, M. Kalanzi, et al, "Autologous Bone Marrow Derived Stem Cell Transfer in Patients with ST-Segment Elevation Myocardial Infarction Double-Blind, Randomized, Controlled Trial," *Lancet* 367 (2006): 113–121; K. Lunde, S. Solheim, S. Aakhus, H. Arneson, M. Abdelnoor, K. Forfgang; ASTAMI Investigators, "Autologous Stem Cell Transplantation in Acute Myocardial Infarction: The ASTAMI Randomized Controlled Trial. Intracoronary Transplantation of Autologous Mononuclear Bone Marrow Cells, Study Design and Safety Aspects," *Scandinavian Cardiovascular Journal* 39 (2005): 150–158.
49. K. R. Chien, "Lost and Found: Cardiac Stem Cell Therapy Revisited," *Journal of Clinical Investigations*, 116 (2006): 1838–1840; S. Dimmler, A. M. Zeiher, M. D. Schneider, "Unchain My Heart: The Scientific Foundations of Cardiac Repair," *Journal of Clinical Investigations* 115 (2005): 572–583; Peggy Peck, "Conflicting Data from Stem Cell Therapy," *American Medical News*, December 19, 2005, 2.
50. Chien, "Making a Play at Regrowing Hearts" (see note 44).
51. National Institutes of Health, "Executive Summary" (see note 3), ES-2, ES-6, ES-9; National Institutes of Health, "Stem Cell Information: Frequently Asked Questions,"October 6, 2006, available at http://stemcells. nih.gov/info/faqs.asp.
52. National Institutes of Health, "Stem Cell Information: Frequently Asked Questions" (see note 51).
53. Christine Soares, "Revving up the Body's Own Stem Cells Could Be the Simplest Route to New Therapies," *Scientific American* 293 (2005): A14.
54. National Institutes of Health, "Adult Stem Cells" (see note 15), 37–38.
55. Ali H. Brivanlou, Fred H. Gage, Rudolph Jaenisch, Thomas Jessell, Douglas Melton, Janet Rossant, "Setting Standards for Human Embryonic Stem Cells," *Science* 300 (2003): 913–916.
56. K. Chadwick, L. Wang, L. Li, P. Menendez, B. Murdoch, A. Rouleau, M. Bhatia, "Cytokines and BMP-4 Promote Hematopoietic Differentiation of Human Embryonic Stem Cells," *Blood* 102 (2003): 906–915; D. S. Kaufman, E. T. Hanson, R. L. Lewis, R. Auerbach, J. A. Thomson, "Hematopoietic Colony-Forming Cells Derived from Human Embryonic Stem Cells," *Proceedings of the National Academy of Sciences USA* 98 (2001): 10716–10721.

57. S. Levenberg, J. S. Golub, M. Amit, J. Itskovitz-Eldor, R. Langer, "Endothelial Cells Derived from Human Embryonic Stem Cells," *Proceedings of the National Academy of Sciences USA* 99 (2002): 4391–4396.

58. C. Mummery, D. Ward, C. E. van den Brink, S. D. Bird, P. A. Doevendans, T. Opthof, A. Brutel de la Riviere, L. Tertoolen, M. van der Heyden, M. Pera, "Cardiomyocyte Differentiation of Mouse and Human Embryonic Stem Cells," *Journal of Anatomy* 200 (2002): 233–242; I. Kehat, D. Kenyagin-Karsenti, M. Snir, H. Segev, M. Amit, A. Gepstein, E. Livine, O. Binah, J. Itskovitz-Eldor, L. Gepstein, "Human Embryonic Stem Cells Can Differentiate into Myocytes with Structural and Functional Properties of Cardiomyocytes," *Journal of Clinical Investigations* 108 (2001): 407–414.

59. B. E. Reubinoff, P. Itsykson, T. Turetsky, M. F. Pera, E. Reinhartz, A. Itzik, T. Ben-Hur, "Neural Progenitors from Human Embryonic Stem Cells," *Nature Biotechnology* 19 (2001): 1134–1140; S. C. Zhang, M. Wernig, I. D. Duncan, O. Brustle, J. A. Thomson, "In Vitro Differentiation of Transplantable Neural Precursors from Human Embryonic Stem Cells," *Nature Biotechnology* 19 (2001): 1117–1118.

60. National Institutes of Health, "Executive Summary" (see note 3), ES-7.

61. S. Assady, G. Maor, M. Amit, J. Itskovitz-Eldor, K. L. Skorecki, M. Tzukerman, "Insulin Production by Human Embryonic Stem Cells," *Diabetes* 50 (2001): 1691–1697.

62. M. Amit, M. K. Carpenter, M. S. Inokuma, C. P. Chiu, C. P. Harris, M. A. Waknitz, Itskovitz-Eldor, J. A. Thomson, "Clonally Derived Human Embryonic Stem Cell Lines Maintain Pluripotency and Proliferative Potential for Prolonged Periods of Culture," *Developmental Biology* 227 (2000): 271–278.

63. Thomson et al., "Embryonic Stem Cell Lines Derived from Human Blastocysts" (see note 1); National Institutes of Health, "3. Human Embryonic Stem Cell" (see note 6), 13.

64. M. Richards, C. Y. Fong, W. K. Chan, P. C. Wong, A. Bongso, "Human Feeders Support Prolonged Undifferentiated Growth of Human Inner Cell Masses and Embryonic Stem Cells," *Nature Biotechnology* 20 (2002): 933–936; B. E. Reubinoff, M. F. Pera, C. Y. Fong, A. Trounson, A. Bongso, "Embryonic Stem Cell Lines from Human Blastocysts: Somatic Differentiation in Vitro," *Nature Biotechnology* 18 (2000): 399–404.

65. Cookson, "Mother of All Cells" (see note 8), A6.

66. Amit et al., "Clonally Derived Human Embryonic Stem Cell Lines" (see note 62); Shamblott et al., "Derivation of Pluripotent Stem Cells" (see note 1).

67. J. S. Odorico, D. S. Kaufman, J. A. Thomson, "Multilineage Differentiation from Human Embryonic Stem Cell Lines," *Stem Cells* 19 (2001): 193–204.

68. M. J. Shamblott, J. Axelman, J. W. Littlefield, P. D. Blumenthal, G. B. Huggins, Y. Cui, L. Cheng, J. D. Gearhart, "Human Embryonic Germ Cell Derivatives Express a Broad Range of Developmentally Distinct Markers and Proliferate Extensively In Vitro," *Proceedings of the National Academy of Sciences USA* 98 (2001): 113–118.

69. M. M. Matalipova, R. R. Rao, D. M. Hoyer, J. A. Johnson, L. F. Meisner, K. L. Jones, S. Dalton, S. L. Stice, "Preserving the Genetic Integrity of Human Embryonic Stem Cells," *Nature Biotechnology* 23 (2005): 19–20;

J. S. Draper, K. Smith, P. Gokhale, H. D. Moore, E. Maltby, J. Johnson, L. Meisner, T. P. Zwaka, J. A. Thomson, P. W. Andrews, "Recurrent Gain of Chromosomes 17q and 12 in Cultured Human Embryonic Stem Cells," *Nature Biotechnology* 22 (2004): 42–43; Nuffield Council on Bioethics, *Stem Cell Therapy: The Ethical Issues—A Discussion Paper*, April 2000, available at http://www.nuffieldbioethics.org/go/print/ourwork/stemcells/introduction.

70. R. Eiges, R. Schuldiner, M. Drukker, O. Yanuka, J. Itskovitz-Eldor, N. Benvenisty, "Establishment of Human Embryonic Stem Cell-Transfected Clones Carrying a Marker for Undifferentiated Cells," *Current Biology* 11 (2001): 514–518; A. Pfeifer, M. Ikawa, Y. Dayn, I. M. Verma, "Transgenesis by Lentiviral Vectors: Lack of Gene Silencing in Mammalian Embryonic Stem Cells and Preimplantation Embryos," *Proceedings of the National Academy of Sciences USA* 99 (2002): 2140–2145; T. P. Zwaka and J. A. Thomson, "Homologous Recombination in Human Embryonic Stem Cells," *Nature Biotechnology* 21 (2003): 319–321.

71. National Research Council and Institute of Medicine of the National Academies, *Guidelines for Human Embryonic Stem Cell Research* (Washington, D.C: National Academy Press, 2002), available at http://www.nap.edu/catalog/11278.html.

72. L. Mishra, R. Derynck, B. Mishra, "Transforming Growth Factor-β Signaling in Stem Cells and Cancer," *Science* 310 (2005): 68–71.

73. National Research Council and Institute of Medicine, *Guidelines* (see note 71), 33.

74. National Institutes of Health, "Human Embryonic Stem Cell" (see note 6), 17.

75. Gretchen Vogel, "Ready or Not? Human ES Cells Head toward the Clinic," *Science* 308 (2005): 1534–1538.

76. Ibid., 1534.

77. Andy Coghlan, "First Embryonic Stem Cell Trials on the Cards," *New Scientist*, June 17, 2006, available at http://www.newscientist.com/article.ns?id=dn9349; Vogel, "Ready or Not?" (see note 75), 1534–1535; Christine Soares, "Problems with Contamination and Genetic Abnormalities May Not Stop Work on Embryonic Stem Cell Therapies," *Scientific American* 293 (2005): A10.

78. H. S. Keirstead, G. Nistor, G. Bernal, M. Totoiu, F. Cloutier, K. Sharp, O. Steward, "Human Embryonic Stem-Cell Derived Oligodendrocyte Progenitor Cell Transplants Remyelinate and Restore Locomotion after Spinal Cord Injury," *Journal of Neuroscience* 25 (2005): 4694–4705.

79. Brivanlou et al., "Setting Standards for Human Embryonic Stem Cells" (see note 55).

80. Vogel, "Ready or Not?" (see note 75), 1536.

81. K. G. Sylvester and M. T. Longaker, "Stem Cells: Review and Update," *Archives of Surgery* 139 (2004): 93–99.

82. Thomson et al., "Embryonic Stem Cell Lines Derived from Human Blastocysts" (see note 1).

83. National Institutes of Health, "Human Embryonic Stem Cell" (see note 6), 18.

84. B. J. Conley, J. C. Young, A. O. Trounson, R. Mollard, "Derivation, Propagation, and Differentiation of Human Embryonic Stem Cells," *International Journal of Biochemistry and Cell Biology* 36 (2004): 555–567.

85. Maria J. Martin, Alysson Muotri, Fred Gage, Ajit Varki, "Human Embryonic Stem Cells Express an Immunogenic Nonhuman Sialic Acid," *Nature Medicine* 11 (2005): 228–232.
86. L. Dawson, A. S. Bateman-House, D. Mueller Agnew, H. Bok, D. W. Brock, A. Chakravarti, M. Greene, et al., "Safety Issues in Cell Based Intervention Trials," *Fertility and Sterility* 80 (2003): 1077–1085.
87. M. Amit, M.E. Winkler, S. Menke, E. Bruning, K. Buscher, J. Denner, A. Haverich, J. Itskovitz-Eldor, U. Martin, "No Evidence for Infection of Human Embryonic Stem Cells by Feeder Cell-Derived Murine Leukemia Viruses," *Stem Cells* 23 (2005): 761–771.
88. National Research Council and Institute of Medicine, *Guidelines* (see note 71), 42.
89. K. Nakashima, S. Colamarino, F. H. Gage, "Embryonic Stem Cells: Staying Plastic on Plastic," *Nature Medicine* 10 (2004): 23–24.
90. M. E. Levenstein, T. E. Ludwig, R. H. Xu, R. A. Llanas, K. VanDenHeuvel-Kramer, D. Manning, J. A. Thomson, "Basic Fibroblast Growth Factor Support of Human Embryonic Stem Cell Self-Renewal," *Stem Cells* 24 (2006): 568–574; T. E. Ludwig, M. E. Levenstein, J. M. Jones, W. T. Berggren, E. R. Mitchen, J. L. Frane, L. J. Crandall, et al., "Derivation of Human Embryonic Stem Cells in Defined Conditions," *Nature Biotechnology* 24 (2006): 185–187; R. Xu, M. Ruthann, D. S. Li, R. Li, G. C. Addicks, C. Glennon, T. P. Zawaka, J. A. Thomson, "Basic FGF and Suppression of BMP Signaling Sustain Undifferentiated Proliferation of Human ES Cells," *Nature Methods* 2 (2005): 185–190; J. Inzunza, K. Gerow, M. A. Stromberg, E. Matilainen, E. Blennow, H. Skottman, S. Wolbank, L. Ahrlund-Richter, O. Hovatta, "Derivation of Human Embryonic Stem Cells Lines in Serum Replacement Medium Using Postnatal Human Fibroblasts as Feeder Cells," *Stem Cells* 23 (2005): 544–549; J. B. Lee, J. E. Lee, J. H. Park, S. J. Kim, M. K. Kim, S. I. Roh, H. S. Yoon, "Establishment and Maintenance of Human Embryonic Stem Cell Lines on Human Feeder Cells Derived from Uterine Endometrium under Serum-Free Condition," *Biology and. Reproduction* 72 (2005): 42–49; A. B. Choo, J. Padmanabhan, A. C. Chin, S. K. Oh, "Expansion of Pluripotent Human Embryonic Stem Cells on Human Feeders," *Biotechnology and Bioengineering* 88 (2004): 321–331; L. Cheng, H. Hammond, Z. Ye, X. Zhan, G. Dravid, "Human Adult Marrow Cells Support Prolonged Expansion of Human Embryonic Cells in Culture," *Stem Cells* 21 (2003): 131–142; Richards et al, "Human Feeders Support Prolonged Undifferentiated Growth of Human Inner Cell Masses and Embryonic Stem Cells" (see note 64); C. Xu, M. S. Inokuma, J. Denham, K. Golds, P. Kundu, J. D. Gold, M. K. Carpenter, "Feeder-Free Growth of Undifferentiated Human Embryonic Stem Cells," *Nature Biotechnology* 19 (2001): 971–974.
91. P. Stojkovic, M. Lako, R. Stewart, S. Przyborski, L. Armstrong, J. Evans, A. Murdoch, T. Strachan, M. Stojkovic, "An Autogenic Feeder Cell System That Efficiently Supports Growth of Undifferentiated Human Embryonic Stem Cells," *Stem Cells* 23 (2005): 306–314.
92. I. Klimanskaya, Y. Chung, L. Meisner, J. Johnson, M. D. West, R. Lanza, "Human Embryonic Stem Cells Derived without Feeder Cells," *Lancet* 365 (2005): 1636–1641; M. Amit, C. Shakiri, V. Margulets, J. Itskovitz-Eldor,

"Feeder Layer and Serum-Free Culture of Human Embryonic Stem Cells," *Biology and Reproduction* 70 (2004): 837–845.

93. John Gearhart, "New Human Embryonic Stem-Cell Lines: More Is Better," *New England Journal of Medicine* 350 (2004): 1275–1276.

94. National Research Council and Institute of Medicine, *Guidelines* (see note 71), 17.

95. National Research Council and Institute of Medicine, *Stem Cells and the Future of Regenerative Medicine* (see note 5), 56.

96. National Institutes of Health, "Stem Cell Information: Frequently Asked Questions (FAQs)" (see note 51).

97. National Institutes of Health, "Executive Summary" (see note 3), ES-10.

98. Ibid.

99. Jason Owen-Smith and Jennifer McCormick, "An International Gap in Human ES Cell Research," *Nature Biotechnology* 24 (2006): 391–392.

100. Ibid., 392.

101. Tracy Hampton, "U.S. Stem Cell Research Lagging," *Journal of the American Medical Association* 295 (2006): 2233–2234; Editorial, "A Matter of Science," *Washington Post*, July 30, 2005, A18; George Q. Daley, "Missed Opportunities in Embryonic Stem-Cell Research," *New England Journal of Medicine* 351 (2004): 627–628; Gearhart, "New Human Embryonic Stem-Cell Lines" (see note 93), 1275–1276; Gareth Cook, "U. S. Stem Cell Research Lagging," *Boston Globe*, May 23, 2004, available at http://www.boston.com/news/science/articles/2004/05/23/us_stem_cell_ research_lagging; Letter dated April 28, 2004 to President Bush from over 200 Members of the House of Representatives, available at http:// www.house.gov/degette/news/releases/040428.pdf; Justin Gillis and Rick Weiss, "NIH: Few Stem Cell Colonies Likely Available for Research," *Washington Post*, March 3, 2004, A3, A13; Raja Mishra, "Scientist at Harvard Boosts Stem Cell Pool," *Boston Globe*, November 15, 2003, A1.

Chapter 2

1. Jason Owen-Smith and Jennifer McCormick, "An International Gap in Human ES Cell Research," *Nature Biotechnology* 24 (2006): 391–392; Tracy Hampton, "U.S. Stem Cell Research Lagging," *Journal of the American Medical Association* 295 (2006): 2233–2234; Editorial, "A Matter of Science," *Washington Post*, July 30, 2005, A18; George Q. Daley, "Missed Opportunities in Embryonic Stem-Cell Research," *New England Journal of Medicine* 351 (2004): 627–628; John Gearhart, "New Human Embryonic Stem-Cell Lines: More Is Better," *New England Journal of Medicine* 350 (2004): 1275–1276; Gareth Cook, "U. S. Stem Cell Research Lagging," *Boston Globe*, May 23, 2004, available at http://www.boston.com/news/ science/articles/2004/05/23/us_stem_cell_research_lagging/; Letter dated April 28, 2004, to President Bush from over 200 Members of the House of Representatives, available at http://www.house.gov/degette/news/ releases/040428.pdf; Justin Gillis and Rick Weiss, "NIH: Few Stem Cell Colonies Likely Available for Research," *Washington Post*, March 3, 2004, A3, A13; Raja Mishra, "Scientist at Harvard Boosts Stem Cell Pool," *Boston Globe*, November 15, 2003, A1.

2. T. E. Ludwig, M. E. Levenstein, J. M. Jones, W. T. Berggren, E. R. Mitchen, J. L. Frane, L. J. Crandall, C. A. Daigh, K. R. Conrad, M. S. Peikarczyk, R. A. Llanas, J. A. Thomson, "Derivation of Human Embryonic Stem Cells in Defined Conditions," *Nature Biotechnology* 24 (2006): 185–187.

3. National Research Council and Institute of Medicine of the National Academies, *Stem Cells and the Future of Regenerative Medicine* (Washington, D.C.: National Academy Press, 2002), 3, available at http://www.nap.edu/catalog/11278.html.

4. President's Council on Bioethics, *Alternative Sources of Human Pluripotent Stem Cells: A White Paper* (Washington, D.C.: President's Council on Bioethics, 2005), 46, available at http://www.bioethics.gov.

5. Cynthia B. Cohen, "Gamete Donation," in *Encyclopedia of Bioethics*, 3rd ed. (New York: Macmillan, 2004), vol. 4, 2283–2290; Cynthia B. Cohen, "Ethical Issues in Reproduction," in *Fletcher's Introduction to Clinical Ethics*, 3rd ed., ed. John C. Fletcher, Edward M. Spencer, Paul A. Lombardo (Hagerstown, Md.: University Publishing, 2005), 235–262, 276.

6. Robert Steinbrook, "Egg Donation and Human Embryonic Stem Cell Research," *New England Journal of Medicine* 354 (2006): 324–326.

7. Ibid.; Cohen, "Gamete Donation" (see note 5), 2284; Cohen, "Ethical Issues in Reproduction" (see note 5), 276.

8. D. I. Hoffman, G. L. Zellman, C. C. Fair, J. F. Mayer, J. G. Zeitz, W. E. Gibbons, T. G. Turner Jr., Society for Assisted Reproductive Technology (SART), RAND, "Cryopreserved Embryos in the United States and Their Availability for Research," *Fertility and Sterility* 79 (2003): 1063–1069.

9. S. Bangsbøll, A. Pinborg, C. Yding Andersen, A. Nyboe Andersen, "Patients' Attitudes towards Donation of Surplus Cryopreserved Embryos for Treatment or Research," *Human Reproduction* 19 (2004): 2415–2419; K. Elford, C. Lawrence, A. Leader, "Research Implications of Embryo Cryopreservation Choices Made by Patients Undergoing In Vitro Fertilization," *Fertility and Sterility* 81 (2004): 1154–1155; Andrea D. Gurmankin, Dominic Sisti, Arthur Caplan, "Embryo Disposal Practices in IVF Clinics in the United States," *Politics and the Life Sciences* 22 (2004): 2–6; Kerstin Bjuresten and Outi Hovatta, "Donation of Embryos for Stem Cell Research: How Many Couples Consent?" *Human Reproduction* 18 (2003): 1353–1355; C. A. McMahon, F. L. Gibson, G. I. Leslie, D. M. Saunders, K. A. Porter, C. C. Tenant, "Embryo Donation for Medical Research: Attitudes and Concerns of Potential Donors," *Human Reproduction* 18 (2003): 871–877; S. C. Klock, S. Sheinin, R. R. Kazer, "The Disposition of Unused Frozen Embryos," *New England Journal of Medicine* 345 (2001): 69–70; J. Oghoetuoma, C. McKeating, G. Horne, D. Brison, B. Liebersman, "Use of In Vitro Fertilization Embryos Cryopreserved for 5 Years or More," *Lancet* (2000): 1336; B. J. Van Voorhis, D. M. Grinstead, A. E. Sparks, J. L. Gerard, R. F. Weir, "Establishment of a Successful Donor Embryo Program: Medical, Ethical, and Policy Issues," *Fertility and Sterility* 71 (1999): 604–608.

10. M. Choudhary, E. Haimes, M. Herbert, M. Stojkovi, A. P. Murdoch, "Demographic, Medical, and Treatment Characteristics Associated with Couples' Decisions to Donate Fresh Spare Embryos for Research," *Human Reproduction* 19 (2004): 2091–2096.

11. G. Q. Daley, "Missed Opportunities in Embryonic Stem-Cell Research," *New England Journal of Medicine* 351 (2004): 627–628; John Gearhart, "Medical Promise of Embryonic Stem Cell Research (Present and Projected)," Testimony before the President's Council on Bioethics, April 25, 2002, available at http://www.bioethics.gov/transcripts/apr02/apr25session1.html.

12. Bernard Lo, Vicki Chou, Marcelle I. Cedars, Elena Gates, Robert N. Taylor, Richard M. Wagner, Leslie Wolf, Keith R. Yamamoto, "Informed Consent in Human Oocyte, Embryo, and Embryonic Stem Cell Research," *Fertility and Sterility* 82 (2004): 559–563, 562.

13. C. A. Cowan, I. Klimanskaya, J. McMahon, J. Atienza, J. Witmyer, J. P. Zucker, S. Wang, "Derivation of Embryonic Stem-Cell Lines from Human Blastocysts," *New England Journal of Medicine* 350 (2004): 1353–1356.

14. Ronald M. Green, *The Human Embryo Research Debates: Bioethics in the Vortex of Controversy* (New York: Oxford University Press, 2001); Alan Trounson, "The Genesis of Embryonic Stem Cells," *Nature Biotechnology* 20 (2002): 237–238.

15. Robert P. George and Patrick Lee, "Acorns and Embryos," *New Atlantis*, Fall 2004/Winter 2005, available at http://www.thenewatlantis.com/archive/7/georgelee.htm.

16. Cynthia B. Cohen, "Use of 'Excess' Human Embryos for Stem Cell Research: Protecting Women's Rights and Health," *Women's Health Issues* 10 (2000): 121–126.

17. Ethics Committee, American Society of Reproductive Medicine, "Donating Spare Embryos for Embryonic Stem-Cell Research," *Fertility and Sterility* 78 (2002): 957–960.

18. Cohen, "Gamete Donation" (see note 5), 2284; Cohen, "Ethical Issues in Reproduction" (see note 5), 276.

19. President's Council on Bioethics, *Reproduction & Responsibility: The Regulation of New Biotechnologies* (Washington, D.C.: President's Council on Bioethics, 2004); Carol A. Tauer, "Responsibility and Regulation: Reproductive Technologies, Cloning, and Embryo Research," in *Cloning and the Future of Human Embryo Research*, ed. Paul Lauritzen (Oxford: Oxford University Press, 2001), 145–161; New York State Task Force on Life and the Law, *Assisted Reproductive Technologies* (New York: New York State Task Force on Life and the Law, 1998), 259–263; Cynthia B. Cohen, "Unmanaged Care: The Need to Regulate New Reproductive Technologies in the United States," *Bioethics* 11 (1997): 348–365; National Advisory Board on Ethics in Reproduction, "Report and Recommendations on Oocyte Donation," in *New Ways of Making Babies: The Case of Egg Donation*, ed. Cynthia B. Cohen (Bloomington: Indiana University Press, 1996), 293–302.

20. S. E. Lazendorf, C. A. Boyd, D. I. Wright, S. Muasher, S. Ochinger, G. D. Hodgen, "Use of Human Gametes Obtained from Anonymous Donors for the Production of Human Embryonic Stem Cell Lines," *Fertility and Sterility* 76 (2001): 132–137.

21. Michael J. Sandel, "The Ethical Implications of Human Cloning," *Perspectives in Biology and Medicine* 48 (2005): 241–247.

22. President's Council on Bioethics, *Human Cloning and Human Dignity: An Ethical Inquiry* (Washington, D.C.: President's Council on Bioethics,

2002), 143–144, 164–165; Steinbrook, "Egg Donation and Human Embryonic Stem-Cell Research" (see note 6).

23. Rudolf Jaenisch, "The Biology of Nuclear Cloning and the Potential of
    Embryonic Stem Cells for Transplantation Therapy," in President's Coun-
    cil on Bioethics, *Monitoring Stem Cell Research* (Washington, D.C.: Pre-
    sident's Council on Bioethics, 2004), 387–417, available at http://
    bioethicsprint.bioethics.gov/background/jaenisch.html.

24. M. Drukker, H. Katchman, G. Katz, S. Evevn-Tov Friedman, E. Shezen,
    E. Hornstein, O. Mandelboim, Y. Reisner, N. Benvenisty, "Human Em-
    bryonic Stem Cells and Their Differentiated Derivatives Are Less Suscep-
    tible for Immune Rejection Than Adult Cells," *Stem Cells* 24 (2006):
    221–229.

25. Konrad Hochedlinger and Rudolf Jaenisch, "Nuclear Transplantation,
    Embryonic Stem Cells, and the Potential for Cell Therapy," *New England
    Journal of Medicine* 349 (2003): 275–286.

26. J. S. Odorico, D. S. Kaufman, D.S., J. A. Thomson, "Multilineage Differ-
    entiation from Human Embryonic Stem Cell Lines," *Stem Cells* 19 (2001):
    750–752.

27. Evan Y. Snyder and Jeanne F. Loring, "Beyond Fraud: Stem Cell Re-
    search Continues," *New England Journal of Medicine* 354 (2006): 321–324.

28. James A. Thomson, "Human Embryonic Stem Cells," in *The Human Embry-
    onic Stem Cell Debate: Science, Ethics, and Public Policy*, ed. S. Holland,
    K. Lebacqz, L. Zoloth (Cambridge, Mass.: MIT Press, 2001), 23.

29. Hochedlinger and Jaenisch, "Nuclear Transplantation, Embryonic Stem
    Cells, and the Potential for Cell Therapy" (see note 25), 281.

30. W. M. Rideout III, K. Hochedlinger, M. Kyba, G. Q. Daley, R. Jaenisch,
    "Correction of a Genetic Defect by Nuclear Transplantation and Com-
    bined Cell and Gene Therapy," *Cell* 109 (2002): 17–27.

31. Hochedlinger and Jaenisch, "Nuclear Transplantation, Embryonic Stem
    Cells, and the Potential for Cell Therapy" (see note 25), 281.

32. Irving Weissman, "Stem Cell Research: Paths to Cancer Therapies and
    Regenerative Medicine," *Journal of the American Medical Association*, 294
    (2005): 1359–1366; Brian Vastage, "U.K. Licenses Human Embryo Cre-
    ation," *Journal of the American Medical Association* 290 (2003): 449–450;
    Hochedlinger and Jaenisch, "Nuclear Transplantation, Embryonic Stem
    Cells, and the Potential for Cell Therapy" (see note 25), 281.

33. George Q. Daley, "Cloning and Stem Cells: Handicapping the Political and
    Scientific Debates," *New England Journal of Medicine* 349 (2003): 3211–3212.

34. K. Hochedlinger and Rudolph Jaenisch, "Monoclonal Mice Generated
    by Nuclear Transfer from Mature B and T Donor Cells," *Nature* 415
    (2002): 1035–1038; Rideout et al., "Correction of a Genetic Defect by
    Nuclear Transplantation and Combined Cell and Gene Therapy" (see note
    30), 17–27; T. Wakayama, V. Tabar, I. Rodriguez, A. C. Perry, L. Studer,
    P. Mombaerts, "Differentiation of Embryonic Stem Cell Lines Generated
    from Adult Somatic Cells by Nuclear Transfer," *Science* 292 (2001):
    740–743; M. J. Munsie, A. E. Michalska, C. M. O'Brien, A. O. Trounson,
    M. F. Pera, P. S. Mountford, "Isolation of Pluripotent Embryonic Stem Cells
    from Reprogrammed Adult Mouse Somatic Cell Nuclei," *Current Biology* 10
    (2000): 989–992.

35. Woo Suk Hwang, Young June Ryu, Jong Hyuk Park, Eui Soon Park, Eu Gene Lee, Ja Min Koo, Hyun Yong Jeon, et al., "Evidence of a Pluripotent Human Embryonic Stem Cell Line Derived from a Cloned Blastocyst," *Science* 303 (2004): 1669–1674.

36. Woo Suk Hwang, Sung Il Roh, Byeong Chun Lee, Sung Keun Kang, Dao Kee Kwon, Sue Kim, Sun Jong Kim, et al., "Patient-Specific Embryonic Stem Cells Derived from Human SCNT Blastocysts," *Science* 308 (2005): 1777–1783.

37. Anthony C. Perry, "Progress in Human Somatic-Cell Nuclear Transfer," *New England Journal of Medicine* 353 (2005): 87–88.

38. Rick Weiss, "Korean Stem Cell Lines Faked," *Washington Post*, December 23, 2005, A1; Choe Sang-Hun, "Panel Discredits Stem Cell Work of South Korean Scientist," *New York Times*, December 29, 2005, available at http://www.nytimes.com/2005/12/29/science/29clonex.html?ex=1143262800&en=952f937826d13af1&ei=5070; Nicholas Wade and Choe Sang-Hun, "Human Cloning Was All Faked, Koreans Report," *New York Times*, January 10, 2006, available at http://select.nytimes.com/gst/abstract.html?res=F60 E12FE3D5B0C738DDDA80894DE404482&n = Top%2fReference%2f Times%20Topics%2fPeople%2fW%2fWade%2c%20Nicholas; Dennis Normile, Gretchen Vogel, and Jennifer Couzin, with reporting by Sei Chong in Seoul, "South Korean Team's Remaining Human Stem Cell Claim Demolished," *Science* 311 (2006): 156; Song Sang-yong, "Whistling While Stem Cells Burn," *Joon Ang Daily*, January 10, 2006, available at http://joongangdaily.joins.com/ 200601/10/200601102208305639900090109012.html.

39. Donald Kennedy, "Editorial Retraction," *Science* 311 (2006): 335.

40. Snyder and Loring, "Beyond Fraud" (see note 27), 322.

41. J. B. Cibelli, A. A. Kiessling, K. Cunniff, C. Richards, R. P. Lanza, M. D. West, "Somatic Cell Nuclear Transfer in Humans: Pronuclear and Early Embryonic Development," *e-biomed: Journal of Regenerative Medicine*, vol. 2 (2001), available at http://www.bedfordresearch.org/articles/cibelli_ jregenmed.pdf; J. B. Cibelli, R. P. Lanza, D. West, C. Ezzell, "The First Human Cloned," *Scientific American* 256 (2002): 44–51; Gary Stix, "What Clones? Widespread Scientific Doubts Greet Word of the First Human Embryo Clones," *Scientific American* 257 (2002): 18–19; Ted Agres and Eugene Russo, "Cloning Controversy Re-emerges in U.S.," *Scientist* 16 (2002): 29; Eliot Marshall and Gretchen Vogel, "Cloning Announcement Sparks Debate and Scientific Skepticism," *Science* 294 (2001): 1802–1803; Joannie Fischer, "Scientists Have Finally Cloned a Human Embryo," *U. S. News and World Report*, December 3, 2001, available at http://www.usnews .com/usnews/biz/interstitials/int.php?title = &pageURL=http://www.usnews .com/usnews/issue/011203/misc/3cloning.htm; Gina Kolata with Andrew Pollack, "A Breakthrough on Cloning? Perhaps, or Perhaps Not Yet," *New York Times*, November 27, 2001, available at http://query.nytimes.com/gst/ fullpage.html?sec=health&res=9E06EED81E3AF934A15752C1A9679C8B 63; Rick Weiss, "First Human Embryos Are Cloned in U.S.," *Washington Post*, November 25, 2001, available at http://www.washingtonpost.com/ac2/ wp-dyn?pagename=article&node=&contentId= A14231-2001Nov25.

42. M. Stojkovic, P. Stojkovic, C. Leary, V. J. Hall, L. Armstrong, M. Herbert, M. Nesbitt, M. Lako, A. Murdoch, "Derivation of a Human Blastocyst

after Heterologous Nuclear Transfer to Donated Oocytes," *Reproductive Biomedicine Online* 11 (2005), 226–231, available at http://www.rbmonline .com/4DCGI/Article/Detail?38%091%09=%201872%09.

43. K. Hochedlinger and R. Jaenisch, "Ectopic Expression of Oct-4 Blocks Progenitor-Cell Differentiation and Causes Dysplasia in Epithelial Tissues," *Cell* 121 (2005): 465–477.

44. Tracy Hampton, "Scientists Confront Cloning Challenges," *Journal of the American Medical Association* 294 (2005): 783–784.

45. President's Council on Bioethics, *Alternative Sources of Human Pluripotent Stem Cells* (see note 4), 46.

46. D. Humpherys, K. Eggan, H. Akutsu, A. Friedman, K. Hochedlinger, R. Yanagimachi, E. S. Lander, T. R. Golub, R. Jaenisch, "Abnormal Gene Expression in Cloned Mice Derived from Embryonic Stem Cell and Cumulus Cell Nuclei," *Proceedings of the National Academy of Sciences USA* 99 (2002): 12889–12894.

47. T. Brambrink, K. Hochedlinger, G. Bell, R. Jaenisch, "ES Cells Derived from Cloned and Fertilized Blastocysts Are Transcriptionally and Functionally Indistinguishable," *Proceedings of the National Academy of Sciences USA* 103(2006): 933–938. See also Rudolf Jaenisch, "Human Cloning: The Science and Ethics of Nuclear Transplantation," *New England Journal of Medicine* 351 (2004): 2787–2791; Hochedlinger and Jaenisch, "Nuclear Transplantation, Embryonic Stem Cells, and the Potential for Cell Therapy" (see note 25), 281; Jaenisch, "Biology of Nuclear Cloning and Potential of Embryonic Stem Cells for Transplantation Therapy" (see note 23), 387–417.

48. Hochedlinger and Jaenisch, "Nuclear Transplantation, Embryonic Stem Cells, and the Potential for Cell Therapy" (see note 25), 281.

49. Brambrink et al., "ES Cells Derived from Cloned and Fertilized Blastocysts Are Transcriptionally and Functionally Indistinguishable" (see note 47), 933.

50. John Gearhart, "Medical Promise of Embryonic Stem Cell Research (Present and Projected)," President's Council on Bioethics, April 25, 2002, available at http://www.bioethics.gov/transcripts/apr02/apr25session1.html.

51. Paul R. McHugh, "Zygote and 'Clonote': The Ethical Use of Embryonic Stem Cells," *New England Journal of Medicine* 351 (2004): 209–211; President's Council on Bioethics, *Human Cloning and Human Dignity* (see note 22), 286.

52. Alexander Morgan Capron, "Placing a Moratorium on Research Cloning to Ensure Effective Control over Reproductive Cloning," *Hastings Law Journal* 53 (2000): 1057–1073, 1057.

53. President's Council on Bioethics, *Human Cloning and Human Dignity* (see note 22), 165.

54. U.S. Food and Drug Administration, "Proposed Approach to Regulation of Cellular and Tissue-Based Products," 1998, available at http://www. fda.gov/oc/ohrt/irbs/irbletr.html; "Statement by Kathryn C. Zoon, Ph.D., Director, Center for Biologics Evaluation and Research, Food and Drug Administration, Department of Health and Human Services Before the Subcommittee on Energy and Commerce, United States House of Representatives, March 28, 2001," available at http://www.fda.gov/ola/2001/

humancloning.html; Rebecca Dresser, "Human Cloning and the FDA," *Hastings Center Report* 33 (2003): 7–8.

55. National Institutes of Health, "Use of Genetically Modified Stem Cells in Experimental Gene Therapies," in *Stem Cells: Scientific Progress and Future Research Directions*, June 2001, updated August 12, 2005, 103–104, available at http://stemcells.nih.gov/info/scireport.

56. National Institute for Biological Standards and Control, "The United Kingdom Stem Cell Bank at NIBSC," available at http://www.ukstemcellbank.org.uk/Overview.html.

57. Ruth R. Faden, Liza Dawson, Alison S. Bateman-House, Dawn Mueller Agnew, Hilary Bok, Dan W. Brock, Aravinda Chakravarti, et al., "Public Stem Cell Banks: Considerations of Justice in Stem Cell Research and Therapy," *Hastings Center Report* 33 (2003): 13–27. See also Craig J. Taylor, Eleanor M. Bolton, Susan Pocock, Linda D. Sharples, Roger A. Pedersen, J. Andrew Bradley, "Banking on Human Embryonic Stem Cells: Estimating the Number of Donor Cell Lines Needed for HLA Matching," *Lancet* 366 (2005): 2019–2025.

58. Cynthia B. Cohen, "Stem Cell Research in the U.S. after the President's Speech of August 2001," *Kennedy Institute of Ethics Journal* 14 (2004): 97–114.

59. N. T. Rogers, E. Hobson, S. Pickering, F. A. Lai, P. Braude, K. Swann, "Phospholipase Czeta Causes Ca^{2+} Oscillations and Parthenogenetic Activation of Human Oocytes," *Reproduction* 129 (2004): 697–702; K. E. Vrana, J. D. Hipp, A. M. Goss, B. A. McCool, D. R. Riddle, S. J. Walker, P. J. Wettstein, et al., "Nonhuman Primate Parthenogenetic Stem Cells," *Proceedings of the National Academy of Sciences USA* 100 (2003): 11911–11916; Trounson, Alan, "The Genesis of Embryonic Stem Cells," *Nature Biotechnology* 20 (2002): 237–238; J. B. Cibelli, K. A. Grant, K. B. Chapman, K. Cunniff, T. Worst, H. L. Green, S. J. Walker, et al., "Parthenogenetic Stem Cells in Nonhuman Primates," *Science* 295 (2002): 779–780.

60. Cibelli et al.,"Somatic Cell Nuclear Transfer in Humans: Pronuclear and Early Embryonic Development" (see note 41); J. B. Cibelli, R. P. Lanza, D. West, C. Ezzell, "The First Human Cloned," *Scientific American* 256 (2002): 44–51.

61. A. A. Kiessling, "Eggs Alone—Human Parthenotes: An Ethical Source of Stem Cells for Therapies?" *Nature* 434 (2005): 145; Ann A. Kiessling, "What Is an Embryo?" *Connecticut Law Review* 36 (2004): 1051–1092; Cibelli et al., "Parthenogenic Stem Cells in Nonhuman Primates" (see note 59); Thomas A. Shannon, "Human Cloning: A Success Story or a Tempest in a Petri Dish?" *America*, February 18, 2002, 15–18; Green, *Human Embryo Research Debates* (see note 14), 110; Harold J. Morowitz and James S. Trefil, *The Facts of Life: Science and the Abortion Controversy* (New York: Oxford University Press, 1992), 193; Germain Grisez, *Abortion: The Myths, the Realities, and the Arguments* (New York: Corpus Books, 1970), 24, 274.

62. Nancy L. Jones and William P. Cheshire, "Can Artificial Techniques Supply Morally Neutral Human Embryos for Research? Part I: Creating Novel Categories of Human Embryos," *Ethics and Medicine* 21 (2005):

29–40; Benedict Ashley and Albert Moraczewski, "Cloning, Aquinas, and the Embryonic Person," *National Catholic Bioethics Quarterly* 1 (2001): 189–201.

63. Cibelli et al., "Parthenogenetic Stem Cells in Nonhuman Primates" (see note 59); see also Vrana et al., "Nonhuman Primate Parthenogenetic Stem Cells" (see note 59).

64. Constance Holden, "Primate Parthenotes Yield Stem Cells," *Science* 295 (2002): 779–780.

65. H. Lin, J. Lei, D. Wininger, M. T. Nguyen, R. Khanna, C. Hartmann, W. L. Yan, S. C. Huang, "Multilineage Potential of Homozygous Stem Cells Derived from Metaphase II Oocytes," *Stem Cells* 21 (2003): 152–161.

66. Sylvia Pagan Westphal, "'Virgin Birth' Method Promises Ethical Stem Cells," *New Scientist*, April 28, 2003, available at http://www.newscientist .com/article.ns?id=dn3654.

67. T. Kono, Y. Obata, Q. Wu, K. Niwa, Y. Ono, Y. Yamamoto, E. S. Park, J. Seo, H. Ogawa, "Birth of Parthenogenetic Mice That Can Develop to Adulthood," *Nature* 428 (2004): 860–864.

68. Rick Weiss, "In a First, Mice Are Made without Fathers," *Washington Post*, April 22, 2004, A13.

69. Davor Solter, Director, Max-Planck Institute of Immunobiology, Freiburg, Germany, personal communication.

70. N. T. Rogers, E. Hobson, S. Pickering, F. A. Lai, P. Baude, K. Swann, "Phospholipase Czeta Causes Ca^{2+} Oscillations and Parthenogenetic Activation of Human Oocytes," *Reproduction* 128 (2004): 697–702.

71. Mark Henderson. "Embryos Open Virgin Territory for Research," *Times* (London), September 10, 2005, available at http://www.timesonline.co.uk/ article/0,,2-1772939,00.html; Jonathan Amos, "'Virgin Conception' First for UK," *BBC News*, September 9, 2005, available at http://news.bbc. co.uk/2/hi/science/nature/4288992.stm.

72. Weiss, "In a First, Mice Are Made without Fathers" (see note 68). However, see K. Kim, P. Lerou, A. Yabuuchi, C. Lengerke, K. Ng, J. West, A. Kirby, M. J. Daly, G. Q. Daley, "Histocompatible Embryonic Stem Cells by Parthenogenesis," *Science* December 2, 2006, Epub ahead of print.

73. D. W. Landry and H. A. Zucker, "Embryonic Death and the Creation of Human Embryonic Stem Cells," *Journal of Clinical Investigation* 114 (2004): 1184–1186.

74. Xin Zhang, Petra Stojkovic, Stefan Przyborski, Michael Cooke, Lyle Armstrong, Majlinda Lako, Miodrag Stojkovic, "Derivation of Human Embryonic Stem Cells from Developing and Arrested Embryos," *Stem Cells* 24 (2006): 2669–2676, available at http://stemcells.alphamedpress .org/cgi/content/full/24/12/2669.

75. Landry and Zucker, "Embryonic Death and the Creation of Human Embryonic Stem Cells" (see note 73).

76. Robert Lanza, "Testimony of Robert Lanza, M.D., to the Senate Appropriations Subcommittee on Labor, Health and Human Services, Education, and Related Agencies, July 12, 2005," available at http://appropriations .senate.gov/hearmarkups/LanzaTestimony.htm.

77. Michael Gazzaniga, "Personal Statement," in President's Council on Bioethics, *Alternative Sources of Human Pluripotent Stem Cells: A White Paper*

(Washington, D.C.: President's Council on Bioethics, 2005), 76, available at http://www.bioethics.gov.

78. Testimony of George Q. Daley, M.D., Ph.D., to the Appropriations Subcommittee on Labor, Health and Human Services, Education Hearing on "An Alternative Method for Obtaining Embryonic Stem Cells," July 12, 2005, available at http://appropriations.senate.gov/hearmarkups/DALEY-Testimony.htm.

79. Janet Rowley, "Personal Statement," in President's Council on Bioethics, *Alternative Sources of Human Pluripotent Stem Cells: A White Paper* (Washington, D.C.: President's Council on Bioethics, 2005), 89, available at http://www.bioethics.gov.

80. I. Klimanskaya, Y. Chung, S. Becker, S.J. Lu, R. Lanza, "Human Embryonic Stem Cell Lines Derived from Single Blastomere," *Nature* 444 (2006): 481–485.

81. Lanza, "Testimony of Robert Lanza, M.D." (see note 76).

82. A. Kuliev and Y. Verlinksy, "Place of Preimplantation Diagnosis in Genetic Practice," *American Journal of Medical Genetics* 134 (2005): 105–110.

83. John A. Robertson, "Blastocyst Transfer (*sic*) Is No Solution," *American Journal of Bioethics* 5 (2005): 18–20.

84. Davor Solter, "Politically Correct Human Embryonic Stem Cells?" *New England Journal of Medicine* 353 (2005): 2321–2323.

85. Ibid., 2323.

86. William B. Hurlbut, "Altered Nuclear Transfer as a Morally Acceptable Means for the Procurement of Human Embryonic Stem Cells," *Perspectives in Biology and Medicine* 48 (2005): 211–228; William B. Hurlbut, "Altered Nuclear Transfer as a Morally Acceptable Means for the Procurement of Human Embryonic Stem Cells," President's Council on Bioethics, *Alternative Sources of Human Pluripotent Stem Cells* (see note 4), 36–37; Gareth Cook, "New Technique Eyed in Stem-Cell Debate," *Boston Globe*, November 21, 2004, available at http://www.boston.com/news/science/articles/2004/11/21/new_technique_eyed_in_stem_cell_debate/.

87. K. Chawengsaksophak, W. de Graaf, J. Rossant, J. Deschamps, F. Beck, "Cdx2 is essential for Axial Elongation in Mouse Development," *Proceedings of the National Academy of Sciences USA* 101 (2004): 7641–7645.

88. Hurlbut, "Altered Nuclear Transfer as a Morally Acceptable Means for the Procurement of Human Embryonic Stem Cells" *Perspectives in Biology and Medicine* (see note 86).

89. President's Council on Bioethics, *Alternative Sources of Human Pluripotent Stem Cells* (see note 4), 37.

90. A. Meissner and R. Jaenisch, "Generation of Nuclear Transfer-Derived Pluripotent ES Cells from Cloned Cdx2-Deficient Blastocysts," *Nature* 439 (2006): 212–215.

91. Davor Solter, "Reply to letter to editor, 'Politically Correct Human Embryonic Stem Cells?'" *New England Journal of Medicine* 354 (2006): 1209–1210.

92. Ibid., 1210.

93. Rudolph Jaenisch, Letter to editor, "Politically Correct Human Embryonic Stem Cells?" *New England Journal of Medicine* 354 (2006): 1208–1209.

94. Solter, "Reply to letter to editor" (see note 91), 1210; Solter, "Politically Correct Human Embryonic Stem Cells?" (see note 84), 2323.
95. Richard Doerflinger, "Comments at meeting of President's Council on Bioethics, December 3, 2004," Session 7: Public Comments, available at http://bioethicsprint.bioethics.gov/transcripts/dec04/session7.html.
96. Douglas A. Melton, George Q. Daley, Charles G. Jennnings, "Altered Nuclear Transfer in Stem-Cell Research: A Flawed Proposal," *New England Journal of Medicine* 351 (2004): 2791–2792, 2792.
97. Ibid., 2792.
98. President's Council on Bioethics, *Alternative Sources of Human Pluripotent Stem Cells* (see note 4), 41.
99. Melton et al., "Altered Nuclear Transfer in Stem-Cell Research" (see note 96).
100. C. A. Cowan, J. Atienza, D. A. Melton, K. Eggan, "Nuclear Reprogramming of Somatic Cells after Fusion with Human Embryonic Stem Cells," *Science* 309 (2005): 1369–1373.
101. Gretchen Vogel, "Embryo-Free Techniques Gain Momentum," *Science* 309 (2005): 240–241.
102. Rick Weiss, "Skin Cells Converted to Stem Cells," *Washington Post*, August 22, 2005, A1, A4.
103. Elizabeth G. Phimister, "A Tetraploid Twist on the Embryonic Stem Cell," *New England Journal of Medicine* 353 (2005): 1646–1647; Ceci Connolly, "Stem Cell Advance Muddles Debate," *Washington Post*, August 23, 2005, A3.
104. President's Council on Bioethics, *Alternative Sources of Human Pluripotent Stem Cells* (see note 4), 52. See also President's Council on Bioethics, "Session 1: Stem Cell Research Update," Meeting of November 16, 2006, available at http://www.bioethics.gov/transcripts/nov06/session1.html, and "Session 2: Stem Cell Research Update and *Alternative Sources of Pluripotent Stem Cells* (May 2005)," Meeting of November 16, 2006, available at http://www.bioethics.gov/transcripts/nov06/session2.html.
105. Daley, "An Alternative Method for Obtaining Embryonic Stem Cells" (see note 78).
106. President's Council on Bioethics, *Alternative Sources of Human Pluripotent Stem Cells* (see note 4), 50.
107. Gazzaniga, "Personal Statement," (see note 77), 77.
108. Bonnie Steinbock, "Alternative Sources of Stem Cells," *Hastings Center Report* 35, no. 4 (2005): 24–25.
109. Bridget M. Kuehn, "Stem Cells Created from Somatic Cells," *Journal of the American Medical Association* 294 (2005): 1475–1476.
110. Paul Berg, George Q. Daley, Lawrence S. B. Goldstein, "Stem Cell 'Alternatives' Fog the Debate," *Washington Post*, July 19, 2005, A 21.
111. Vogel, "Embryo-Free Techniques Gain Momentum" (see note 101), 24.
112. Gazzaniga, "Personal Statement" (see note 77), 76.

Chapter 3

1. Gilbert Meilaender, "Some Protestant Reflections," in *The Human Embryonic Stem Cell Debate*, ed. Suzanne Holland, Karen Lebacqz, Laurie Zoloth (Cambridge, Mass.: MIT Press, 2001), 141–147, 142.

2. I do not use the term "moral status" to refer to the moral significance of the early human embryo because this term, which first came into the use in the 1970s and whose use was modeled after the notion of having legal standing, has since been given a variety of meanings associated with a spectrum of sometimes conflicting ethical theories and ethical requirements. See Mary Anne Warren, *Moral Status: Obligations to Persons and Other Living Things* (Oxford: Oxford University Press, 1997), 3–23. It would raise questions for the reader about which of these theories and requirements I had in mind were I to use the term.

3. Robert P. George, *The Clash of Orthodoxies: Law, Religion, and Morality in Crisis* (Wilmington, Del.: ISI Books, 2001), 320.

4. John T. Noonan Jr., "An Almost Absolute Value in History," in *The Morality of Abortion: Legal and Historical Perspectives*, ed. John T. Noonan Jr. (Cambridge, Mass.: Harvard University Press, 1972), 57.

5. President's Council on Bioethics, *Human Cloning and Human Dignity* (New York: Public Affairs, 2002), 173–175.

6. National Institutes of Health, Stem Cell Information: "Early Development," available at http://stemcells.nih.gov/info/scireport/appendixA.asp (accessed September 14, 2005).

7. Helen Pearson, "Your Destiny from Day One," *Nature* 414 (2002): 14–15; Richard M. Doerflinger, "The Ethics of Funding Embryonic Stem Cell Research: A Catholic Viewpoint," *Kennedy Institute of Ethics Journal* 9 (1999): 137–150.

8. K. Piotrowska, F. Wianny, R. A. Pedersen, M. Zernicka-Goetz, "Blastomeres Arising from the First Cleavage Division Have Distinguishable Fates in Normal Mouse Development," *Development* 128 (2001): 3739–3748; R. L. Gardner, "Specification of Embryonic Axes Begins before Cleavage in Normal Mouse Development," *Development* 128 (2001): 839–847; R. L. Gardner, "The Early Blastocyst is Bilaterally Symmetrical and Its Axis of Symmetry Is Aligned with the Animal-Vegetal Axis of the Zygote in the Mouse," *Development* 124 (1997): 289–301. Additional articles have subsequently been published in support of the claim that the zygote exhibits such polarity. I list a representative sample of them sequentially according to date of publication. See B. Plusa, A. K. Hadjantonakis, D. Gray, K. Piotrowska-Nitsche, A. Jedrusik, V. E. Papaioannou, D. M. Glover, M. Zernicka-Goetz, "The First Cleavage of the Mouse Zygote Predicts the Blastocyst Axis," *Nature* 434 (2005): 391–395; M. Zernicka-Goetz, "Developmental Cell Biology: Cleavage Pattern and Emerging Asymmetry of the Mouse Embryo," *Nature Reviews Developmental Biology* 6 (2005): 919–928; R. L. Gardner and T. J. Davies, "An Investigation of the Origin and Sgnificance of Bilateral Symmetry of the Pronuclear Zygote in the Mouse," *Human Reproduction* 21 (2006): 492–502; R. L. Gardner, "Weakness in the Case against Prepatterning in the Mouse," *Reproductive Biomedicine Online* 12 (2006): 144–149; Deb Kaushik, Mayandi Sivaguru, Hwan Yul Yong, R. Michael Roberts, "Cdx2 Gene Expression and Trophectoderm Lineage Specification in Mouse Embryos," *Science* 311 (2006): 992–996. The editor of *Science* has published "Editorial Expression of Concern" *Science* 314 (2006): 592 regarding the article by Kaushik et al., and a report in *Science* suggests that that article

will be retracted; see "Fraud Investigation Clouds Paper on Early Cell Fate," *Science* 314 (2006): 1368–1369.

9. Norman M. Ford, *The Prenatal Person* (Oxford: Blackwell, 2002), 63.
10. Doerflinger, "Ethics of Funding Embryonic Stem Cell Research" (see note 7).
11. C. A. Bedate and R. C. Cefalo, "The Zygote: To Be or Not to Be a Person," *Journal of Medicine and Philosophy* 14 (1989): 635–649, 638.
12. Lewis Wolpert, *The Triumph of the Embryo* (Oxford: Oxford University Press, 1991), 31–32, 37–40, 84, 199–202.
13. Ronan O'Rahilly and Fabiola Müller, *Human Embryology & Teratology* (New York: Wiley-Liss, 1992), 6.
14. Board of Social Responsibility, Church of England, *Personal Origins,* 2nd rev. ed., (London: Church House Publishing, 1996), 34.
15. William J. Larsen, *Human Embryology*, 2nd ed. (New York: Churchill Livingstone, 1997), 42; Keith L. Moore and T. V. N. Persaud, *The Developing Human: Clinically Oriented Embryology*, 6th ed. (Philadelphia: W. B. Saunders, 1998), 37.
16. Larsen, *Human Embryology* (see note 15), 42.
17. Errol R. Norwitz, Danny J. Shust, Susan J. Fisher, "Implantation and the Survival of Early Pregnancy," *New England Journal of Medicine* 345 (2001): 1400–1408; K. Hardy, S. Spanos, D. Becker, P. Iannelli, R. M. Winston, J. Stark, "From Cell Death to Embryo Arrest: Mathematical Models of Human Preimplantation Embryo Development," *Proceedings of the National Academy of Sciences USA* 98 (2001): 1655–1660; A. J. Wilcox, C. R. Weinberg, J. F. O'Connor, et al., "Incidence of Early Loss of Pregnancy," *New England Journal of Medicine* 319 (1988): 189–194.
18. D. Wells and B. Levy, "Cytogenetics in Reproductive Medicine: The Contribution of Comparative Genomic Hybridization," *Bioessays* 25 (2003): 289–300.
19. Harold J. Morowitz and James S. Trefil, *The Facts of Life: Science and the Abortion Controversy* (New York: Oxford University Press, 1992), 51.
20. Bruce Carlson, *Human Embryology and Developmental Biology*, 2nd ed. (St. Louis, Mo.: Mosby, 1999), 46–48.
21. M. G. Bulmer, *The Biology of Twinning in Man* (Oxford: Clarendon Press, 1970), 98.
22. G. E. M. Anscombe, "Were You a Zygote?" *Philosophy* 18 (1984 suppl.): 11–16.
23. Peter van Inwagen, *Material Beings* (Ithaca, N.Y.: Cornell University Press), 154.
24. Jean Porter, "Individuality, Personal Identity, and the Moral Status of the Preembryo: A Response to Mark Johnson," *Theological Studies* 56 (1995): 767.
25. T. Hiiragi and D. Solter, "Fatal Flaws in the Case for Prepatterning in the Mouse Egg," *Reproductive Biomedicine Online* 12 (2006): 144–149; Nami Motosugi, Jens-Erik Dietrich, Zbigniew Polanski, Davor Solter, Takashi Hiiragi, "Space Asymmetry Directs Preferential Sperm Entry in of Polarity in the Mouse Oocyte," *PLoS* (*Public Library of Science*) *Biology* 4 (2006): e135, available at http://biology.plosjournals.org/perlserv/?request=get-document&doi=10.1371/journal.pbio.0040135; N. Motosugi, T. Bauer, Z. Polanski, D. Solter, T. Hiiragi, "Polarity of the Mouse Embryo Is Established

at Blastocyst and Is Not Prepatterned," *Genes and Development* 19 (2005): 1081–1092; V. B. Alarcon and Y. Marikawa, "Unbiased Contribution of the First Two Blastomeres to Mouse Blastocyst Development," *Molecular Reproductive Development* 72 (2005); 354–361; T. Hiiragi and D. Solter, "Mechanism of First Cleavage Specification in the Mouse Egg: Is Our Body Plan Set at Day 0?" *Cell Cycle* 4: (2005): 661–664; S. Louvet-Valee, S. Vinot, B. Maro, "Mitotic Spindles and Cleavage Plnes Are Oriented Radomly in the Two-Cell Mouse Embryo," *Current Biology* 15 (2005): 464–469; T. Hiiragi and D. Solter, "First Cleavage Plane of the Mouse Egg Is Not Predetermined but Defined by the Topology of the Two Apposing Pronuclei," *Nature* 430 (2004): 360–364.

26. Gretchen Vogel, "Embryologists Polarized over Early Cell Fate Determination," *Science* 308 (2005): 782–783.

27. Motosugi et al., "Polarity of the Mouse Embryo" (see note 25), 1089.

28. Alfonso Gómez-Lobo, "On the Ethical Evaluation of Stem Cell Research: Remarks on a Paper by N. Knoepfflcr," *Kennedy Institute of Ethics Journal* 14 (2004): 75 80, 79.

29. Norman M. Ford, *When Did I Begin? Conception of the Human Individual in History, Philosophy and Science* (Cambridge: Cambridge University Press, 1988), 168–177.

30. Larsen, *Human Embryology* (see note 15), 49–53.

31. For further discussion of various views of the moral significance of human embryos after day fourteen, see, for example, Bonnie Steinbock, *Life before Birth: The Moral and Legal Status of Embryos and Fetuses* (New York: Oxford University Press, 1992), 43–88.

32. Human Embryo Research Panel, National Institutes of Health, *Report of the Human Embryo Research Panel* (Bethesda, Md.: National Institutes of Health, 1994), 2.

33. Ibid., 3.

34. President's Council on Bioethics, *Human Cloning and Human Dignity* (see note 5), 153.

35. Ibid., 157.

36. John A. Robertson, "Symbolic Issues in Embryo Research," *Hastings Center Report* 25, no. 1 (1995): 37–38. See also John A. Robertson, "Ethics and Policy in Embryonic Stem Cell Research," *Kennedy Institute of Ethics Journal* 9 (1999): 109–136.

37. Daniel Callahan, "The Puzzle of Profound Respect," *Hastings Center Report* 25, no. 1 (1995): 39–40.

38. President's Council on Bioethics, *Human Cloning and Human Dignity* (see note 5), 175.

39. Ibid., 157.

40. Michael J. Meyer and Lawrence J. Nelson, "Respecting What We Destroy: Reflections on Human Embryo Research," *Hastings Center Report* 31, no. 1 (2001): 16–23.

41. Robertson, "Symbolic Issues in Embryo Research" (see note 36), 38.

42. National Institutes of Health, *Report of the Human Embryo Research Panel* (see note 32), 4.

43. Bonnie Steinbock, "Respect for Human Embryos," in *Cloning and the Future of Human Embryo Research*, ed. Paul Lauritzen (Oxford: Oxford University Press, 2001), 21–33.

44. Robert P. Lanza, Arthur L. Caplan, Lee M. Silver, Jose B. Cibelli, Michael D. West, Ronald M. Green, "The Ethical Validity of Using Nuclear Transfer in Human Transplantation," *Journal of the American Medical Association* 284 (2000): 3175–3179.

45. President's Council on Bioethics, *Human Cloning and Human Dignity* (see note 5), 176–177.

46. Ibid., 176.

47. Teresa Iglesias, "In Vitro Fertilisation: The Major Issues," *Journal of Medical Ethics* 10 (1984): 32–46, 34.

48. Michael Tooley, *Abortion and Infanticide* (Oxford: Clarendon Press, 1983), 165–166.

49. John Harris, *The Value of Life: An Introduction to Medical Ethics* (London: Routledge and Kegan Paul, 1985), 11–12.

50. John Andrew Fisher, "Why Potentiality Does Not Matter: A Reply to Stone," *Canadian Journal of Philosophy* 24 (1994): 261–280; Jim Stone, "Why Potentiality Still Matters," *Canadian Journal of Philosophy* 24 (1994): 281–294.

51. Stephen Buckle, "Arguing from Potential," *Bioethics* 2 (1988): 227–253.

52. Ibid., 233.

53. Derek Parfit, *Reasons and Persons* (Oxford: Clarendon Press, 1982), 201–202.

54. Buckle "Arguing from Potential" (see note 51), 233.

55. Ibid., 239.

56. President's Council on Bioethics, *Human Cloning and Human Dignity* (see note 5), 168.

57. Ibid., 169.

58. Ibid., 168.

59. Ibid., 168–169.

60. Ibid., 167.

61. Ibid., 157, 175.

62. Peter Singer, *Practical Ethics*, 2nd ed. (Cambridge: Cambridge University Press, 1993), 87.

63. Peter Singer, *Rethinking Life and Death: The Collapse of Our Traditional Ethics* (Oxford: Oxford University Press, 1995), 181.

64. Ibid., 182.

65. Singer, *Practical Ethics* (see note 62), 118.

66. Cynthia B. Cohen, "Creating Human-Animal Chimeras: Of Mice and Men," *American Journal of Bioethics* 3 (2003): W4–W5.

67. Jane English, "Abortion and the Concept of a Person," *Canadian Journal of Philosophy* 5 (1975): 233–243.

68. Singer, *Rethinking Life and Death* (see note 63), 182.

69. Gene Outka, "The Ethics of Stem Cell Research," *Kennedy Institute of Ethics Journal* 12 (2002): 175–214.

70. Maura Ryan, "Creating Embryos for Research: On Weighing Symbolic Costs," in *Cloning and the Future of Human Embryo Research*, ed. Paul Lauritzen (Oxford: Oxford University Press, 2001), 50–66.

71. Ibid., 58.

72. Ibid.

73. Michael J. Sandel, "The Ethical Implications of Human Cloning," *Perspectives in Biology and Medicine* 48 (2005): 241–247, 245.

74. Ryan, "Creating Embryos for Research" (see note 70), 63.

Chapter 4

1. Robert Audi, "The Separation of Church and State and the Obligations of Citizenship," *Philosophy and Public Affairs* 18 (1989): 278.
2. Cynthia B. Cohen, "Religion, Public Reason, and Embryonic Stem Cell Research," *Handbook of Bioethics and Religion*, ed. David Guinn (New York: Oxford University Press, 2006), 129–143.
3. James F. Childress, "The Challenges of Public Ethics: Reflections on NBAC's Report," *Hastings Center Report* 27 (1997): 9–11, 10.
4. Courtney S. Campbell, "Prophecy and Policy," *Hastings Center Report* 27, no. 5 (1997): 15–17.
5. Judith Jarvis Thomson, "A Defense of Abortion," *Philosophy and Public Affairs* 1 (1971): 47–66.
6. Jeremy Waldron, "Religious Contributions in Public Deliberation," *San Diego Law Review* 30 (1993): 838.
7. Michael J. Perry, *Morality, Politics and Law* (Oxford: Oxford University Press, 1988), 181.
8. Cynthia B. Cohen, "Religious Belief, Politics, and Public Bioethics: A Challenge to Political Liberalism," *Second Opinion* 6 (2001): 37–52.
9. Kevin Phillips, *The Peril and Politics of Radical Religion, Oil, and Borrowed Money in the 21st Century* (New York: Viking, 2006); Jim Wallis, *God's Politics: Why the Right Gets It Wrong and the Left Doesn't Get It* (San Francisco: Harper, 2005); "A Hot Line to Heaven: Is George Bush Too Religious?" *Economist*, December 16, 2004, available at http://www.religionandsocialpolicy.org/news/article.cfm?id=2186; Howard Fineman, "Bush and God," *Newsweek*, March 10, 2003, 22–28; Martin E. Marty, "The Sin of Pride," *Newsweek*, March 10, 2003, 32.
10. Cynthia B. Cohen, "Culture Wars Erupt over Use of Stem Cells," *Science &Theology News*, May 2006, 20.
11. National Bioethics Advisory Commission, *Ethical Issues in Human Stem Cell Research*, Vol. 3: *Religious Perspectives* (Rockville, Md.: National Bioethics Advisory Commission, 2000).
12. Childress, "Challenges of Public Ethics" (see note 3), 11.
13. Jeffrey Stout, *Democracy and Tradition* (Princeton, N.J.: Princeton University Press, 2004), 64.
14. Mark J. Hanson, "Cloning for Therapeutic Purposes: Ethical and Policy Considerations," in *Human Cloning: Papers from a Church Consultation*, ed. Roger A. Willer (Minneapolis, Minn.: Augsburg Fortress, 2001), 58–65.
15. Cynthia B. Cohen, "The Image of God, the Eggs of Women, and Therapeutic Cloning," *University of Toledo Law Review* 32 (2001): 367–374.
16. Image of God," in *Cyclopedia of Biblical, Theological, and Ecclesiastical Literature*, ed. John McClintock (Grand Rapids, Mich.: Baker Academic, 1982), vol. 4, 499–501.
17. Stephen Beasley, "Contraception and the Moral Status of the Early Human Embryo," in *Conceiving the Embryo: Ethics, Law and Practice in Human Embryology*, ed. Donald Evans (The Hague: Martinus Nijhoff, 1996), 93.
18. James C. Peterson, *Genetic Turning Points: The Ethics of Human Genetic Intervention* (Grand Rapids, Mich.: Eerdmans, 2001), 114.

19. Oliver O'Donovan, *The Christian and the Unborn Child* (Bramcote, Eng.: Grove Books, 1986), 15.

20. David Atkinson, "Some Theological Perspectives on the Human Embryo (Part 2)," *Ethics and Medicine: A Christian Perspective* 2 no. 23 (1986): 23–32.

21. Peterson, *Genetic Turning Points* (see note 18), 114–115.

22. Anthony Dyson, "At Heaven's Command? The Churches, Theology, and Experiments on Embryos," in *Experiments on Embryos*, ed. A. Dyson and J. Harris (London: Routledge, 1992), 82–104.

23. David Jones et al., "A Theologians' Brief on the Place of the Human Embryo within the Christian Tradition," *Ethics & Medicine*, 2001, available at http://www.ethicsandmedicine.com/contents/17/fall01_commentary2.html.

24. Gilbert Meilaender, *Bioethics: A Primer for Christians* (Grand Rapids, Mich.: Eerdmans, 1996), 29.

25. G. R. Dunstan, "The Moral Status of the Human Embryo: A Tradition Recalled," *Journal of Medical Ethics* 1 (1984): 38–44; Norman M. Ford, *When Did I Begin? Conception of the Human Individual in History, Philosophy and Science* (Cambridge: Cambridge University Press, 1988), 39–51, 57–64.

26. Translation from David Feldman, *Marital Relations, Birth Control and Abortion in Jewish Law* (New York: Schocken Books, 1987), 255.

27. Immanuel Jakobovits, "Jewish Views on Abortion," in *Abortion, Society, and Law*, ed. D. Walbert and J. Butler (Cleveland: Press of Case Western University, 1973), 103–121.

28. Translation from G. Bonner, "Abortion and Early Christian Thought," in *Abortion and the Sanctity of Human Life*, ed. J. H. Channer (Exeter, Eng.: Paternoster Press, 1985), 93–122, 114.

29. Aristotle, *On the Soul*, trans. H. Lawson-Tancred (Hammondsworth: Penguin, 1987), 402a–416b; Aristotle, *On the Generation of Animals*, trans. A. Platt in *The Works of Aristotle Translated into English*, vol. 5, ed. J. A. Smith and W. D. Ross (Oxford: Clarendon Press, 1912), 729a–744b; J. Needham, *A History of Embryology* (Cambridge: Cambridge University Press, 1959), 37–60.

30. Aristotle, *The History of Animals*, trans. D. W. Thomson, in *The Works of Aristotle Translated into English*, vol. 4, ed. J. A. Smith and W. D. Ross (Oxford: Clarendon Press, 1912), book VII, chapter 3, 583b.

31. Carol Tauer, "Abortion," in *The HarperCollins Encyclopedia of Catholicism*, ed. Richard P. McBrien (New York: HarperCollins, 1995), 4–8.

32. Tertullian, *On the Soul*, trans. P. Holmes, in *Latin Christianity: Its Founder, Tertullian, the Ante-Nicene Fathers,* ed. Alexander Roberts and James Donaldson (Grand Rapids, Mich,: Eerdmans, 1973), vol. 3, 217–218.

33. Gregory of Nyssa, *On the Making of Man*, in *Nicene and Post-Nicene Fathers*, Series 2, vol. 5, chap 29, ed. Philip Schaff and Henry Wace (Peabody, Mass.: Hendrickson, 1956), 320.

34. Augustine of Hippo, *On Exodus* 21.80, cited in John T. Noonan Jr., *Contraception: A History of Its Treatment by the Catholic Theologians and Canonists* (Cambridge, Mass.: Belknap Press of Harvard University, 1986), 90.

35. Augustine, *Enchiridion*, in *Confessions and Enchiridion*, trans. and ed. Albert C. Outler, *Library of Congress Classics*, vol. 7 (Philadelphia: Westminster Press, 1955), chapter 23, 85.

36. Augustine, *The City of God*, trans Marcus Dods (New York: Modern Library, 1950), 14–16.

37. Basil, Epistle 188 *Ad Amphilochium II*, cited in Dunstan, "Moral Status of the Human Embryo" (see note 25), 40.

38. Jones, "Theologian's Brief" (see note 23), 3.

39. Aquinas, Thomas. *Summa Theologica,* trans. Fathers of the English Dominican Province (New York: Thomas More, 1981), 2a2ae: 64.1–76.3.

40. John Noonan, "An Almost Absolute Value in History," in *The Morality of Abortion: Legal and Historical Perspectives,* ed. John Noonan (Cambridge, Mass.: Harvard University Press, 1970), 38; Gordon Dunstan, "The Moral Status of the Human Embryo," in *Philosophical Ethics in Reproductive Medicine,* ed. David R. Bronham, Maureen E. Dalston, Jennifer C. Jackson (Manchester: University Press, 1988), 5.

41. John Connery, *Abortion: The Development of the Roman Catholic Perspective* (Chicago: Loyola University Press, 1977), 306.

42. V. Nutton, "The Anatomy of the Soul in Early Renaissance Medicine," in *The Human Embryo: Aristotle and the Arabic and European Traditions*, ed. G. R. Dunstan (Exeter: University of Exeter Press, 1990), 43–59.

43. Martin Luther, "Commentary on Galatians," in *Martin Luther: Selections from His Writings*, ed. J. Dillenberger (London: Anchor Books, 1961), 128.

44. David C. Steinmetz, "What Luther Got Wrong," *Christian Century* 122, no. 17 (2005): 23–26, 24.

45. Martin Luther, *Luther's Work: Lectures on Genesis*, ed. Jaroslav Jan Pelikan, Hilton C. Oswald, Helmut T. Lehmann (St. Louis: Concordia, 1964), vol. 4, 304. 46. John Calvin, *Commentary on the Four Last Books of Moses Arranged in the Form of a Harmony* (Grand Rapids, Mich.: Eerdmans, 1950), 43.

47. John Calvin, *Commentary on Psalms* (Grand Rapids, Mich.: Christian Classics Ethereal Library, 1999), vol. 5, 25.

48. John Calvin, "Sermons on Job, 12," in W. Bouwsma, *John Calvin: A Sixteenth Century Portrait* (Oxford: Oxford University Press, 1988), 78.

49. C. D. O'Malley and J. B. de C. M. Saunders, *Leonardo da Vinci on the Human Body: The Anatomical, Physiological, and Embryological Drawings of Leonardo da Vinci* (New York: Greenwich House, 1982), 470–485.

50. Noonan, *Contraception* (see note 34), 89; Jane Maienschein, *Whose View of Life? Embryos, Cloning, and Stem Cells* (Cambridge, Mass.: Harvard University Press, 2003), 24–27.

51. Needham, *History of Embryology* (see note 29), 133–153.

52. Peter Bowler, "Preformation and Pre-existence in the Seventeenth Century: A Brief Analysis," *Journal of the History of Biology* 4 (1971): 221–244.

53. S. Roe, *Matter, Life, and Generation: Eighteenth-Century Embryology and the Haller-Wolff Debate* (Cambridge: Cambridge University Press, 1981); C. Pinto-Correia, *The Ovary of Eve* (Chicago: University of Chicago Press, 1997).

54. H. Alexandre, "A History of Mammalian Embryological Research," *International Journal of Developmental Biology* 45 (2001): 457–467.

55. Noonan, "An Almost Absolute Value in History" (see note 40), 38–39.

56. Noonan, "An Almost Absolute Value in History" (see note 40), 39.
57. Carol Tauer, "The Tradition of Probabilism and the Moral Status of the Early Embryo," *Theological Studies* 45 (1984): 3–33.
58. Bernard Häring, *Medical Ethics* (Notre Dame, Ind.: Fides Publishers, 1973), 80.
59. Congregation for the Doctrine of the Faith, *Declaration on Procured Abortion* (Washington, D.C.: United States Catholic Conference, 1974), 13.
60. Congregation for the Doctrine of the Faith, *Donum Vitae* (Washington, D.C.: United States Catholic Conference, 1987), part I, no. 1.
61. Nicole Winfield, "Pope Says Pre-Implanted Embryo Is Sacred," *Boston Globe*, February 27, 2006, available at http://www.boston.com/news/science/articles/2006/02/27/pope_says_pre_implanted_embryo_is_sacred/.
62. Margaret Farley, "Roman Catholic Views on Research Involving Human Embryonic Stem Cells," in National Bioethics Advisory Commission, *Ethical Issues in Human Stem Cell Research*, Vol. 3: *Religious Perspectives* (Rockville, Md.: National Bioethics Advisory Commission, 2000), D3–5, D3.
63. Ibid., D4.
64. Demetrios Demopoulos, "An Eastern Orthodox View of Embryonic Stem Cell Research," in National Bioethics Advisory Commission, *Ethical Issues in Human Stem Cell Research*, Vol. 3: *Religious Perspectives* (Rockville, Md.: National Bioethics Advisory Commission, 2000), B3–4.
65. Cynthia B. Cohen, "Bioethics," in *Christianity: The Complete Guide*, ed. John Bowden (London: Continuum, 2005), 158–164.
66. Southern Baptist Convention, "Resolution on Human Embryonic and Stem Cell Research," June 1999, available at http://www.sbc.net/resolutions/amResolution.asp?ID=620.
67. Report of a Working Party on Human Fertilisation and Embryology of the Board of Social Responsibility, Church of England, *Personal Origins*, 2nd rev. ed. (London: Church House Publishing, 1996), 32–45; Dunstan, "Moral Status of the Human Embryo" (see note 25); Dunstan, "Moral Status of the Human Embryo" (see note 40); G. R. Dunstan, "The Embryo, from Aristotle to Alton," *History Today* 38, no. 4 (1988): 6–8; Dyson, "At Heaven's Command?" (see note 22); Cynthia B. Cohen, "The Moral Status of Early Embryos and New Genetic Interventions," in *A Christian Response to the New Genetics*, ed. David H. Smith and Cynthia B. Cohen (Lanham, Md.: Rowman and Littlefield, 2003), 105–130.
68. General Assembly, Presbyterian Church (USA), "Overture 01-50. On Adopting a Resolution Enunciating Ethical Guidelines for Fetal Tissue and Stem Cell Research—From the Presbytery of Baltimore. Attachment A: Statement on the Ethical and Moral Implications of Stem Cell and Fetal Tissue Research," 2001, available at http://www.pcusa.org/oga/actions-of-213.htm.
69. Ronald Cole-Turner, "Testimony," in National Bioethics Advisory Commission, *Ethical Issues in Human Stem Cell Research*, Vol. 3: *Religious Perspectives* (Rockville, Md.: National Bioethics Advisory Commission, 2000), A3–4, A3.
70. United Church of Christ Committee on Genetics, "Statement on Human Cloning," in *Human Cloning: Religious Responses*, ed. Ronald Cole-Turner (Louisville, Ky.: Westminster John Knox Press, 1997), 149–151.

71. Roland de Vaux, *Ancient Israel*, Vol. 1: *Social Institutions* (New York: McGraw-Hill, 1965), 34–37; Elliot N. Dorff and Arthur Rosett, *A Living Tree: The Roots and Growth of Jewish Law* (Albany: State University of New York Press, 1988), 485–486; Peter Brown, *The Body and Society: Men, Women, and Sexual Renunciation in Early Christianity* (New York: Columbia University Press, 1988), 61–65.

72. Laurie Zoloth, "The Ethics of the Eighth Day: Jewish Bioethics and Research on Human Embryonic Stem Cells," in *The Human Embryonic Stem Cell Debate*, ed. Suzanne Holland, Karen Lebacqz, Laurie Zoloth (Cambridge, Mass.: MIT Press, 2001), 95.

73. Immanuel Jakobovitz, *Jewish Medical Ethics* (New York: Bloch, 1975), 275; Zoloth, "Ethics of the Eighth Day" (see note 72), 98.

74. Moshe Dovid Tendler, "Stem Cell Research and Therapy: A Judeo-Biblical Perspective," in National Bioethics Advisory Commission, *Ethical Issues in Human Stem Cell Research*, Vol. 3: *Religious Perspectives* (Rockville, Md.: National Bioethics Advisory Commission, 2000), H3–4.75. Elliot N. Dorff, "Testimony," in National Bioethics Advisory Commission, *Ethical Issues in Human Stem Cell Research*, Vol. 1: *Report and Recommendations of the National Bioethics Advisory Commission* (Rockville, Md.: National Bioethics Advisory Commission, 1999), 50.

76. Union of Orthodox Jewish Congregations of America and the Rabbinical Council of America, "Cloning Research, Jewish Tradition, and Public Policy: A Joint Statement," Washington, D.C., 2002, available at http://www.ou.org/public/Publib/cloninglet.htm.

77. Mark Washofsky, "Why Judaism Supports Stem Cell Research," *Reform Judaism*, Fall 2005, 38.

78. M. Bucaille, "Human Reproduction," in *The Bible, the Qur'an and Science* (Indianapolis: North American Trust Publications, 1979), 198–210.

79. Abdulaziz Sachedina, "Islamic Perspectives on Cloning," G-4, available at http://www.people.virginia.edu/~aas/issues/cloning.htm.

80. Imad-ad-Dean-Ahmad, "Federal Funding for Stem Cell Research?" August 2001, *IslamOnline.net,* available at http://198.65.147.194/English/Views/2001/08/article6.shtml.

81. M. A. Al Bar, *Human Development as Revealed in the Holy Qur'an and Hadith* (Jeddah: Saudi Arabia Publishing and Distributing House, 1986); M. A. Al Bar, "Conception and Abortion: An Islamic View," in *Contemporary Topics in Islamic Medicine*, ed. M. A. Al Bar (Jeddah: Saudi Arabia Publishing and Distributing House, 1995), 147–153.

82. M. A. Al Bar, "When Is the Soul Inspired?" In *Contemporary Topics in Islamic Medicine,* ed. M. A. Al Bar (Jeddah: Saudi Arabia Publishing and Distributing House, 1995), 131–136.

83. Abdulaziz Sachedina, "Islamic Bioethics," in *Religious Perspectives in Bioethics*, ed John F. Peppin, Mark J. Cherry, Ana Iltis (London: Taylor and Francis, 2004), 153–171.

84. Abdulaziz Sachedina, "Islamic Perspectives on Research with Human Embryonic Stem Cells," in National Bioethics Advisory Commission, *Ethical Issues in Human Stem Cell Research*, Vol. 3: *Religious Perspectives* (Rockville, Md.: National Bioethics Advisory Commission, 2000), G3–6, G3.

85. Damien Keown, "Buddhism and Bioethics," in *Religious Perspectives in Bioethics*, ed. John F. Peppin, Mark J. Cherry, Ana Iltis (London: Taylor and Francis, 2004), 183. See also Damien Keown, *Buddhism and Bioethics* (London: Macmillan, 1995), 91.

86. Michael G. Barnhart, "Buddhism and the Morality of Abortion," *Journal of Buddhist Ethics* 5 (1998): 282, 293.

87. Cromwell Crawford, "Hindu Bioethics," in *Religious Perspectives in Bioethics*, ed John F. Peppin, Mark J. Cherry, Ana Iltis (London: Taylor and Francis, 2004), 200.

88. Sripati Chandrasekhar, *Abortion in a Crowded World: The Problem of Abortion with Special Reference to India* (Seattle: University of Washington Press, 1974), 47–48.

89. S. Cromwell Crawford, *Dilemmas of Life and Death: Hindu Ethics in North American Context* (New York: State University of New York Press, 1995).

90. Cynthia B. Cohen, "Religion, Public Reason, and Embryonic Stem Cell Research" (see note 2); Cynthia B. Cohen, "Open Possibilities, Close Concerns: The Import of Religious Views on the Future of Stem Cell Research," *Park Ridge Center Bulletin*, January/February 2000, 12.

91. Aristotle, *Nichomachean Ethics*, trans. Martin Oswald (Indianapolis: Bobbs-Merrill, 1962), book IX, chapter 1167a,b, 255–258.

92. Amy Gutmann and Dennis Thompson, *Why Deliberative Democracy?* (Princeton, N.J.: Princeton University Press, 2004).

93. Cynthia B. Cohen, "Religion, Public Reason, and Embryonic Stem Cell Research" (see note 2); Lisa Sowle Cahill, "Theology's Role in Public Bioethics," *Handbook of Bioethics and Religion*, ed. David Guinn (New York: Oxford University Press, 2006), 37–57.

Chapter 5

This chapter draws from sections of the following two articles and adds new material: Phillip Karpowicz, Cynthia B. Cohen, Derek Van der Kooy, "Developing Human-Nonhuman Chimeras in Human Stem Cell Research: Ethical Issues and Boundaries," *Kennedy Institute of Ethics Journal* 15 (2005): 107–134; Phillip Karpowicz, Cynthia B. Cohen, Derek Van der Kooy, "It Is Ethical to Transplant Human Stem Cells into Nonhuman Embryos," *Nature Medicine* 10 (2004): 331–335. I am indebted to my co-authors, Phillip Karpowicz and Derek Van der Kooy, for their observations about and contributions to several of the arguments presented in this chapter.

1. Homer, *The Iliad*, trans. Richard Lattimore (Chicago: University of Chicago Press, 1961), book VI, 179–182; cf. Robert Graves, *The Greek Myths* (New York: Penguin, 1960), 1, 252–256.

2. H. G. Wells, *The Island of Dr. Moreau* (Garden City, N.Y.: Garden City Publishing, 1896), 125.

3. C. B. Fehilly, S. M. Willasden, E. M. Tucker, "Interspecific Chimaerism between Sheep and Goat," *Nature* 307 (1984): 634–636; V. J. Polzin, D. L. Anderson, G. B. Anderson, R. H. BonDurant, J. E. Butler, R. L. Pashen, C. T. Penedo, J. D. Rowe, "Production of Sheep-Goat," *Journal of Animal Science* 65 (1987): 325–330.

4. E. Balaban, M.-A. Teillet, N. Le Douarin, "Application of the Quail-Chick Chimera System to the Study of Brain Development and Behavior," *Science* 241 (1988): 1339–1342.

5. J. E. Dick, G. Guenechea, O. I. Gan, C. Dorrell, "Distinct Classes of Human Stem Cells That Differ in Proliferative and Self-Renewal Potential," *Nature Immunology* 1 (2001): 75–82; S. Raychaudhuri, M. Sanyal, S. K. Raychaudhuri, S. Dutt, E. M. Farber, "Severe Combined Immunodeficiency Mouse-Human Skin Chimeras: A Unique Animal Model for the Study of Psoriasis and Cutaneous Inflammation," *British Journal of Dermatology* 144 (2001): 931–939; R. Kauffman, V. Mielke, J. Reimann, C. E. Klein, W. Sterry, "Cellular and Molecular Composition of Human Skin in Long-term Xenografts on SCID Mice," *Experimental Dermatology* 2 (1993): 209–216; S. Kamel-Reid and J. E. Dick, "Engraftment of Immune-Deficient Mice with Human Hematopoietic Stem Cells," *Science* 242 (1988): 1706–1709.

6. Sylvia Pagan Westphal, "Humanised Organs Can Be Grown in Animals," *New Scientist* December 17, 2003, available at http://www.newscientist.com/article.ns?id=dn4492; E. D. Zanjani, F. R. Mackintosh, M. R. Harrison, "Hematopoietic Chimerism in Sheep and Nonhuman Primates by In Utero Transplantation of Fetal Hematopoietic Stem Cells," *Blood Cells* 17 (1991): 349–363, discussion 364–366.

7. Gaia Vince, "Pig-Human Chimeras Contain Cell Surprise," *New Scientist* January 13, 2004, available at http://www.newscientist.com/article.ns?id=dn4558.

8. V. Ourednik, J. Ourednik, J. D. Flax, W. M. Zawada, C. Hutt, C. Yang, K. I. Park, S. U. Kim, R. L. Sidman, E. Y. Snyder, "Segregation of Human Neural Stem Cells in the Developing Primate Forebrain," *Science* 293 (2001): 1820–1824.

9. Jack Price, "Neural Stem Cells: Where Are You?" *Nature Medicine* 7 (2001): 998–999.

10. R. S. Goldstein, M. Drukker, B. E. Reubinoff, N. Benvenisty, "Integration and Differentiation of Human Embryonic Stem Cells Transplanted to the Chick Embryo," *Developmental Dynamics* 225 (2002): 80–86.

11. Nell Boyce, "Mixing Species—and Crossing a Line?" *U.S. News & World Report,* October 27, 2003, 58–60.

12. Natalie DeWitt, "Biologists Divided over Proposal to Create Human-Mouse Embryos," *Nature* 420 (2002): 255.

13. N. Uchida, D. W. Buck, D. He, M. J. Reitsma, M. Masek, T. V. Phan, A. S. Tsukamoto, F. H. Gage, I. L. Weissman, "Direct Isolation of Human Central Nervous System Stem Cells," *Proceedings of the National Academy of Sciences USA* 97 (2000): 14720–14725.

14. Lisa M. Krieger, "Treading New Ethical Ground: Scientists Put a Bit of Man into a Mouse," *Mercury News,* December 8, 2002, available at http://www.siliconvalley.com/mld/siliconvalley/4700100.htm?template=contentModules.

15. Uchida et al., "Direct Isolation of Human Central Nervous System Stem Cells" (see note 13); S. Kelly, T. M. Bliss, A. K. Shah, G. H. Sun, M. Ma, W. C. Foo, J. Masel, et al., "Transplanted Human Fetal Neural Stem Cells Survive, Migrate, and Differentiate in Ischemic Rat Cerebral Cortex,"

Proceedings of the National Academy of Sciences USA 101 (2004): 11839–11844.

16. Clive Cookson, "Brain Cells Research Fuels Debate," *Financial Times* (London), February 23, 2001, 22; Krieger, "Treading New Ethical Ground" (see note 14).

17. DeWitt, "Biologists Divided over Proposal to Create Human-Mouse Embryos" (see note 12).

18. Krieger, "Treading New Ethical Ground" (see note 14); Boyce, "Mixing Species—and Crossing a Line?" (see note 11).

19. Henry Greely, Stanford University Law School, chair of advisory committee, April 1, 2006, personal communication.

20. Lisa M. Krieger, "Stanford Gets OK to Try Human Cells in Mouse Brain," *Mercury News*, February 14, 2005, B1.

21. A. R. Muotri, K. Nakashima, N. Toni, V. M. Sandler, F. H. Gage, "Development of Functional Human Embryonic Stem Cell-Derived Neurons in the Mouse Brain," *Proceedings of the National Academy of Sciences USA* 102 (2005): 18638–18643.

22. Ibid., 18638, 18641–18643.

23. "Mice Born with Human Brain Cells," Associated Press, December 13, 2005, available at http://www.cbsnews.com/stories/2005/12/13/tech/printable1120129.shtml; Rick Weiss, "Human Brain Cells Are Grown in Mice," *Washington Post*, December 13, 2005, A3.

24. William F. Hurlbut, "Ethical Considerations in Creating Human-Nonhuman Chimeras in Stem Cell Research," presentation at Public Workshop on Guidelines for Human Embryonic Stem Cell Research of the National Academies and Institute of Medicine, Washington, D.C., October 13, 2004.

25. Patricia Tippett, "Human Chimeras," in *Chimeras in Developmental Biology*, ed. Nicole Le Douarin and Anne McLaren (Orlando: Academic Press, 1984).

26. Leon F. Kass, Teleology, Darwinism, and the Place of Man: Beyond Chance and Necessity?" in *Toward a More Natural Science: Biology and Human Affairs* (New York: Free Press, 1985), 249–275.

27. Michael Crowe, *The Changing Profile of the Natural Law* (The Hague: Martinus Nijhoff, 1977), 192–245; A. P. d'Entreves, *Natural Law: An Introduction to Legal Philosophy*, 2nd rev. ed. (London: Hutchinson, 1970).

28. Kass, *Toward a More Natural Science* (see note 26).

29. Thomas Aquinas, *Summa Theologica*, trans. Blackfriars (New York: McGraw-Hill, 1968), 2a2ae, 154.

30. Owen J. Flanagan Jr., *Varieties of Moral Personality: Ethics and Psychological Realism* (Cambridge, Mass.: Harvard University Press, 1991); Leon F. Kass, *Toward a More Natural Science: Biology and Human Affairs* (New York: Free Press, 1985); Mary Midgely, *Beast and Man: The Roots of Human Nature* (New York: Meridian, 1978).

31. Jean Porter, *Natural and Divine Law: Reclaiming the Tradition for Christian Ethics* (Grand Rapids, Mich.: William B. Eerdmans, 1999.)

32. Kass, *Toward a More Natural Science* (see note 26).

33. President's Council on Bioethics, Meeting of October 16, 2003, available at http://bioethics.gov/transcripts/oct03/session2.html; Mary Midgely, "Biotechnology and Monstrosity: Why We Should Pay Attention to the "Yuk Factor." *Hastings Center Report* 30, no. 5 (2000): 7–15.

34. Julian Savulescu, "Human-Animal Transgenesis and Chimeras Might Be an Expression of Our Humanity" *American Journal of Bioethics* 3 (2003): 3–5.
35. Phillip Karpowicz, Cynthia B. Cohen, Derek Van der Kooy, "Developing Human-Nonhuman Chimeras in Human Stem Cell Research: Ethical Issues and Boundaries," *Kennedy Institute of Ethics Journal* 15 (2005): 107–134.
36. P. E. Griffiths, "Squaring the Circle: Natural Kinds with Historical Essences," in *Species: New Interdisciplinary Essays*, ed. R. A. Wilson (Cambridge, Mass.: MIT Press, 1999), 210–228.
37. Ibid.; R. Boyd, "Homeostasis, Species and Higher Taxa," in *Species: New Interdisciplinary Essays*, ed. R. A. Wilson (Cambridge, Mass.: MIT Press, 1999), 141 185; D. L. Hull, "On the Plurality of Species: Questioning the Party Line," in *Species: New Interdisciplinary Essays,* ed. R. A. Wilson. (Cambridge, Mass.: MIT Press, 1999), 23–48; R. A. Wilson, "Realism, Essence, and Kind: Resuscitating Species Essentialism?" in *Species: New Interdisciplinary Essays*, ed. R. A. Wilson. (Cambridge, Mass.: MIT Press, 1999), 188–207.
38. John D. Lotke and Moshe D. Tendler, "Revisiting the Definition of *Homo sapiens,*" *Kennedy Institute of Ethics* 12 (2002): 343–350.
39. Ronald de Sousa, "The Natural Shiftiness of Natural Kinds," *Canadian Journal of Philosophy* 14, no. 4 (1984): 561–581; Karpowicz et al., "Developing Human-Nonhuman Chimeras in Human Stem Cell Research" (see note 35).
40. Marc Ereshefsky, "Species and the Linnean Hierarchy," in *Species: New Interdisciplinary Essays*, ed. R. A. Wilson. (Cambridge, Mass.: MIT Press, 1999), 285–306.
41. Ernst Mayr, *Toward a New Philosophy of Biology: Observations of an Evolutionist* (Cambridge, Mass.: Harvard University Press, 1988).
42. de Sousa, "Natural Shiftiness of Natural Kinds" (see note 39).
43. R. L. Mayden, "A Hierarchy of Species Concepts: The Denouement in the Saga of the Species Problem," in *Species: The Units of Diversity*, ed. M. F. Claridge, H. A. Dawah, M. R. Wilson (London: Chapman and Hall, 1997), 381–424.
44. Jason Scott Robert and Françoise Baylis, "Crossing Species Boundaries," *American Journal of Bioethics* 3, no. 3 (2003): 1–13.
45. Ibid., 10.
46. Bernard E. Rollin, "Ethics and Species Integrity," *American Journal of Bioethics* 3, no. 3 (2003): 15–17; Louis C. Charland, "Are There Answers?" *American Journal of Bioethics* 3, no. 3 (2003): W 1–2; Robert Streiffer, "In Defense of the Moral Relevance of Species Boundaries," *American Journal of Bioethics* 3, no. 3 (2003): 37–38.
47. National Bioethics Advisory Commission, Letter to President Clinton, *Ethical Issues in Human Stem Cell Research* (Rockville, Md.: National Bioethics Advisory Commission, 1999), vol. 1, 91–92.
48. Charland, "Are There Answers?" (see note 46), 38.
49. Leon F. Kass, "The Wisdom of Repugnance," *New Republic* 2 (1997): 20.
50. Kass quoted in President's Council on Bioethics, Meeting of October 16, 2003 (see note 33).

51. Leon F. Kass, "Why We Should Ban Human Cloning Now: Preventing a Brave New World," *New Republic*, 2001, available at http://www.thenewrepublic.com/052101/kass052101_print.html; Kass, "Wisdom of Repugnance" (see note 49), 20.

52. Midgely, "Biotechnology and Monstrosity" (see note 33).

53. John Kekes, "Moral Intuition," *American Philosophical Quarterly* 23 (1986): 83–93.

54. W. D. Ross, *The Right and the Good* (Oxford: Oxford University Press, 1930).

55. Claude Levi-Strauss, *Myth and Meaning* (London: Routledge and Kegan Paul, 1978); Mary Douglas, *Purity and Danger* (London: Routledge and Kegan Paul, 1966).

56. Karpowicz et al., "Developing Human-Nonhuman Chimeras in Human Stem Cell Research" (see note 35), 112.

57. Jeffrey Stout, *Ethics after Babel: The Languages of Morals and Their Discontents* (Boston: Beacon Press, 1988).

58. Ibid., 149–150.

59. Y. Cao, J. P. Vacanti, K. T. Paige, J. Upton, C. A. Vacanti, "Transplantation of Chondrocytes Utilizing a Polymer-Cell Construct to Produce a Tissue-Engineered Cartilage in the Shape of a Human Ear," *Plastic Reconstructive Surgery* 100, no. 2 (1997): 297–302.

60. Karpowicz et al., "Developing Human-Nonhuman Chimeras in Human Stem Cell Research" (see note 35), 113; Phillip Karpowicz, Cynthia B. Cohen, Derek Van der Kooy, "It Is Ethical to Transplant Human Stem Cells into Nonhuman Embryos," *Nature Medicine* 10 (2004): 331–335.

61. Sarah Franklin, "Drawing the Line at Not-Fully-Human: What We Already Know," *American Journal of Bioethics* 3, no. 3 (2003): W 25–27.

62. Timothy Caulfield and Roger Brownsword, "Human Dignity: A Guide to Policy Making in the Biotechnology Era?" *Nature* 7 (2006): 72–76. See also President's Council on Bioethics, "Human Dignity as a Bioethical Concept," Meeting of December 8, 2005, available at http://www.bioethics.gov/transcripts/dec05/session5.html, "The Concept of Human Dignity," Meeting of February 2, 2006, available at http://www.bioethics.gov/transcripts/feb06/session1.html, and "Session 2: The Concept of Human Dignity (cont'd)," available at http://www.bioethics.gov/transcripts/feb06/session2.html.

63. Leon F. Kass, *Life, Liberty, and the Defense of Dignity: The Challenge for Bioethics* (San Francisco: Encounter Books, 2002), 18.

64. Ruth Macklin, "Dignity Is a Useless Concept," *British Medical Journal* 327 (2003): 1419–1420; see also Ruth Macklin, "Reflections on the Human Dignity Symposium: Is Dignity a Useless Concept?" *Journal of Palliative Care* 20 (2004): 212–216.

65. John Harris, "Cloning and Human Dignity," *Cambridge Quarterly of Healthcare Ethics* 7 (1998): 163–167, 166.

66. Immanuel Kant, *Critique of Practical Reason*, trans. Lewis White Beck (Indianapolis: Bobbs-Merrill, 1956); T. E. Hill Jr., *Dignity and Practical Reason in Kant's Ethical Theory* (Ithaca, N.Y.: Cornell University Press, 1992), 10, 47–50, 56, 166–167, 178, 202–217, 246–247; Cynthia B. Cohen, "Selling Bits and Pieces of Humans to Make Babies: 'The Gift of the Magi' Revisited," *Journal of Medicine and Philosophy* 24 (1999): 288–306.

67. Hill, *Dignity and Practical Reason in Kant's Ethical Theory* (see note 66), 176.

68. Immanuel Kant, *Groundwork of the Metaphysics of Morals*, trans. H. J. Paton (New York: Harper and Row, 1964), 92.

69. Alan Gewirth, "Human Dignity as the Basis of Rights," in *The Constitution of Rights: Human Dignity and American Values*, ed. Michael J. Meyer and William A. Parent (Ithaca, N.Y.: Cornell University Press, 1992), 1–9; Alan Gewirth, *Human Rights* (Chicago: University of Chicago Press, 1982).

70. Karpowicz et al., "Developing Human-Nonhuman Chimeras in Human Stem Cell Research" (see note 35), 120; Cynthia B. Cohen, "Creating Human-Animal Chimeras: Of Mice and Men," *American Journal of Bioethics* 3 (2003): W 3–5; Cohen, "Selling Bits and Pieces of Humans to Make Babies," (see note 66).

71. Ludwig Wittgenstein, *Philosophical Investigatons,* 3rd ed., trans. G. E. M. Anscombe (New York: Macmillan, 1958), secs. 65–66.

72. Daryl Pullman, "Death, Dignity and Moral Nonsense," *Journal of Palliative Care* 20 (2004): 171–178.

73. Gewirth, *Human Rights* (see note 69), 27–28.

74. Karpowicz et al., "Developing Human Nonhuman Chimeras in Human Stem Cell Research" (see note 35), 120–121.

75. Walter Glannon, "Free Will and Moral Responsibility in the Age of Neuroscience," *Lahey Clinic Medical Ethics Newsletter* 13, no. 2 (2006): 1–2.

76. Helga Kuhse, "Is There a Tension between Autonomy and Dignity?" in *Bioethics and Biolaw*, Vol. 2: *Four Ethical Principles*, ed. Peter Kemp, Jacob Rendtorff, Niels Mattson Johansen (Copenhagen: Rhodos International Science and Art Publishers and Centre for Ethics and Law, 2000), 69–70.

77. Robert Streiffer, "At the Edge of Humanity: Human Stem Cells, Chimeras, and Moral Status," *Kennedy Institute of Ethics Journal* 15 (2005): 347–370.

78. Deryck Beyleveld and Roger Brownsword, *Human Dignity in Bioethics and Biolaw* (Oxford: Oxford University Press, 2001), 23.

79. Frans de Waal, *Good Natured: The Origins of Right and Wrong in Humans and Other Animals* (Cambridge, Mass.: Harvard University Press, 1996), 210.

80. Ourednik et al., "Segregation of Human Neural Stem Cells" (see note 8).

81. Uchida et al., "Direct Isolation of Human Central Nervous System Stem Cells" (see note 13); Kelly et al., "Transplanted Human Fetal Neural Stem Cells Survive, Migrate, and Differentiate" (see note 15).

82. Karpowicz et al., "Developing Human-Nonhuman Chimeras in Human Stem Cell Research" (see note 35), 125–126; Cohen, "Creating Human-Animal Chimeras," (see note 70), W4; Karpowicz et al., "It Is Ethical to Transplant Human Stem Cells into Nonhuman Embryos" (see note 60), 334.

83. Ibid., "It Is Ethical to Transplant Human Stem Cells into Nonhuman Embryos" (see note 60), 125–126.

84. Ibid., "Developing Human-Nonhuman Chimeras in Human Stem Cell Research" (see note 35), 124.

85. Ibid., 125–126.

86. Karpowicz et al., 126–127; Karpowicz et al., "It Is Ethical to Transplant Human Stem Cells into Nonhuman Embryos" (see note 60), 334.
87. Fehilly et al., "Interspecific Chimaerism between Sheep and Goat" (see note 3); Polzin et al., "Production of Sheep-Goat" (see note 3).
88. Balaban et al., "Application of the Quail-Chick Chimera System" (see note 4).
89. Karpowicz et al, "Developing Human-Nonhuman Chimeras in Human Stem Cell Research" (see note 35), 128–129. See also Mark Greene, Kathryn Schill, Shoji Takahashi, Alison Bateman-House, Tom Beauchamp, Hilary Bok, Dorothy Cheney, et al., "Moral Issues of Human-Non-Human Primate Neural Grafting," *Science* 309 (1995): 385–386.
90. Goldstein et al., "Integration and Differentiation of Human Embryonic Stem Cells Transplanted to the Chick Embryo" (see note 10).
91. Muotri et al., "Development of Functional Human Embryonic Stem Cell-Derived Neurons in the Mouse Brain" (see note 21).
92. National Research Council and the Institute of Medicine of the National Academies, *Stem Cells and the Future of Regenerative Medicine* (Washington, D.C.: National Academies, 2002), 50.
93. Ibid., 40–41.
94. Ibid., 57.
95. Ibid., 41.
96. Cohen, "Creating Human-Animal Chimeras: Of Mice and Men" (see note 70).
97. National Advisory Board on Ethics in Reproduction, "Report and Recommendations on Oocyte Donation by the National Advisory Board on Ethics in Reproduction," in *New Ways of Making Babies,* ed. Cynthia B. Cohen (Bloomington: Indiana University Press, 1996), 233–302; Cynthia B. Cohen, "Ethical Issues in Reproduction," in *Fletcher's Introduction to Clinical Ethics*, 3rd ed., ed. John C. Fletcher, Edward M. Spencer, Paul A. Lombardo (Hagerstown, Md.: University Press, 2005), 263–282.
98. National Research Council and Institute of Medicine, *Stem Cells and the Future of Regenerative Medicine* (see note 92), 58.

Chapter 6

1. Rosario M. Isasi and Bartha M. Knoppers, "Beyond the Permissibility of Embryonic and Stem Cell Research: Substantive Requirements and Procedural Safeguards," *Human Reproduction* 21 (2006): 2472–2481; Rosario M. Isasi and Bartha M. Knoppers, "Mind the Gap: Policy Approaches to Embryonic Stem Cell and Cloning Research in 50 Countries," *European Journal of Health Law* 13 (2006): 9–26; LeRoy Walters, "Human Embryonic Stem Cell Research: An International Perspective," *Kennedy Institute of Ethics Journal* 14 (2004): 3–38.
2. Rosario M. Isasi, Bartha M. Knoppers, Peter A. Singer, Abdallah S. Daar, "Legal and Ethical Approaches to Stem Cell and Cloning Research: A Comparative Analysis of Policies in Latin America, Asia, and Africa," *Journal of Law, Medicine & Ethics* 32 (2004): 626–640.
3. Mary Warnock, *A Question of Life: The Warnock Report on Human Fertilisation & Embryology* (Oxford: Basil Blackwell, 1985).
4. Ibid., 4.
5. Ibid., "Introduction," xvi.

6. Mary Warnock, *A Question of Life: The Warnock Report on Human Fertilisation & Embryology* (Oxford: Basil Blackwell, 1985), "Introduction," xiv.
7. Ibid., xv.
8. Ibid., Section 11.18 at 64.
9. Ibid., Section 11.20–21 at 65–66.
10. Ibid., Section 11.22 at 66.
11. Ibid., Section 11.24 at 66–67.
12. Ibid., Section 11.29 at 68.
13. Ibid., Section 11.30 at 69.
14. Ibid., viii.
15. Reported in Mary Warnock, *Making Babies: Is There a Right to Have Children?* (Oxford: Oxford University Press, 2002), 34.
16. Thomas Banchoff, "Path Dependence and Value-Driven Issues: The Comparative Politics of Stem Cell Research," *World Politics* 57 (2005): 200–230.
17. Michael Mulkay, *The Embryo Research Debate: Science and the Politics of Reproduction* (Cambridge: Cambridge University Press, 1997).
18. Human Fertilisation and Embryology Act, 1990, c. 37 (Eng.) (1990), available at http://www.opsi.gov.uk/acts/acts1990/Ukpga_19900037_en_1.htm.
19. Human Fertilisation and Embryology Authority, Code of Practice, 6th edition, 2004, available at http://www.hfea.gov.uk/cps/rde/xbcr/SID-3F57D79B-43E09108/hfea/Code_of_Practice_Sixth_Edition_-_final.pdf. The HFEA will be merged with the Human Tissue Authority to create the Regulatory Authority for Tissue and Embryos (RATE) in 2008. RATE will be responsible for regulating the use in treatment and research of all human tissues, embryos, cells (including sperm and eggs), blood, and organs. See "How Fertility Laws Might Change," *BBC News*, available at http://news.bbc.co.uk/1/hi/health/4155372.stm.
20. Anne McLaren, "Formulating Effective Policy in ART: Where Do We Go from Here?" Workshop on Evidence Based Assisted Reproductive Technologies, Food and Drug Administration, September 19, 2002, available at http://www.fda.gov/cber/minutes/art091902.htm.
21. Department of Health, *Stem Cell Research: Medical Progress with Responsibility, A Report from the Chief Medical Officer's Expert Group Reviewing the Potential of Developments in Stem Cell Research and Cell Nuclear Replacement to Benefit Human Health*, Rec. 2 (2000), available at http://staminali.aduc.it/donaldson_eng.pdf.
22. Danuta Mendelson, "Regulating Embryonic Stem Cell Research in the United Kingdom," *Journal of Law and Medicine* 9 (2002): 380–381.
23. Human Reproductive Cloning Act, 2001, c. 23 (Eng.) (Dec. 4, 2001), available at http://www.hmso.gov.uk/acts/acts2001/20010023.htm.
24. Michael Schirber, "U.K. Doubles Stem Cell Funding," *Science* 310 (2005): 1599.
25. Clive Cookson, "Country Report: United Kingdom," *Scientific American/ Financial Times* 293 (2005): A23.
26. Rick Weiss, "The Power to Divide: Stem Cells," *National Geographic*, July 2005, 17.
27. M. Stojkovic, P. Stojkovic, C. Leary, V. J. Hall, L. Armstrong, M. Herbert, M. Nesbitt, M. Lako, A. Murdoch, "Derivation of a Human Blastocyst after Heterologous Nuclear Transfer to Donated Oocytes," *Reproductive*

Biomedicine Online 11 (2005): 226–231, available at http://www.rbmonline.com/4DCGI/Article/Detail?38%091%09=%201872%09.

28. Brian Vastag, "UK Licenses Human Embryo Creation, 'Dolly' Cloner to Create Embryos for Research," *Journal of the American Medical Association* 290 (2003): 449–450.

29. Gretchen Vogel, "Pioneering Stem Cell Bank Will Soon Be Open for Deposits," *Science* 297 (2002): 1784.

30. U.K. Stem Cell Bank, *Code of Practice for the Use of Human Stem Cell Lines*, section 5, available at http://www.mrc.ac.uk/Utilities/Documentrecord/index.htm?d=MRC003132.

31. U.K. Stem Cell Bank, "Mission Statement," available at http://www.ukstemcellbank.org.uk.

32. Poll, *Daily Telegraph*. August 2005, available at http://www.telegraph.co.uk/news/graphics/2005/08/29/nabor129big.gif; Poll, Human Fertilisation and Embryology Authority, July 2005, available at http://www.hfea.gov.uk/cps/rde/xchg/hfea/hs.xsl/488.html.

33. "Developmental Biology in Germany," *International Journal of Developmental Biology* 40, no. 1 (1996), available at http://www.ijdb.ehu.es/9601contents.htm; John A. Robertson, "Reproductive Technology in Germany and the United States: An Essay in Comparative Law and Bioethics," *Columbia Journal of Transnational Law* 43 (2004): 189–227.

34. Nicole Richardt, "A Comparative Analysis of the Embryological Research Debate," *Social Politics* 110 (2003): 102–114.

35. Kathrin Braun, "Not Just for Experts: The Public Debate about Reprogenetics in Germany," *Hastings Center Report* 35, no. 3 (2005): 42–49, 43.

36. Angela Campbell, "Ethos and Economics: Examining the Rationale Underlying Stem Cell and Cloning Research Politics in the United States, Germany, and Japan," *American Journal of Law and Medicine* 31 (2005): 47–86, 74.

37. Eric Brown, "The Dilemmas of German Bioethics," *New Atlantis*, Spring 2004, 4, available at http://www.thenewatlantis.com/archive/5/brownprint.htm.

38. Cynthia B. Cohen, " 'Quality of Life' and the Analogy with the Nazis," *Journal of Medicine and Philosophy* 8 (1983): 113–135, reprinted in *Quality of Life: The New Medical Dilemma*, ed. James. J. Walter and Thomas A. Shannon (New York: Paulist Press, 1990), 61–77.

39. Grundgesetz der Bundesrepublik Deutschland. 1949, article 1.

40. Robertson, "Reproductive Technology in Germany and the United States" (see note 33), 195–196.

41. Ibid., 197; Gerald L. Neuman, "Casey in the Mirror: Abortion, Abuse and the Right to Protection in the United States and Germany," *American Journal of Comparative Law* 43 (1995): 273–279.

42. Robertson, "Reproductive Technology in Germany and the United States" (see note 33), 197–199; Neuman, "Casey in the Mirror" (see note 41), 280.

43. Robertson, "Reproductive Technology in Germany and the United States" (see note 33), 203; Brown, "Dilemmas of German Bioethics" (see note 37), 5.

44. Bettina Schöne-Seifert and Klaus-Peter Rippe, "Silencing the Singer: Antibioethics in Germany," *Hastings Center Report* 21, no. 6 (1991): 20–27.

45. Peter Singer, *Practical Ethics*, 2nd ed. (Cambridge: Cambridge University Press, 1993), 85–87, 123.

46. Schöne-Seifert and Rippe, "Silencing the Singer" (see note 44), 21; Brown, "Dilemmas of German Bioethics" (see note 37), 7.
47. Embryonenschutzgesetz (Embryo Protection Act), Grundgesetz der Bundesrepublik Deustchland, *Bundesgesetzblatt* (1990) I, 2746–2753, art. 8.
48. Silvia Sanides, "Stem Cell Pioneer," *Scientist* 17 (2003): 52–53.
49. Grundgesetz der Bundesrepublik Deutschland, article 5.
50. Braun, "Not Just for Experts" (see note 35), 43–44.
51. Deutsche Forschungsgemeinschaft, "Empfehlungen der Deutschen Forschungsgemeinschaft zur Forschung mit menschlichen Stammzellen," in *Jahrbuch für Wissenschaft und Ethik*, ed. L. Honnefelder and C. Streffer (Berlin: Deutsche Forschungsgemeinschaft, 2001), vol. 6, 349–385.
52. Jan P. Beckmann, "On the German Debate on Human Embryonic Stem Cell Research," *Journal of Medicine and Philosophy* 29 (2004): 603–621.
53. Ibid., 605.
54. Gretchen Vogel, "Germany Dithers over Stem Cells, While Sweden Gives Green Light," *Science* 294 (2001): 2262. See also German National Council on Ethics, "Opinion on the Import of Embryonic Stem Cells" (2001), available at http://www.ethikrat.org/_english/publications/stem_cells/Opinion_Import-HESC.pdf.
55. Robert Koenig and Gretchen Vogel, "Embryonic Stem Cells: German Leaders Spar over Bioethics," *Science* 292 (2001): 1811–1812.
56. Stammzellgesetz (Stem Cell Act). Grundgesetz der Bundesrepublik Deustchland, *Bundesgesetzblatt* (2002): I, 2277–2280, articles 5, 6, and 8, available at http://www.bmbf.de/pub/stammzellgesetz.pdf.
57. Thomas Heinemann and Ludger Honnefelder, "Principles of Ethical Decision-Making Regarding Embryonic Stem Cell Research in Germany," *Bioethics* 16 (2002): 530–543, 540.
58. Gretchen Vogel, "German Researchers Get Green Light, Just," *Science* 295 (2002): 943.
59. Brown, "Dilemmas of German Bioethics" (see note 37), 9.
60. Ibid.
61. Sanides, "Stem Cell Pioneer" (see note 48), 53.
62. Schöne-Seifert and Rippe, "Silencing the Singer" (see note 44), 21.
63. Brown, "Dilemmas of German Bioethics" (see note 37).
64. "Schroeder Urges Stem Cell Easing," *BBC News*, June 14, 2005, available at http://news.bbc.co.uk/1/hi/world/europe/4093082.stm.
65. Ibid.
66. Ned Stafford, "Stem Cells Trickle into Germany: Only a Handful of Groups Have Applied to Import Embryonic Stem Cells under Stringent Rules," *Scientist*, October 31, 2003, available at http://www.the-scientist.com/article/display/21746.
67. David A. Scott, personal communication, September 7, 2005.
68. Ned Stafford, "German Minister Rebukes Stem Cell Research," *Scientist*, January 5, 2006, available at http://www.the-scientist.com/news/display/22923.
69. William LaFleur, *Liquid Life: Abortion and Buddhism in Japan* (Princeton, N.J.: Princeton University Press, 1992), 38–39.
70. Ibid., 11.
71. Ibid., 2.

72. Elizabeth G. Harrison, "Strands of Complexity: The Emergence of *Mizuko Kuyō* in Postwar Japan," *Journal of the American Academy of Religion* 67 (1999): 769–796, 779.

73. Elizabeth G. Harrison, " 'I Can Only Move My Feet towards *mizuko kuyō*': Memorial Services for Dead Children in Japan," in *Buddhism and Abortion*, ed. Damien Keown (London: Macmillan, 1999), 93–120; LaFleur, *Liquid Life* (see note 69), 23.

74. Harrison, "Strands of Complexity" (see note 72), 770.

75. LaFleur, *Liquid Life* (see note 69), 26.

76. Harrison, " 'I Can Only Move My Feet' " (see note 73), 94.

77. Harrison "Strands of Complexity" (see note 72), 779; Harrison " 'I Can Only Move My Feet' " (see note 73), 94.

78. Harrison, "Strands of Complexity" (see note 72), 778–779.

79. Ibid., 783.

80. Ibid., 784; LaFleur, *Liquid Life* (see note 69), 206.

81. Shinryo N. Shinagawa, "A Short History of Reproductive Medical Problems in Japan," *Eubios Journal of Asian and International Bioethics* 6 (1996): 158–159, available at http://www.csu.edu.au/learning/eubios/EJ66/EJ66D.html.

82. Harrison, " 'I Can Only Move My Feet' " (see note 73), 94–95.

83. Lynn D. Wardle, " 'Crying Stones:' A Comparison of Abortion in Japan and the United States," *New York Law School Journal of International and Comparative Law* 14 (1993): 195.

84. LaFleur, *Liquid Life* (see note 69), 11.

85. Ibid., 12.

86. Robert J. Smith, *Ancestor Worship in Contemporary Japan* (Palo Alto, Calif.: Stanford University Press, 1971).

87. Harrison, "Strands of Complexity" (see note 72), 777.

88. Harrison, " 'I Can Only Move My Feet" (see note 73), 93.

89. Harrison, "Strands of Complexity" (see note 72), 775.

90. Campbell, "Ethos and Economics" (see note 36), 84.

91. Harrison, "Strands of Complexity" (see note 72), 771.

92. Ibid., 772.

93. Shinagawa, "Short History of Reproductive Medical Problems in Japan" (see note 81), 159.

94. Ibid.

95. Stephen Endicott and Edward Hagerman, *The United States and Biological Warfare: Secrets from the Early Cold War and Korea* (Bloomington: Indiana University Press, 1988), 37–41; Herbert P. Hix, *Hirohito and the Making of Modern Japan* (New York: HarperCollins, 2000), 616–617.

96. Jing-Bao Nie, "The United States Cover-Up of Japanese Wartime Medical Atrocities: Complicity Committed in the National Interest and Two Proposals for Contemporary Action," *American Journal of Bioethics* 6, no. 3 (2006): W 21.

97. Japan Ministry of Education, Culture, Sports, Science and Technology, "The Guidelines for Derivation and Utilization of Human Embryonic Stem Cells" (September 25, 2001), available at http://www.mext.go.jp/a_menu/shinkou/seimei/2001/es/020101.pdf.

98. "Japan Set to Embrace Stem Cell Research," *BBC News*, August 1, 2001, available at http://news.bbc.co.uk/2/hi/science/nature/1468518.stm.

99. Law Concerning Regulation Relating to Human Cloning Techniques and Other Similar Techniques, Law No. 146 of 2001, available at http://www.mext.go.jp/a_menu/shinkou/seimei/eclone.pdf.

100. Jiro Nudeshima, "Human Cloning Legislation in Japan," *Eubios Journal of Asian and International Bioethics* 11 (2001): 2, available at http://www2.unescobkk.org/eubios/EJ111/ej111b.htm; Dennis Normile, "Japan: Human Cloning Ban Allows Some Research," *Science* 290 (2000): 1872.

101. "Japan Allows Stem Cell Research," *Age*, December 14, 2003, available at http://www.theage.com.au/articles/2003/12/14/1071336795092.html?one-click=true.

102. Dennis Normile, "Japan Faces Decision as Moratorium Expires," *Science* 304 (2004): 1729.

103. David Cyranoski, "Research Cloning Gets Green Light from Japanese Ethicists," *Nature* 430 (2004): 5.

104. Masakazu Inaba and Darryl Macer, "Attitudes to Biotechnology in Japan in 2003," *Eubios Journal of Asian and International Bioethics* 13 (2003): 78–90, available at http://www2.unescobkk.org/eubios/EJ133/ej133b.htm.

105. Campbell, "Ethos and Economics" (see note 36), 81.

106. "Isolation of the First Domestic hESC in Japan," *CellNews*, June 3, 2003, available at http://www.geocities.com/giantfideli//art/CellNEWS_Japan_first_hESC.html.

107. Matthew Herper, "Japan's Stem-Cell Bid Lures U.S. Researchers, *Forbes*, March 4, 2002, available at http://www.forbes.com/2002/03/04/0304japan_print.html; Campbell, "Ethos and Economics" (see note 36); David Cyranoski, "Japan Sets Rules for Stem Cell Research," *Nature Medicine* 10 (2004): 763.

108. Ella De Trizio and Christopher A. Brennan, "The Business of Human Embryonic Stem Cell Research and an International Analysis of Relevant Laws," *Journal of Biolaw and Business* 7 (2004): 1–23

109. David Cyranoski, "Japan's Embryo Experts Beg for Faster Ethical Reviews," *Nature* 438 (2005): 263.

110. International Stem Cell Forum Ethics Working Party, "Ethics Issues in Stem Cell Research," *Science* 312 (2006): 366–367.

111. The Hinxton Group, An International Consortium on Stem Cells, Ethics and Law, "Consensus Statement," 2006, available at http://www.hopkins-medicine.org/bioethics/finalsc.doc.

112. David B. Resnik, "The Need for International Stem Cell Agreements," *Nature Biotechnology* 22 (2004): 1207; A. H. Brivanlou, F. H. Gage, R. Jaenisch, et al., "Setting Standards for Human Embryonic Stem Cells," *Science* 300 (2003): 913–916.

Chapter 7

1. William J. Clinton, Executive Order 12975: "Protection of Human Research Subjects and Creation of National Bioethics Advisory Commission,"

1995, available at http://www.georgetown.edu/research/nrcbl/nbac/about/eo 12975.htm.

2. National Bioethics Advisory Commission, *Ethical Issues in Human Stem Cell Research* (Rockville, Md.: U.S. Government Printing Office, 1999), 89, available at http://www.georgetown.edu/research/nrcbl/nbac/pubs.html.

3. Cynthia B. Cohen, "Promises and Perils of Public Deliberation: Contrasting Two National Bioethics Commissions on Embryonic Stem Cell Research," *Kennedy Institute of Ethics Journal* 15 (2005): 269–288.

4. National Bioethics Advisory Commission, Charter, 1995, available at http://www.georgetown.edu/research/nrcbl/nbac.

5. Eliot Marshall, "Ethicists Back Stem Cell Research, White House Treads Cautiously," *Science* 285 (1999): 502–503.

6. Nicholas Wade, "Primordial Cells Fuel Debate on Ethics," *New York Times*, November 10, 1998, F1.

7. The original rider can be found in Section 128 of P.L. 104–99; for subsequent fiscal years, the rider is found attached to the following public laws: 1997, P.L. 104-208; 1998, P.L. 105-78; 1999, P.L. 105-277; 2000, P.L. 106-113; 2001, P.L. 106-554; 2002, P.L. 107-116; 2003, P.L. 108-7; 2004, P.L. 108-199; 2005, P.L. 108-447; 2006, P.L. 109-149. The Dickey-Wicker Amendment reads as follows:

> Sec. 511. (a) None of the funds made available in this Act may be used for—(1) the creation of a human embryo or embryos for research purposes; or (2) research in which a human embryo or embryos are destroyed, discarded, or knowingly subjected to risk of injury or death greater than that allowed for research on fetuses in utero under 45 CFR 46.208(a)(2) and section 498(b) of the Public Health Service Act (42 U.S.C. 289g(b)).
>
> (b) For purposes of this section, the term "human embryo or embryos" includes any organism, not protected as a human subject under 45 CFR 46 as of the date of the enactment of this Act, that is derived by fertilization, parthenogenesis, cloning, or any other means from one or more human gametes or human diploid cells.

8. Department of Health and Human Services, Public Health Service, National Institutes of Health, "Draft National Institutes of Health Guidelines for Research Involving Human Pluripotent Stem Cells," *Federal Register* 64 (231): 67576–67579.

9. National Bioethics Advisory Commission, *Ethical Issues in Human Stem Cell Research* (see note 2), 50.

10. Ronald Dworkin, *Life's Dominion: An Argument about Abortion, Euthanasia, and Individual Freedom* (New York: Alfred A. Knopf, 1993), 52–53.

11. National Bioethics Advisory Commission, *Ethical Issues in Human Stem Cell Research* (see note 2), 52.

12. Ibid., 68–71, 72–73, 74, 71–72.

13. Cohen, "Promises and Perils of Public Deliberation" (see note 3), 271–276.

14. National Institutes of Health, "Guidelines for Research Using Human Pluripotent Stem Cells," *Federal Register* 65 (166): 51975, August 25, 2000, available at http://stemcells.nih.gov/staticresources/news/newsArchives/fr25au00-136.asp.

15. Rick Weiss, "Bush Administration Order Halts Stem Cell Meeting: NIH Planned Session to Review Fund Requests," *Washington Post*, April 21, 2001, A2.

16. Rick Weiss, "Bush Administration Order Halts Stem Cell Meeting: NIH Planned Session to Review Fund Requests," *Washington Post*, April 21, 2001, A2.

17. Karen Tumulty, "Why Bush's Ban Could Be Reversed," *Time*, May 23, 2005, 26–30.

18. George W. Bush, "Remarks by the President on Stem Cell Research," August 9, 2001, available at http://www.whitehouse.gov/news/releases/2001/08/200108 09-2.html.

19. White House, "Fact Sheet on Embryonic Stem Cell Research," August 9, 2001, available at http://www.whitehouse.gov/news/releases/2001/08/2001-0809-1.html.

20. National Institutes of Health, "Notice of Criteria for Federal Funding of Research on Existing Human Embryonic Stem Cells and Establishment of NIH Human Embryonic Stem Cell Registry," November 7, 2001, available at http://grants.nih.gov/grants/guide/notice-files/NOT-OD-02-005.html.

21. Bush, "Remarks by the President on Stem Cell Research" (see note 18).

22. For discussion of this theory, see Jan C. Heller, "Complicity in Embryonic and Fetal Stem Cell Research and Applications: Exploring and Extending Catholic Responses," in *Stem Cell Research*, ed. James M. Humber and Robert F. Almeder (Totowa, N. J.: Humana Press, 2004), 123–147; M. C. Kaveny, "Appropriation of Evil: Cooperation's Mirror Image," *Theological Studies* 61 (2000): 280–313; E. E. Smith, "The Principle of Cooperation in Catholic Thought," in *The Fetal Tissue Issue: Medical and Ethical Aspects*, ed. P. J. Cataldo and A. S. Moraczewski (Braintree, Mass.: Pope John Center, 1994), 81–92; Daniel C. Maguire, "Cooperation with Evil," in *Dictionary of Christian Ethics*, 2nd ed., ed. James F. Childress and John Macquarrie (Philadelphia: Westminster Press, 1986), 129.

23. Pontifical Academy for Life, "Declaration on the Production and the Scientific and Therapeutic Use of Human Embryonic Stem Cells," August 2000, available at http://www.vatican.va/roman_curia/pontifical_academies/acdlife/documents/rc_pa_acdlife_doc_20000824_cellule-staminali_en.html.

24. Richard M. Doerflinger, "The Ethics of Funding Embryonic Stem Cell Research: A Catholic Viewpoint," *Kennedy Institute of Ethics Journal* 9 (1999): 137–150, 141.

25. For example, John A. Robertson, "Causative vs. Beneficial Complicity in the Embryonic Stem Cell Debate," *Connecticut Law Review* 36 (2004): 1099–1113; Ronald M. Green, "Benefiting from 'Evil': An Incipient Moral Problem in Human Stem Cell Research," *Bioethics* 16 (2002): 544–556; Stephen G. Post, "The Echo of Nuremberg: Nazi Data and Ethics," *Journal of Medical Ethics* 17 (1991): 42–44; Dorothy E. Vawter, Warren Kearney, Karen G. Gervais, Arthur L. Caplan, Daniel Garry, Carol Tauer, *The Use of Human Fetal Tissue: Scientific, Ethical, and Public Policy Concerns* (Minneapolis: University of Minnesota, 1990): 251–271; Richard B. Miller, "On Transplanting Human Fetal Tissue: Presumptive Duties and the Task of Casuistry," *Journal of Medicine and Philosophy* 14 (1989): 617–640; Arthur L. Caplan, "The Meaning of the Holocaust for Bioethics," *Hastings Center Report* 19 (1989): 2–3; John A. Robertson, "Fetal Tissue Transplants," *Washington University Law Quarterly* 66 (1988): 443–498; Benjamin Freedman, "The Ethics of Using Human Fetal Tissue," *IRB: Ethics & Human Research* 10, no. 4 (1988): 7–11.

26. Thomas B. Edsall, "Catholics Differ on Stem Cell Issue," *Washington Post*, July 30, 2001, A3.

27. See, for instance, Richard Land, "Interview with Richard Land, *Frontline*, April 29, 2004, available at http://www.pbs.org/wgbh/pages/frontline/shows/jesus/interviews/land.html.

28. Richard Brownstein and Aaron Zitner, "Compromise in Works for Embryo Cells," *Los Angeles Times*, June 28, 2001, A14.

29. Aaron Zitner, "Catholic Leaders Say Stem Cell Research Compromise Possible," *Los Angeles Times*, July 8, 2001, A14.

30. Edsall, "Catholics Differ on Stem Cell Issue" (see note 26).

31. C. Ben Mitchell, "NIH, Stem Cells, and Moral Guilt," Center for Bioethics and Human Dignity, August 21, 2000, available at http://www.cbhd.org/resources/stemcells/nitchell_2000-08-24.htm; Land, "Interview with Richard Land" (see note 27).

32. Cynthia B. Cohen, "Stem Cell Research in the U.S. after the President's Speech of August 2001," *Kennedy Institute of Ethics Journal* 14 (2004): 97–114.

33. Rachel Zoll, "Catholics Angered by Bush Decision," Associated Press, 2001, available at http://www.wwrn.org/article.php?idd=2006&sec=24 &con=4.

34. Zitner, "Catholic Leaders Say Stem Cell Research Compromise Possible" (see note 29).

35. Ibid.

36. National Institutes of Health, "Stem Cell Information: Information on Eligibility Criteria for Federal Funding of Research on Human Embryonic Stem Cells," October 6, 2006, available at http://stemcells.nih.gov/research/registry/eligibilityCriteria.asp.

37. United States Conference of Catholic Bishops, "President Bush's Stem Cell Decision," August 13, 2001, available at http://www.usccb.org/prolife/issues/bioethic/fact801.htm; American Life League, "Broken Promises," August 2002, available at http://www.all.org/article.php?id=10136.

38. National Institutes of Health, "Human Embryonic Stem Cell Registry," October 6, 2006, available at http://stemcells.nih.gov/research/registry.

39. Judith A. Johnson and Erin Williams, Congressional Research Service, "Stem Cell Research: Federal Funding and Oversight," August 24, 2006, available at http://www.popenvironment.org/NLE/CRSreports/06Aug/RL33540.pdf.

40. A. Maitra, D. E. Arking, N. Shivapurkar, M. Ikeda, V. Stastny, K. Kassauei, G. Sui, et al., "Genomic Alterations in Cultured Human Embryonic Stem Cells," *Nature Genetics* 37 (2005): 1099–2003.

41. Ella De Trizio and Christopher S. Brennan, "The Business of Human Embryonic Stem Cell Research and an International Analysis of Relevant Laws," *Journal of Biolaw and Business* 7 (2004): 3–11, 5.

42. Gareth Cook, "U.S. Stem Cell Research Lagging: Without Aid, Work Moving Overseas," *Boston Globe*, May 23, 2004, available at http://www.pulitzer.org/year/2005/explanatory-reporting/works/cook2.html.

43. Gareth Cook, "Harvard Provost OKs Procedure," *Boston Globe*, March 20, 2005, A29.

44. National Institutes of Health, "Stem Cell Information: Frequently Asked Questions, Funding," questions 3–4, 6–8, October 6, 2006, available at http://stemcells.nih.gov/info/faqs.asp.

45. George W. Bush, Executive Order 13237, "Creation of the President's Council on Bioethics," November 28, 2001, available at http://www.whitehouse.gov/news/releases/2001/11/20011128-13.html.

46. President's Council on Bioethics, *Monitoring Stem Cell Research* (Washington, D.C.: President's Council on Bioethics, 2004).

47. President's Council on Bioethics, *Human Cloning and Human Dignity: An Ethical Inquiry* (Washington, D.C.: President's Council on Bioethics, 2002), 117–171.

48. Ibid., 128.

49. Ibid., xxxii; see also 150, 167.

50. Ibid., 207–208.

51. Stem Cell Research Enhancement Act of 2005 (HR 810), available at http://www.govtrack.us/congress/bill.xpd?bill=h109-810; Stem Cell Research Enhancement Act of 2005 (S 471), available at http://www.nyamr.org/bills/S471.pdf.

52. George W.Bush, "Message to the House of Representatives," July 2006, available at http://www.whitehouse.gov/news/releases/2006/07/20060719-5.html.

53. National Conference of State Legislatures, "State Embryonic and Fetal Research Laws," August 14, 2006, available at http://www.ncsl.org/programs/health/Genetics/embfet.htm; Gregory M. Lamb, "State Laws Bypass Research Ban," *Christian Science Monitor*, February 1, 2006, available at http://www.csmonitor.com/2006/0201/p13s01-stss.htm.

54. Eugene Russo, "Follow the Money: The Politics of Embryonic Stem Cell Research," *PLoS* (*Public Library of Science*) *Biology* 3 (2005): e324, available at http://biology.plosjournals.org/perlserv/?request=get-document&doi=10.1371%2Fjournal.pbio.0030234.

55. Kenneth Giacin, quoted in Ed Silverman, "Legislating Stem Cells," *Scientist* 19, no. 6 (2005): 39–41, 41.

56. South Dakota Codified Laws § 34-14-16 (2000).

57. Judith A. Johnson and Erin D. Williams, *Congressional Research Service Report for Congress: Stem Cell Research* (see note 39).

58. Jeff Chu, "California Leads, but a Pack Follows," *Time*, May 23, 2005, 28–29; Peter Slevin, "Missouri May Vote on Stem Cell Research," *Washington Post*, December 25, 2005, A4.

59. National Conference of State Legislatures, "State Embryonic and Fetal Research Laws" (see note 53); Johnson and Williams, *Congressional Research Service Report for Congress: Stem Cell Research* (see note 39).

60. William Hathaway, "Stem Cell Grants Now Available," *Hartford Courant*, May 10, 2006, available at http://www.uchc.edu/ocomm/features/stories/stories06/feature_stemcellgrants.html.

61. National Conference of State Legislatures, "State Embryonic and Fetal Research Laws" (see note 53).

62. Ibid.; Johnson and Williams, *Congressional Research Service Report for Congress: Stem Cell Research* (see note 39).

63. Proposition 71, California Stem Cell Research and Cures Bond Act, available at http://www.cirm.ca.gov/prop71/pdf/prop71.pdf.

64. Constance Holden, "California Institute: Most Systems Go," *Science* 309 (2005): 241.

65. Judith A. Johnson and Erin Williams, *Congressional Research Service Report for Congress: Stem Cell Research* (see note 39); Anne Harding, "California Stem Cell Plans Stalled, but Alive," *Scientist*, February 8, 2006, available at http://www.thescientist.com/news/display/23097; Steve Johnson, "Lawsuits Will Delay Stem-Cell Research," *Mercury News*, August 2, 2005, 1; Paul Elias, "Suits Filed to Invalidate California's $3 Billion Stem Cell Institute," Associated Press, February 23, 2005, available at http://sfgate.com/cgi-bin/article.cgi?file=/n/a/2005/02/23/state/n001132S34.DTL.

66. Harding, "California Stem Cell Plans Stalled, but Alive" (see note 65); Johnson, "Lawsuits Will Delay Stem-Cell Research" (see note 65); Elias, "Suits Filed to Invalidate California's $3 Billion Stem Cell Institute" (see note 65).

67. Andrew Pollack, "Trial over California Stem Cell Research Ends," *New York Times*, March 3, 2006, available at http://www.nytimes.com/2006/03/03/national/03calif.html?ei=5070&en=20a2240ea10101; Constance Holden, "Stem Cells by the Sea," *Science* 311 (2006): 1537.

68. Jocelyn Kaiser, "Court Rules in Favor of California Stem Cell Institute," *Science* 312 (2006): 509; Tracy Hampton, "US Stem Cell Research Lagging," *Journal of the American Medical Association* 295 (2006): 2233–2234; Maria L. La Ganga, "State OKs Loan to Aid Stem Cell Research Center," *Los Angeles Times*, November 21, 2006, available at http://www.latimes.com/features/health/medicine/la-me-stemcell21nov21,1,6451593.story?coll=la-health-medicine.

69. "Monash and ASCC Join International Stem Cell Powerhouse," Monash University press release, April 11, 2006, available at http://monash.edu.au/news/newsline/story/822.

70. National Research Council and Institute of Medicine of the National Academies, *Guidelines for Human Embryonic Stem Cell Research* (Washington, D.C.: National Academies Press, 2005), available at http://www.nap.edu/catalog/11278.html.

71. J. Mark Waxman, "The Stem Cell Legislative Process," *Health Lawyer* 17 (2005): 23–27.

72. Chad A. Cowan, Irina Klimanskaya, Jill McMahon, Jocelyn Atienza, Jeannine Witmeyer, Jacob P. Zucker, Shunping Wang, Cynthia C. Morton, Andrew P. McMahon, Doug Powers, Douglas A. Melton, "Derivation of Embryonic Stem-Cell Lines from Human Blastocysts," *New England Journal of Medicine* 350 (2004): 1353–1356.

73. Gareth Cook, "Harvard Provost OKs Procedure," *Boston Globe*, March 20, 2005, A29.

74. Kevin Kelleher, "Banking on Biotechnology," *Popular Science*, December 2004, 21–22.

75. Stephen A. Bent, "Under the Microscope," *Scientist* 19, no. 13 (2005): 22–23.

76. Ibid., 22; Nuala Moran, "Tough Cell to Investors," *Scientific American/Financial Times* 293, no. 1 (2005): A32–34; Gretchen Vogel, "Stem Cells Lose Market Luster," *Science* 299 (2003): 1830–1831.

77. Moran, "Tough Cell to Investors" (see note 76), A32.

78. Ibid., A34.

79. Antonio Regalado, "Big Companies Quietly Pursue Research on Embryonic Stem Cells," *Wall Street Journal*, April 2, 2005, A1.

80. MedMarket Diligence, "Worldwide Tissue Engineering, Cell Therapy and Transplantation: Products, Technologies and Market Opportunities, 2001–2014," April 2005, available at http://www.mediligence.com/rpt-s515.htm.

81. Pilar Ossorio, "Legal and Ethical Issues in Biotechnology Patenting," in *A Companion to Bioethics*, ed. Justine Burley and John Harris (Malden, Mass.: Blackwell, 2002).

82. Robert P. Merges, "Property Rights Theory and the Commons: The Case of Scientific Research," in *Scientific Innovation, Philosophy, and Public Policy*, ed. Ellen Frankel, Fred D. Miller Jr., Jeffrey Paul (Cambridge: Cambridge University Press, 1996), 145–167.

83. Patrick L. Taylor, "Closing the Ethics Gap: Coordinating Review of Legal, Ethical and Scientific Issues in Human Embryonic Stem Cell Research," *Health Lawyer* 17, no. 2 (2005): 1–11.

84. National Institutes of Health, "Stem Cell Information: Information on Eligibility Criteria for Federal Funding of Research on Human Embryonic Stem Cells" (see note 36).

85. *Madey v. Duke University*, 307 F. 3d 1351, 1362 (Fed. Cir. 2002), available at http://cyber.law.harvard.edu/people/tfisher/2002Madeyedit.html.

86. United States Patent and Trademark Office, available at http://www.uspto.gov.

87. Kenneth S. Taymor, Christopher Thomas Scott, Henry T. Greely, "The Paths around Stem Cell Intellectual Property," *Nature Biotechnology* 24 (2006): 411–413; Jeanne F. Loring and Cathryn Campbell, "Intellectual Property and Human Embryonic Stem Cell Research," *Science* 311 (2006): 1716–1717.

88. WiCell Research Institute, "Unlocking the Potential of Human Embryotic Stem Cells," available at http://www.Wicell.org.

89. Loring and Campbell, "Intellectual Property and Human Embryonic Stem Cell Research" (see note 87), 1717, 1719.

90. Taylor, "Closing the Ethics Gap" (see note 83), 6–7.

91. Taymor et al., "Paths around Stem Cell Intellectual Property" (see note 87), 411; Taylor, "Closing the Ethics Gap" (see note 83), 7.

92. Loring and Campell, "Intellectual Property and Human Embryonic Stem Cell Research" (see note 87), 1717.

93. For instance, see the materials transfer agreement used for the transfer of the new stem cell lines created by Howard Hughes–funded investigator Douglas Melton at Harvard University, available through http://www.mcb.harvard.edu/melton/hues/HUES_MTA.html.

94. Arti K. Rai and Rebecca S. Eisenberg, "Bayh-Dole Reform and the Progress of Biomedicine," *Law and Contemporary Problems* 66 (2003): 289–325, 303.

95. Taymor et al., "Paths around Stem Cell Intellectual Property" (see note 87), 411–413.

96. Taylor, "Closing the Ethics Gap" (see note 83), 7.

97. Eli Kintisch, "Groups Challenge Key Stem Cell Patents," *Science* 313 (2006): 281; California Stem Cell Report, "Wisconsin to CIRM: Cough Up Some Cash," March 14, 2006, available at http://californiastemcellreport.blogspot.com/2006/03/wisconsin-to-cirm-cough-up-some-cash.html.

98. Baruch Brody, "Intellectual Property and Biotechnology: The U.S. Internal Experience—Part I," *Kennedy Institute of Ethics Journal* 16 (2006): 1–37; Peter Mikhail, "Hopkins v. CellPro: An Illustration that Patenting and Exclusive Licensing of Fundamental Science Is Not Always in the Public Interest" *Harvard Journal of Law and Technology* 13 (2000): 375–394; M. T. Hella and R. S. Eisenberg, "Can Patents Deter Innovation? The Anticommons in Biomedical Research," *Science* 280 (1998): 698.

99. Hella and Eisenberg, "Can Patents Deter Innovation?" (see note 98).

100. National Institutes of Health, "Principles and Guidelines for Recipients of NIH Research Grants and Contracts on Obtaining and Disseminating Biomedical Research Resources: Final Notice," *Federal Register* 64, No. 246 (December 23, 1999): 72090, available at http://grants.nih.gov/grants/intell-property_64FR72090.pdf.

101. Mikhail, "Hopkins v. CellPro" (see note 98), 388.

102. Rai and Eisenberg, "Bayh-Dole Reform and the Progress of Biomedicine" (see note 95).

103. National Research Council, Committee on Intellectual Property Rights in Genomic and Protein Research and Regulation, *Reaping the Benefits of Genomic and Proteomic Research: Intellectual Property Rights, Innovation, and Public Health* (Washington, D.C.: National Academies Press, 2006).

104. Taylor, "Closing the Ethics Gap" (see note 83), 8.

105. "Baying for Blood or Doling Out Cash?" *Economist*, December 20, 2005, available at http://www.economist.com/science/displaystory.cfm?story_id=5327661&no_na_tran=1.

106. Jason Owen-Smith and Jennifer McCormick, "An International Gap in Human ES Cell Research," *Nature Biotechnology* 24 (2006): 391–392.

107. National Research Council and Institute of Medicine, *Guidelines* (see note 70).

108. Angus Reid Consultants, "Support for Stem Cell Research up in U.S.," May 22, 2006, available at http://www.angus-reid.com/polls/index.cfm/fuseaction/viewItem/itemID/11958.

109. Harris Interactive, "New Harris Poll Finds Different Religious Groups Have Very Different Attitudes to Some Health Policies and Programs," October 20, 2005, available at http://www.harrisinteractive.com/harris_poll/index.asp?PID=608.

Chapter 8

1. Ned Shaw, "Body by Science," *Scientist* 17 (2003): 34–37; Charles Vacanti, "Cells for Building," *Scientist* 18 (2004): 22–23; Fabrizio Gelain, Daniele Bottai, AngeloVescovi, Shuguang Zhang, "Designer Self-Assembling Peptide Nonfiber Scaffolds for Adult Mouse Neural Stem Cell 3-Dimensional Cultures," *PLoS One*, December 27, 2006, available at http://www. plosone.org/article/fetchArticle.action?article URI=info%3A doi%2F10.1371%2Fjournal.pone.0000119.

2. F. J. Muller, E. Y. Snyder, J. F. Loring, "Gene Therapy: Can Neural Stem Cells Deliver?" *Nature Reviews Neurosciences* 7 (2006): 75–84.

3. Bruce Jennings, "Serving the Public Interest: Conducting Human Embryonic Stem Cell Research in a Democratic Society," presentation at Public Workshop on Guidelines for Human Embryonic Stem Cell Research of

the National Research Academy and Institute of Medicine of the National Academies, Washington, D.C., October 13, 2004; Daniel Callahan, "Ethical Responsibility in Science in the Face of Uncertain Consequences," *Annals of the New York Academy of Sciences* 265 (1976): 1–12.

4. Lori P. Knowles, "Science, Policy and the Law: Reproductive and Therapeutic Cloning," *New York University Journal of Legislation and Public Policy* 4 (2000–2001): 13–22. See also National Bioethics Advisory Commission, *Ethical Issues in Human Stem Cell Research* (Rockville, Md.: U.S. Government Printing Office, 1999), 74–77.

5. "Summary of the Meeting of NIH Stem Cell Task Force, September 20, 2002, available at http://stemcells.nih.gov/policy/taskForce/tfSummaries/ 09_20_02.asp

6. National Institutes of Health, "Notice of Criteria for Federal Funding of Research on Existing Human Embryonic Stem Cells and Establishment of NIH Human Embryonic Stem Cell Registry" (November 7, 2001), available at http://grants.nih.gov/grants/guide/notice-files/NOT-OD-02-005.html.

7. Angus Reid Consultants, "Support for Stem Cell Research up in U.S.," May 22, 2006, available at http://www.angus-reid.com/polls/index.cfm/ fuseaction/viewItem/itemID/11958; Harris Interactive, "New Harris Poll Finds Different Religious Groups Have Very Different Attitudes to Some Health Policies and Programs," October 20, 2005, available at http:// www.harrisinteractive.com/harris_poll/index.asp?PID=608.

8. 45 C.F.R. (*Code of Federal Regulations*) §46.102–115.

9. 45 C.F.R. §46.102(f).

10. David Magnus and Mildred K. Cho, "Issues in Oocyte Donation for Stem Cell Research," *Science* 308 (2005): 1747–1748.

11. 45 C.F.R. §46.116 (a)(5–7).

12. U.S. Food and Drug Administration, "Proposed Approach to Regulation of Cellular and Tissue-Based Products," February 28, 1997, available at http://www.fda.gov/cber/gdlns/celltissue.pdf; 21 C.F.R. §1271, 3d; Patrick L. Taylor, "Closing the Ethics Gap: Coordinating Review of Legal, Ethical and Scientific Issues in Human Embryonic Stem Cell Research," *Health Lawyer* 17, no. 2 (2005): 1–11.

13. 21 C.F.R. §1271; Dina Gould Halme and David A. Kessler, "FDA Regulation of Stem-Cell-Baed Therapies," *New England Journal of Medicine* 355 (2006): 1730–1735.

14. National Research Council and Institute of Medicine of the National Academies, *Guidelines for Human Embryonic Stem Cell Research* (Washington, D.C.: National Academies, 2002), 72, available at http://www.nap.edu/ catalog/11278.html; Simon B. Auerbach, "Taking Another Look at the Definition of an Embryo: President Bush's Criteria, and the Problematic Application of Federal Regulations to Human Embryonic Stem Cells," *Emory Law Journal* 51 (2002): 1557–1604; Cynthia B. Cohen, "Leaps and Boundaries: Expanding Oversight of Human Stem Cell Research," in *The Human Embryonic Stem Cell Debate: Science, Ethics, and Public Policy*, ed. Suzanne Holland, Karen Lebacqz, Laurie Zoloth (Cambridge, Mass.: MIT Press, 2001), 209–222.

15. Angus Reid Consultants, "Support for Stem Cell Research up in U.S." (see note 7); Harris Interactive, "New Harris Poll Finds Different Religious Groups Have Very Different Attitudes to Some Health Policies and

Programs" (see note 7); CBS News, "Poll: Stem Cell Use Gains Support," May 24, 2005, available at http://www.cbsnews.com/stories/2005/05/24/opinion/polls/main697546.shtml. See also Rick Weiss, "Senate to Consider Stem Cell Proposals," *Washington Post*, June 30, 2006, A5.

16. Carol A. Tauer, "Responsibility and Regulation: Reproductive Technologies, Cloning, and Embryo Research," in *Cloning and the Future of Human Embryonic Research*, ed. Paul Lauritzen (New York: Oxford University Press, 2001), 145–161; Cynthia B. Cohen, "Unmanaged Care: The Need to Regulate New Reproductive Technologies in the United States," *Bioethics* 11 (1997): 348–365.

17. National Research Council and Institute of Medicine, *Guidelines* (see note 14).

18. Ethics Committee, American Society for Reproductive Medicine, "Donating Spare Embryos for Embryonic Stem-Cell Research," *Fertility and Sterility* 78 (2002): 957–960.

19. Bernard Lo, Vicki Chou, Marcelle I. Cedars, Elena Gates, Robert N. Tatlor, Richard M. Wagner, Leslie Wolf, Keith R. Yamamoto, "Informed Consent in Human Oocyte, Embryo, and Embryonic Stem Cell Research," *Fertility and Sterility* 82 (2004): 559–563.

20. Practice Committee of the American Society for Reproductive Medicine, "Ovarian Hyperstimulation Syndrome," *Fertility and Sterility* 80 (2003): 1309–1314.

21. Monash IVF, "Ovarian Hyperstimulation Syndrome," available at http://www.monashivf.edu.au/default.asp?action=article&ID=21718.

22. R. Orvieto, "Can We Eliminate Severe Ovarian Hyperstimulation Syndrome?" *Human Reproduction* 20 (2005): 320–322; B. Hedon, H. J. Out, J. N. Hughes, B. Camier, J. Cohen, P. Lopes, J. R. Zorn, B. van der Heijden, H. J. Coelingh Bennink, "Efficacy and Safety of Recombinant Follicle Stimulating Hormone (Puregon) in Infertile Women Pituitary-Suppressed with Triptorelin Undergoing In-Vitro Fertilization: A Prospective, Randomized, Assessor-Blind, Multicentre Trial," *Human Reproduction* 10 (1995): 3102–3106; Practice Committee of the American Society for Reproductive Medicine, "Ovarian Hyperstimulation Syndrome" (see note 20).

23. Mark V. Sauer, "Egg Donor Solicitation Problems Exist, but Do Abuses?" *American Journal of Bioethics* 1 (2001): 1–2; M. J. MacDougall, S. L. Tan, H. S. Jacobs, "In-Vitro Fertilization and the Ovarian Hyperstimulation Syndrome," *Human Reproduction* 7 (1992): 597–600.

24. Arthur Leader, M.D., University of Ottawa, personal communication.

25. Ibid.

26. S. C. Klock, "Embryo Disposition: The Forgotten 'Child' of In Vitro Fertilization," *International Journal of Fertility and Women's Medicine* 49 (2004): 19–23.

27. D. L. Hoffman, G. L. Zellman, C. C. Fair, J. F. Mayer, J. G. Zeitz, W. E. Gibbons, T. G. Turner, "Cryopreserved Embryos in the United States and Their Availability for Research," *Fertility and Sterility* 79 (2003): 1063–1069.

28. Andrea D. Gurmankin and Doninc Sisti, "Embryo Disposal Practices in IVF Clinics in the United States," *Politics and the Life Sciences* 22, no. 2 (2004): 2–6; B. Van Voorhees, D. Grinstead, A. Sparks, J. Gerard, R. Weir,

"Establishment of a Successful Donor Embryo Program: Medical, Ethical and Policy Issues," *Fertility and Sterility* 71 (1999): 604–608.

29. Ethics Committee, "Donating Spare Embryos for Embryonic Stem-Cell Research" (see note 18), 959.

30. National Research Council and Institute of Medicine, *Guidelines* (see note 14), 9.

31. Lo et al., "Informed Consent in Human Oocyte, Embryo, and Embryonic Stem Cell Research" (see note 19), 562.

32. Ethics Committee, "Donating Spare Embryos for Embryonic Stem-Cell Research" (see note 18), 959.

33. National Bioethics Advisory Commission, *Ethical Issues in Human Stem Cell Research* (see note 4), 53, 72.

34. National Research Council and Institute of Medicine, *Guidelines* (see note 12), 88.

35. Lo et al., "Informed Consent in Human Oocyte, Embryo, and Embryonic Stem Cell Research" (see note 19), 561.

36. Cynthia B. Cohen, "Ethical Issues in Reproduction," in *Fletcher's Introduction to Clinical Ethics*, 3rd ed., ed. John C. Fletcher, Edward M. Spencer, Paul A. Lombardo (Hagerstown, Md.: University Press, 2005), 263–282; Gurmankin and Sisti, "Embryo Disposal Practices in IVF Clinics in the United States" (see note 28); V. Soderstrom-Anttila, T. Foudila, U. Ripati, R. Siegberg, "Embryo Donation: Outcome and Attitudes among Embryo Donors and Recipients," *Human Reproduction* 16 (2001): 1120–1128.

37. National Research Council and Institute of Medicine, *Guidelines* (see note 14), 101–102.

38. Ibid., 89–90.

39. Suzi Leather, Chair, Human Fertilisation and Embryology Authority, presentation to the President's Council on Bioethics, Session 6, "Regulation 9: International Models (United Kingdom)," October 18, 2002, available at http://www.bioethics.gov/transcripts/oct02/session6.html.

40. LeRoy Walters and Julie Gage Palmer, *The Ethics of Human Gene Thearpy* (New York: Oxford University Press, 1997), 143–153.

41. Cohen, "Leaps and Boundaries: Expanding Oversight of Human Stem Cell Research" (see note 14).

42. National Bioethics Advisory Commission, *Ethical Issues in Human Stem Cell Research* (see note 4).

43. National Institutes of Health, "Guidelines for Research Using Human Pluripotent Stem Cells and Notification of Request for Emergency Clearance," *Federal Register* 65, no. 166 (August 25, 2000): 51975 , available at http://stemcells.nih.gov/staticresources/news/newsArchives/fr25au00-136.asp.

44. National Institutes of Health, "Notice: Withdrawal of NIH Guidelines for Research Using Pluripotent Stem Cells Derived from Human Embryos," *Federal Register* 66, no. 220 (November 14, 2001): 5107, available at http://stemcells.nih.gov/staticresources/news/newsArchives/fr14no01-95.asp.

45. Geron Ethics Advisory Board, "Research with Human Embryonic Stem Cells: Ethical Considerations," *Hastings Center Report* 29, no. 2 (1999): 31–36.

46. Ronald M. Green, Kier Olsen DeVries, Judith Bernstein, Kennth W. Goodman, Robert Kaufmann, Ann A. Kiessling, Susan R. Levin, Susan L. Moss, Carol A. Tauer, "Overseeing Research on Therapeutic Cloning:

A Private Ethics Board Responds to Its Critics," *Hastings Center Report* 32, no. 3 (2002): 27–33.

47. National Research Council and Institute of Medicine, *Guidelines* (see note 14), 70, 107.

48. National Bioethics Advisory Commission, *Ethical Issues in Human Stem Cell Research* (see note 4), 76–79.

49. National Institutes of Health, "Guidelines for Research Using Human Pluripotent Stem Cells" (see note 43).

50. Geron Ethics Advisory Board, "Research with Human Embryonic Stem Cells" (see note 45), 32.

51. Green et al., "Overseeing Research on Therapeutic Cloning" (see note 46).

52. National Academies, "Committee Named to Update Stem Cell Research Guidelines," available at http://www.nationalacademies.org/morenews/ 20060502.html.

53. National Research Council and Institute of Medicine, *Guidelines* (see note 14), 79.

54. National Bioethics Advisory Commission, *Ethical Issues in Human Stem Cell Research* (see note 4), 59.

55. National Institutes of Health, "Guidelines for Research Using Human Pluripotent Stem Cells" (see note 43).

56. Geron Ethics Advisory Board, "Research with Human Embryonic Stem Cell" (see note 45), 31; Laurie Zoloth, "Jordan's Banks: A View from the First Years of Human Embryonic Stem Cell Research," *American Journal of Bioethics* 2 (2002): 3–11.

57. Green et al., "Overseeing Research on Therapeutic Cloning" (see note 46), 25.

58. National Research Council and Institute of Medicine, *Guidelines* (see note 14), 107.

59. Nicholas Wade, "Science Academy Creating Panel to Monitor Stem-Cell Research," *New York Times*, February 16, 2006, available at http://www .nytimes.com/2006/02/16/science/16stem.html?_r=1&oref=slogin.

60. National Academies, "Committee Named to Update Stem Cell Research Guidelines" (see note 52).

61. Center for Genetics and Society and Center for Science in the Public Interest, "Public Interest Groups Call for 'Needed Balance' on Stem Cell Research Oversight Committee," May 24, 2006, available at http://www .genetics-and-society.org/resources/cgs/20060524_naletter_press.html.

62. National Bioethics Advisory Commission, *Ethical Issues in Human Stem Cell Research* (see note 4), 51.

63. Ibid., 52–53.

64. John Rawls, *Political Liberalism* (New York: Columbia University Press, 1993), 212–254.

65. John Rawls, "The Idea of Public Reason Revisited," *University of Chicago Law Review* 64 (1997): 765–807.

66. National Bioethics Advisory Commission, *Ethical Issues in Human Stem Cell Research* (see note 4), 53; see also ii, iii, 3, 51, 52, 66, 67, 81.

67. Cynthia B. Cohen, "Promises and Perils of Public Deliberation: Contrasting Two National Bioethics Commissions on Embryonic Stem Cell Research," *Kennedy Institute of Ethics Journal* 15 (2005): 269–288.

68. Leon R. Kass, "Chairman's Vision," January 17, 2002, available at http://www.bioethics.gov/about/chairman.html.
69. President's Council on Bioethics, *Human Cloning and Human Dignity: An Ethical Inquiry* (Washington, D.C.: President's Council on Bioethics, 2002), ix, xix, xi.
70. Ibid., ix.
71. Steven Smith, *Reading Leo Strauss: Politics, Philosophy, Judaism* (Chicago: University of Chicago Press, 2006); Irving Kristol, *Neoconservatism: The Autobiography of an Idea* (New York: Free Press, 1995); Robert B. Pippin, "The Modern World of Leo Strauss," *Political Theory* 20 (1992): 448–472.
72. Leo Strauss, *What Is Political Philosophy? And Other Studies* (Chicago: University of Chicago Press, 1988); Leo Strauss, *Natural Right and History* (Chicago: University of Chicago Press, 1974); Leo Strauss, "Epilogue," in *Essays on the Scientific Study of Politics,* ed. Herbert Storing (New York: Holt, 1962), 325.
73. Leo Strauss, *The City and the Man* (University of Chicago Press, 1978).
74. President's Council on Bioethics, *Human Cloning and Human Dignity* (see note 69), 128.
75. Ibid., 167.
76. Ibid., 207–208.
77. Ibid., 214.
78. Cohen, "Promises and Perils of Public Deliberation" (see note 67).
79. Mary Anderlik Majumder, "Respecting Difference and Moving beyond Regulation: Tasks for U.S. Bioethics Commissions in the Twenty-First Century," *Kennedy Institute of Ethics Journal* 15 (2005): 289–303; Jonathan D. Moreno and Alex John London, "Consensus, Ethics, and Politics in Cloning and Embryo Research," in *Cloning and the Future of Human Embryonic Research*, ed. Paul Lauritzen (New York: Oxford University Press, 2001), 162–177.
80. Green et al., "Overseeing Research on Therapeutic Cloning" (see note 46).
81. Office of the Secretary, *The Belmont Report Ethical Principles and Guidelines for the Protection of Human Subjects of Research*, National Commission for the Protection of Human Subjects of Biomedical and Behavioral Research, April 18, 1979, available at http://www.hhs.gov/ohrp/humansubjects/guidance/belmont.htm.
82. National Bioethics Advisory Commission, *Ethical Issues in Human Stem Cell Research* (see note 4), 75.
83. Ibid., 7.

Glossary

ADULT STEM CELL: A cell found in any tissue of the body that can both renew itself and differentiate to yield the specialized cell types of the tissue from which it originated (*see also* embryonic stem cell).

ALTERED NUCLEAR TRANSFER: A process of modifying a somatic cell so that it lacks one or more genes that an embryo needs to develop, transferring this cell to an egg whose nucleus has been removed, and fusing the two together in a process that mimics somatic cell nuclear transfer; the resulting cluster of cells cannot survive beyond a week or two, it has been hypothesized, due to the initial genetic modification (*see also* cloning and somatic cell nuclear transfer).

ASSISTED REPRODUCTION: Medical treatment that involves the use of laboratory techniques such as in vitro fertilization to aid in initiating pregnancy.

BIOTECHNOLOGY: The use of living organisms, their components, or their products to improve human or animal lives, agriculture, and the environment.

BLASTOCYST: A hollow ball of 30 to 150 cells that develops at about five days after fertilization; it is made up of an outer layer of cells that can develop into membranes, such as the placenta, and an inner cell mass composed of a cluster of embryonic stem cells.

BONE MARROW: The tissue that fills most bone cavities and that contains hematopoietic stem cells from which all blood cells develop, as well as mesenchymal stem cells from which cartilage-producing cells evolve.

CELL: The basic structural and functional unit of all living matter.

CHIMERA: An organism consisting of cells derived from at least two genetically different entities that may be of different species (e.g., human-nonhuman); the genetic matter from each of the different entities remains distinct within the individual cells (*see also* hybrid).

CLONING: In relation to stem cell research, a process of making multiple identical copies of a cell, group of cells, embryo, or organism through the process of somatic cell nuclear transfer—that is, transferring the nucleus of a somatic cell into an unfertilized egg from which the nucleus has been removed and fusing them.; there are two sorts of cloning: research cloning (also known as research or therapeutic cloning) and reproductive cloning.

DEDIFFERENTIATION: A process of inducing a specialized cell to revert to an unspecialized pluripotent state in which it has the capacity, under the appropriate conditions, to develop into almost every cell type of the body (*see also* differentiation, redifferentiation).

DIFFERENTIATION: A process by which an unspecialized early embryonic cell forms more specialized cell types, such as those of the heart, liver, or muscles (*see also* dedifferentiation, redifferentiation).

DNA (deoxyribonucleic acid): A chemical that constitutes the primary genetic material in cells and carries the instructions for making all the structures that the body needs to function.

EMBRYO: In humans, the developing organism from the time of fertilization until the end of the eighth week of gestation that is marked by very small size and the absence of bodily form and specialized tissues and organs (*see also* fetus, zygote).

EMBRYONIC GERM CELL: A cell that could eventually become the ovaries or testes; it is found in the part of the fetus known as the gonadal ridge.

EMBRYONIC STEM CELL: An undifferentiated cell derived from the inner cell mass of the blastocyst with the capacity to develop into almost every cell type of the body (*see also* adult stem cell).

ENUCLEATED CELL: A cell from which the nucleus has been removed.

FEEDER CELL LAYER: The group of cells that are used to maintain pluripotent stem cells in culture through a supply of nutrients.

FERTILIZATION: The fusion of two gametes (egg and sperm) to form a zygote or an embryo.

FETUS: An organism from the end of the embryonic stage up to birth (*see also* embryo, zygote).

GAMETE: A mature reproductive cell (germ cell); the male gamete is a sperm, and the female gamete is an ovum or egg (*see also* oocyte).

GENE: The basic unit of inheritance that is a segment of DNA.

GENOME: The complete genetic material of an organism.

GERM CELL: A sperm or an egg, or a cell that can become a sperm or an egg (*see also* gamete, ooctye).

HEMATOPOIETIC STEM CELL: A stem cell from which red and white blood cells and platelets form; it is found mainly in the bone marrow.

HUMAN CELL TYPE: One of over 200 different types of cells in the human body: for example, blood cells, liver cells, and neural cells; each of these different cell types has specific characteristics that allow it to serve a specific function in the body.

HYBRID: An organism consisting of cells derived from at least two genetically different entities that may be of different species (e.g., horse and donkey combine to make a mule); the genetic matter from the two different species is fused in individual cells (*see also* chimera).

INNER CELL MASS: The cluster of cells inside the blastocyst capable of giving rise to the embryo proper.

IN VITRO: Studies carried out in a laboratory dish, test tube, or other artificial environment, rather than a living organism (literally means "in glass").

IN VITRO FERTILIZATION (IVF): A method of assisted reproduction in which an egg is fertilized by sperm in a laboratory dish outside the body of a woman.

IN VITRO: Studies carried out in living organisms (literally means "in a living body").

MESENCHYMAL STEM CELLS: Stem cells found in the regions of bone marrow that can give rise to bone and cartilage.

MULTIPOTENT: Capable of developing into a limited number of specialized cells or tissues of an organism (*see also* pluripotent, totipotent).

NEURAL STEM CELL: A stem cell found in adult neural tissue that can give rise to neurons and other cells of the nervous system.

NUCLEUS: The portion of the cell that encloses its genetic material.

OOCYTE: The female egg; a large and immobile cell (*see also* gamete).

PARTHENOGENESIS: The process of artificially stimulating an unfertilized egg to begin the earliest stages of cell division without involvement of sperm.

PLASTICITY: The ability of stem cells from one adult tissue to develop into specialized cell types of another tissue.

PLURIPOTENT: Under the appropriate conditions, capable of developing into almost every cell type of the body except extraembryonic tissues such as the placenta and the umbilical cord (*see also* multipotent, totipotent).

PREIMPLANTATION GENETIC DIAGNOSIS (PGD): A way of screening embryos that involves removing one cell from an eight-cell embryo that has been developed through in vitro fertilization and assessing its genetic composition.

PRIMITIVE STREAK: A band of cells that appears at about fourteen days after fertilization whose formation marks the onset of gastrulation, the process in which the early embryo is transformed into a body consisting of multiple cell and tissue types.

PROTEOMICS: The study of the structure and functions of proteins.

REGENERATIVE MEDICINE: Medical treatments that use stem cells, among other means, to repair or replace diseased or injured tissue and organs.

REPRODUCTIVE CLONING: A process in which the nucleus of a somatic cell is fused with an unfertilized egg whose nucleus has been removed to form a reconstructed embryo that is then transferred to a woman's uterus in an attempt to develop an offspring that is genetically identical to the donor of the nucleus. (In scientific terms, the process in which this reconstructed embryo is formed is known as "somatic cell nuclear transfer.")

RESEARCH CLONING (also known as "therapeutic cloning"): A process in which the nucleus of a somatic cell is fused with an unfertilized egg whose nucleus has been removed to form a reconstructed embryo that serves as a source of embryonic stem cells for research and therapeutic applications (in scientific terms, the process in which this reconstructed embryo is formed is known as "somatic cell nuclear transfer")

SINGLE-CELL EMBRYO BIOPSY: Removing one cell from an early embryo at the six-to-eight-cell stage and deriving embryonic stem cell lines from it.

SOMATIC CELL: A cell of the body other than those that give rise to sperm and egg (*soma* means "body").

SOMATIC CELL NUCLEAR TRANSFER (SCNT): A process in which the nucleus of a somatic cell is fused with an unfertilized egg whose nucleus has been removed to form a reconstructed embryo that is also referred to as "cloning." (*see also* cloning, reproductive cloning, research cloning, altered nuclear transfer).

SPARE EMBRYOS: Embryos originally created by means of in vitro fertilization for reproductive purposes that remain after in vitro fertilization treatments have ended.

STEM CELL: A cell that has two definitive characteristics: cell division and cell differentiation: that is, the ability to divide and make copies of itself for indefinite periods of time in culture and the ability to give rise to a variety of specialized cells in the body.

STEM CELL LINE: A group of stem cells that come from a common ancestor cell and that can be grown in culture in the laboratory indefinitely; human stem cell lines may be derived from different sources, such as adult, placental, fetal, or embryonic tissue.

TERATOMA: A nonlethal tumor composed of tissue from the three embryonic germ layers; it is produced experimentally in animals by injecting them with pluripotent stem cells in order to determine the ability of the stem cells to differentiate into various types of tissues.

THERAPEUTIC CLONING: *see* research cloning.

TOTIPOTENT: Having the capacity to become every organ or tissue of the body, as well as the placenta and extraembryonic tissues, and thus able to form an entire organism under the appropriate conditions; the zygote and the cells of the very early embryo are totipotent, but no stem cell line has been shown to have this capacity (*see also* multipotent, pluripotent).

UNDIFFERENTIATED: Not having transformed into a specialized cell.

UNIVERSAL STEM CELL LINE: A stem cell line that would be immunologically compatible with most patients and therefore would not trigger rejection in them.

ZYGOTE: A fertilized egg formed as a result of the union of the sperm and the egg (*see also* embryo, fetus).

Index

abortion
  and donation of embryonic germ
    cells for stem cell research, 13
  and ethics of human embryonic
    stem cell research, 59–60
  Roman Catholic *Declaration on
    Procured Abortion*, 102
  Singer, Peter, view of, 82
access to stem cell therapies. *See* stem
  cell research, and justice
additional sources of human
  embryonic stem cells besides
  in vitro fertilization, 5, 28–29,
  34–58. *See also* altered nuclear
  transfer; dead human embryos;
  dedifferentiation of adult cells;
  in vitro fertilization (IVF);
  parthenogenesis; research
  cloning; single-cell embryo
  biopsy
adult stem cells, 3, 10, 13, 14–19, 25–26
  advantages and limitations of using
    in research and therapy, 18–19
  compared with embryonic stem
    cells, 25–26
  federal funding of research on, 172
  plasticity, 15–17, 26
  therapeutic uses of, 17–18
Advanced Cell Technology, 37,
  44–45, 48, 49

ethics advisory board for stem cell
  research, 211, 212, 215
altered nuclear transfer, 5, 51–54, 57
American Society for Reproductive
  Medicine, 32, 197
  guidelines for informed consent for
    embryo donation, 203–204,
    205–208
amniotic fluid, stem cells found in,
  246 *n* 21
animal-human chimeras. *See* human-
  nonhuman chimeras
Aquinas, Thomas, 98, 116
Aristotle, 95–97, 98, 99, 100, 108,
  116, 118
Audi, Robert, 89
Augustine, 97–98
Austria, stem cell research policy, 140

Barnhart, Michael G., 107
Baylis, Françoise, 119–120
Belmont Report. *See* National
  Institutes of Health
blastocyst. *See* embryos,
  early human
Bongso, Ariff, 13
Buckle, Stephen, 76, 77
Buddhist tradition, moral significance
  of early human embryos,
  106–107, 157

religion and the development of
public policy, 88, 89–92, 108–109
religious views of moral significance
of early human embryos, 6,
88–109. *See also specific religious
traditions*
reproductive cloning, 38, 39–41, 43, 124
proposed federal legislation
regarding, 182
See also under Japan; United
Kingdom
repugnance, 111, 112, 120–123
research cloning (somatic cell nuclear
transfer), 5, 24, 34–43, 44, 57
and "clonote," 39
proposed federal legislation
regarding, 182–183
South Korean (false) scientific
reports about, 37
as step toward reproductive
cloning, 4, 38, 39–41, 43
See also under Japan; United
Kingdom
respect for embryos. *See* embryos,
early human, special respect
owed to
Robert, Jason Scott, 119–120
Robertson, John A., 70, 71
Roman Catholic tradition
moral significance of early human
embryos in, 98, 101, 102–103.
See also under Christian tradition
Pontifical Academy for Life, 175
Pope Benedict XVI, 102
Pope Pius IX, 101
theory of complicity. *See*
complicity with evil, Roman
Catholic theory of
Roslin Institute, 46, 145. *See also*
United Kingdom, development
of stem cell research policy
Rowley, Janet, 48–49
Ryan, Maura, 85

Sachedina, Abdulaziz, 106
Sandel, Michael, 85

Scientific Revolution, 99–101
and epigenetic theory of
fertilization, 100
and preformation theory of
fertilization, 100
Scott, David A., 154
secular views of moral significance of
early human embryos, 3–4, 6, 28,
31–32, 33, 39, 43, 58, 59–87
fourteen-day or later view, 59, 60,
61, 64, 65, 66, 67–73, 78, 79, 81,
84, 85, 87
group of cells view, 60, 61, 78–81,
84, 87
person view, 60, 61, 80–83,
84, 149
potentiality view, 60, 61, 73–78, 79,
84, 87
time of fertilization view, 59, 60,
61–67, 68, 70, 72, 73, 78, 84, 87
See also under National Bioethics
Advisory Commission;
President's Council on Bioethics;
Germany; Japan; United
Kingdom
Singapore, stem cell research policy,
139, 197
Singer, Peter, 81–83, 149
single-cell embryo biopsy, 49–51
Snyder, Evan, 37, 112
social taboos, 120–123, 137, 138
Solter, Davor, 50, 52–53
somatic cell nuclear transfer (SCNT).
See research cloning
South Korea, stem cell research
policy, 139
Southern Baptist Convention, moral
significance of early human
embryos, 103. *See also under*
Christian tradition
Spain, stem cell research policy, 139
spare embryos remaining at IVF
clinics. *See* in vitro fertilization
(IVF)
species, 111, 118–120, 138
speciesism, 81, 127, 128